AF184154

Brutal treatments

Manchester University Press

SOCIAL HISTORIES OF MEDICINE

Series Editors
David Cantor, Anne Hanley and Elaine Leong
Editorial Board
Diego Armus, Swarthmore College, PA, USA
Rana Hogarth, University of Illinois, Urbana-Champaign, USA
Angela Ki Che Leung, University of Hong Kong, China
Ian Miller, Ulster University, Northern Ireland

Social Histories of Medicine is concerned with all aspects of health, illness and medicine, from prehistory to the present, in every part of the world. The series covers the circumstances that promote health or illness, the ways in which people experience and explain such conditions, and what, practically, they do about them. Practitioners of all approaches to health and healing come within its scope, as do their ideas, beliefs, and practices, and the social, economic and cultural contexts in which they operate. Methodologically, the series welcomes relevant studies in social, economic, cultural, and intellectual history, as well as approaches derived from other disciplines in the arts, sciences, social sciences and humanities. The series is a collaboration between Manchester University Press and the Society for the Social History of Medicine.

To buy or to find out more about the books currently
available in this series, please go to:
https://manchesteruniversitypress.co.uk/series/
social-histories-of-medicine/

Brutal treatments

Medicine and colonial violence at the end of empire

Russell T. Moul

MANCHESTER UNIVERSITY PRESS

Copyright © Russell T. Moul 2025

The right of Russell T. Moul to be identified as the author of
this work has been asserted in accordance with the
Copyright, Designs and Patents Act 1988.

Published by Manchester University Press
Oxford Road, Manchester, M13 9PL

www.manchesteruniversitypress.co.uk

British Library Cataloguing-in-Publication Data
A catalogue record for this book is available from the British Library

ISBN 978 1 5261 6751 4 hardback

First published 2025

The publisher has no responsibility for the persistence or
accuracy of URLs for any external or third-party internet
websites referred to in this book, and does not guarantee
that any content on such websites is, or will remain, accurate
or appropriate.

EU authorised representative for GPSR:
Easy Access System Europe, Mustamäe tee 50, 10621 Tallinn, Estonia
gpsr.requests@easproject.com

Typeset by Newgen Publishing UK

Contents

Acknowledgements

This book was only possible with the help and support of many people who deserve far more praise than I can record here. Firstly, I would like to thank Dr Giacomo Macola for his advice and guidance over the years. His extensive knowledge of colonial history was invaluable and helped set the basis for this book. Thanks are also owed to Dr Julie Anderson and Dr Claire Jones for their advice during the early phase of this work. Without their guidance I would not have been able to get this project off the ground.

Over the last few years, I have also had the privilege of working with and being supported by my peers at the University of Kent and wider academia. These wonderful people have not only provided valuable conversation and intellectual support, but also a sliver of a social life that has helped to enrich this experience. Firstly, and most importantly, I want to thank Dr Alfredo Carpeneti for his bulletproof resolve and consistent assurances. Many people have contributed to this book's completion, but you have been a stalwart anchor in the stormiest of seas. I would also like to thank Dr Peter Good and Dr Declan Kavanagh who, between them, helped this fledgling academic stay in flight. And to my 'academic big sister', Dr Alice White, thank you for your sustained reassurances and sage advice throughout my research and beyond. I owe you all so much.

I am extremely pleased that this book is going to appear in the Manchester University Press (MUP) *Social Histories of Medicine* series. Their team have been extremely supportive and patient throughout the process of creating this book. I would also like to thank the reviewer for suggesting new avenues and ideas to strengthen this work.

Special thanks should also go to the Royal Historical Society for financially supporting my field research in Kenya; this project, as well as my own research experience, has greatly benefitted from this aid. I would also like to thank the staff at the British Institute in East Africa for the logistical support they provided me with prior to and during my time in Kenya. Thanks also to the archives of the International Committee of the Red Cross in Geneva and especially Fabrizio Bensi for his interest in my work and his assistance with my archive hunting.

This project has made use of archives contained in many libraries and institutions; thank you to the staff at the Wellcome Trust; the British Library; the School of Tropical Medicine; the British National Archives; the Rhodes House Commonwealth and African collection at the Bodleian Library, Oxford; the Service historique de la Défense; the Sciences Po Archives; the Bibliothèque nationale de France; the Kenya National Archives; the archives of the World Medical Association; and finally the Templeman Library, University of Kent.

I am forever grateful to family and friends who have helped me maintain perspective throughout the last few years. The road to completing this work was not always a straight one and their gentle and patient support has kept me going when I did not feel I could. Thank you to my parents, Fran and Gary, for their unconditional reassurance throughout this work, for their faith in my ability to see it through and their patience over the long gaps between my visits. Duncan Beer has been a bastion of cheer throughout my work. I am extremely grateful for his ability to drag me (willingly or otherwise) to social events, but also for his comments on various drafts. Hannah Huxley has had the challenge of living with me throughout this slow birthing process. Thank you for the cups of tea, letting me bounce ideas off you (at all hours) and for offering your thoughts on the whole book-writing process. And I would like to extend a heartfelt thank you to Brendon Treeby and Daniel Brett for providing many fantastic and fantastical distractions over the last few years, many of which have helped keep me sane and entertained. You two have been the greatest of friends when I have needed it the most.

Abbreviations

ALN	Armée de libération nationale
BMA	British Medical Association, London
BMJ	*British Medical Journal*
CICRC	International Commission Against Concentration Camps
CMS	Colonial Medical Service
CRUA	Comité révolutionnaire d'unité et d'action
CSDIC	Combined Services Detailed Interrogation Centre
CTT	*Centre de tri et transit*
ECHR	European Convention on Human Rights
FCO	Foreign and Commonwealth Office, London
FLN	Front de libération nationale
IBEAC	Imperial British East Africa Company
ICRC	International Committee of the Red Cross, Geneva
KAR	King's African Rifles
KCA	Kikuyu Central Association
KCU	Kikuyu African Union
KNA	Kenya National Archives, Nairobi
KPR	Kenya Police Reserves
LNHO	League of Nations Health Organization
LSD	Lysergic acid diethylamide
MNLA	Malayan National Liberation Army
MTLD	Mouvement pour le triomphe des libertés démocratiques
OAS	Organisation de l'armée secrète
OS	Organisation spéciale
PCA	Parti communiste algérien

PoW	Prisoner of war
PPA	Parti du peuple algérien
SAS	*Sections administratives spécialisées*
SMC	Service médical de colonisation
SOAS	School of Oriental and African Studies, London
TNA	The National Archives, London
WHO	World Health Organization, Geneva
WMA	World Medical Association, Ferney-Voltaire

Maps

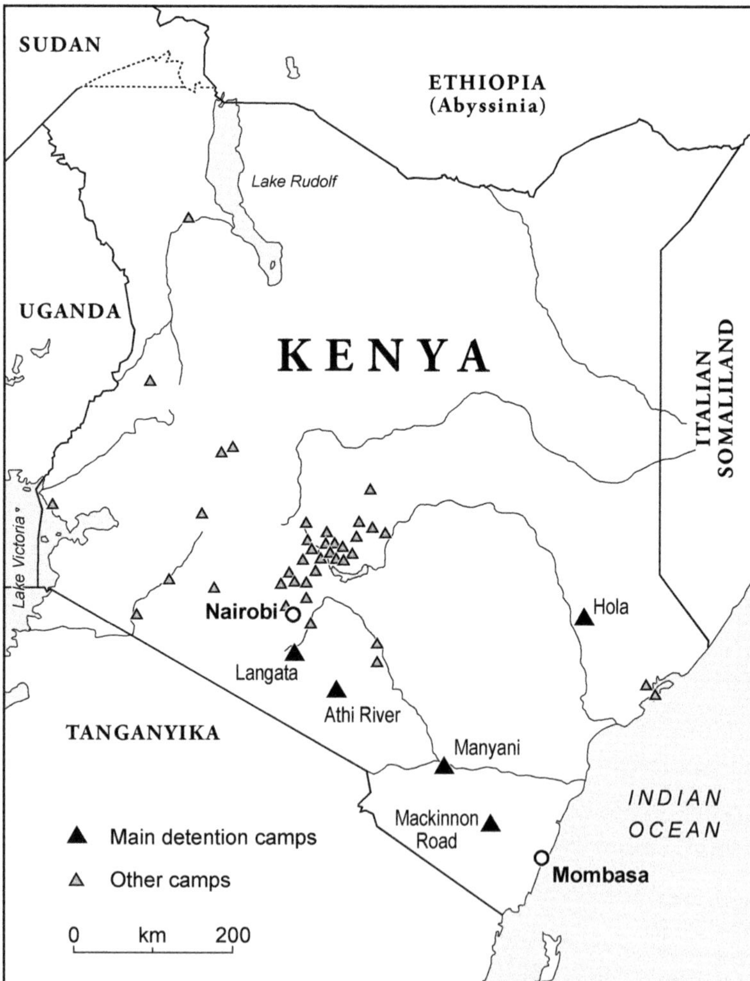

Map 1 Main detention camps in Kenya, 1959. Produced with data from The Museum of British Colonialism.

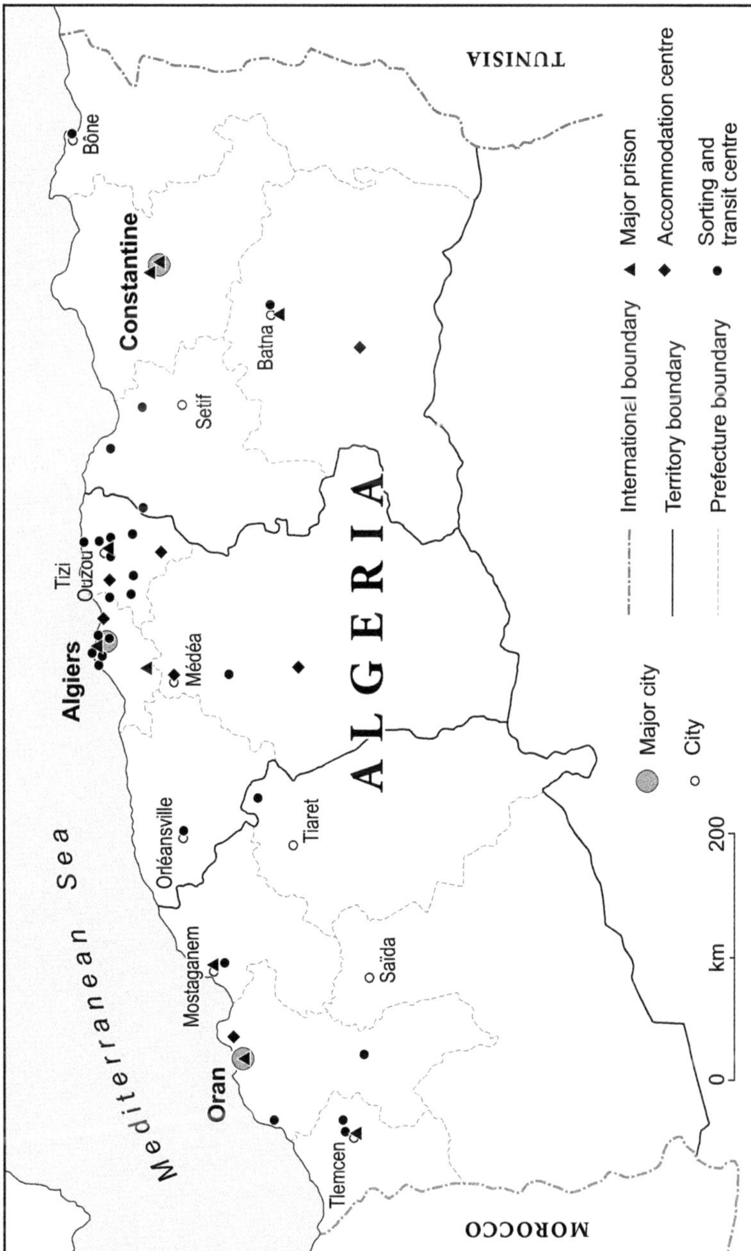

Map 2 Main detention centres in Algeria, 1962.

Introduction

In October 1975, the World Medical Association (WMA) met in Tokyo as part of their 29th annual assembly. Among the items on the agenda for this international meeting of medical experts was one issue that made the whole profession uncomfortable: how should doctors respond when asked to participate in acts of torture and other forms of violence? Far from being a hypothetical situation, the realities of this thorny question were very much alive. A few years earlier, the interrogation tactics employed by the British security forces against suspected members of the Irish Republican Army in Northern Ireland fell under criticism for their alleged brutality. As a result, committees were assembled to investigate the nature of these claims and the extent to which the tactics employed should remain as authorised practices. These efforts resulted in the 1971 Compton Report and the 1972 *Parker Report*, respectively.[1] The latter report noted that the controversial tactics – which included forced standing in stressed positions, hooding, continuous noise, sleep deprivation and heavily restricted diets – had been developed after the Second World War and were tested in various counterinsurgency campaigns in former British colonies, including Palestine, Malaya, Kenya, Cyprus and Aden. Ultimately, so the Majority Report concluded, 'there is no reason to rule out these techniques on moral grounds and that it is possible to operate them in a manner consistent with the highest standards of our society'.[2]

What was needed were strong safeguards to prevent abuse, and it was one of these suggested measures that alarmed the medical community. Paragraph 41 of the Majority Report stated:

> We think that a doctor with some psychiatric training should be present at all times at the interrogation centre and should be in a position

> to observe the course of oral interrogation. It is not suggested he should be himself responsible for stopping the interrogation – rather that he should warn the controller if he felt that the interrogation was being pressed too far having regard to the demeanour of the detainee, leaving the decision to the controller. This should be some safeguard both for the constitutionally vulnerable detainee and at the same time for the interrogator.[3]

The official suggestion that doctors be present to oversee interrogation which, whether authorised or not, was designed to cause harm and discomfort was a dizzying prospect for many doctors. Even weighed against the harsh 'necessities' of an effective counterterrorism campaign, where any tactic was surely justified to identify the site of the next bombing, as proponents of this response argue, could a doctor become embroiled in acts of violence?[4] But then again, if a doctor is present to observe, are they failing in their duty of care towards a patient who could be seriously injured or even killed as a result? Moreover, was it morally right to provide treatment to a detainee knowing that it was merely sustaining them so they could undergo further torture? The nature of this problem struck deep at the profession, raising the sinister spectre of the human rights abuses perpetrated by Nazi doctors during the Second World War. As a response, the British and Irish medical associations sought clarification from the WMA who, in turn, established a committee in 1974 to draft a new international declaration to protect medical professionals faced by these ethical challenges.

It was this draft declaration that was under consideration at the WMA's meeting in Tokyo in 1975.[5] The document, known as the Declaration of Tokyo, provides guidelines for doctors concerning torture and other cruel, inhuman or degrading treatment or punishments within detention or imprisonment. Although inspired by the events in Ireland, the declaration was designed to remind all doctors that, as the *British Medical Journal* (*BMJ*) wrote ahead of the meeting in Tokyo, their duty is towards their patient and 'to have nothing to do with any kind of cruel or inhumane or degrading treatment or the threat of it'.[6]

The adoption of the Declaration of Tokyo at the assembly represented a significant moment for the medical community. The document was the first set of ethical guidelines to explicitly address physicians encountering contexts where they or their medical knowledge could be manipulated by a third party – the State, the police or the military – for torture and abuse. The sentiment underpinning this achievement was summarised by Sir William Refshauge, the then Secretary General of the WMA, who stated that 'in the past year, it is the international community that has, in effect turned to us for moral guidance' at a time when societies' values were changing. Within this context, he added, the WMA's moral authority would not only be derived from its 'international forum', which was 'free from the political influences of Governments', but, most importantly, 'from the fact that it speaks for a profession which, more than any other, has responsibilities to mankind which transcend all other considerations'.[7] Refshauge concluded that 'I think that I need not remind you that this has been the case since the remotest antiquity'.

Despite its laudable goals, the Declaration of Tokyo has not always been successful in keeping members of the medical community away from torture. Since its creation, accusations of medical participation in human rights violations have emerged from various contexts including Russia, Uruguay, Chile, Kuwait, South Africa, the former Yugoslavia, Turkey and, more recently, Iraq and Afghanistan.[8] As such, it seems that Refshauge's more sanguine assertions about the benevolence and beneficence of the medical profession was misplaced. But what is it that makes doctors participate in state-sponsored violence? Is it always the result of coercion, be it from a demanding government or corrupt institution? Or, alternatively, is this type of collusion between medicine and the police or military simply the actions of a few malicious individuals who willingly abandoned their professional ethics for personal gain? Neither of these answers is satisfying, but they are often the ones offered in defence of the medical community as a whole whenever the subject of torture is raised. But could there instead be something else going on in these contexts that may help account for why some doctors, members of a profession associated with healing, can become entangled in institutions and activities that purposefully cause harm?

This is the purpose of this book. It examines two near contemporary cases where medical expertise and professionals were entangled in the excessive violences of two counterinsurgency campaigns. Specifically, it focuses on the role doctors and the institutions of medicine played in supporting the perpetration of violence by European security forces in the Algerian War of Independence and the Kenya Emergency, or the Mau Mau uprising as it is often referred to. In both examples, doctors employed by the state – and it is nearly always white male doctors rather than female doctors, members of the indigenous communities, or other medical professionals such as nurses – operated in direct proximity to the exercise of torture and other forms of violence in detention facilities controlled by the imperial powers.

This book represents the first in-depth comparative historical investigation into this subject. It explores how certain doctors in 1950s North and East Africa were involved in a variety of violent interventions that sought to coerce troublesome populations into complying with colonial rule and its demands.[9] In the following pages, I will show that, in these two contexts, a range of medical experts undertook activities that supported human rights violations and other forms of repressive force. Remarkably, the role medical professionals can play in counterinsurgency efforts, especially in relation to the perpetration of actual violence during official states of emergency, has received little cogent historical attention. This is especially true for the final years of the colonial era when both Britain and France encountered violent challenges to their authority. In these two historical cases, the colonial authorities used wide-ranging emergency powers to establish networks of detention centres, camps and resettlement villages to interrogate and hold suspected terrorists and troublesome populations. Within these centres, detainees experienced harsh conditions and a pervasive atmosphere of violence which was, to a lesser or greater degree, monitored and sustained by medical experts working for the state. This historical blind spot is thus regrettable, as research into these practices offers valuable comparative perspectives for understanding more recent experiences with counterterrorist campaigns, such as the War on Terror, and current debates surrounding medical and scientific participation in state-engineered repression.[10]

To be sure, the subject of medicine and violence in Algeria and Kenya has not been completely overlooked. Both David Anderson and Caroline Elkins, as well as others, have touched upon the role of particular doctors involved in the Kenya Emergency when discussing the health of detainees held in the 'pipeline', the series of detention centres, work camps and resettlement villages established to hold and process Mau Mau adherents and suspects.[11] But these references are incidental, brief and used primarily as additional illustrations of the atrocious conditions experienced by detainees during their confinement. In contrast, Raphaëlle Branche is one of the few to offer a direct consideration of doctors within the wider history of the Algerian War of Independence. Although Branche's discussion is limited to a few dozen pages or so of *La Torture et l'armée pendant la guerre d'Algérie*, it represents virtually the only attempt to examine the activities of specific doctors and the ways that medicine in Algeria was subverted to military need. Branche's pioneering efforts have not yet found a Kenyan counterpart, despite the release of the so-called Migrated Archives in 2012 that provided hitherto unknown but long-suspected evidence of colonial violence, some of which situates several doctors within range of torture and other abuses in Kenya.[12]

With the release of the Migrated Archives in Britain, scholars have started to ask comparative questions about Britain's use of violence in other overseas territories.[13] Similarly, in 2013, Laleh Khalili called for comparative discussions about violence in various contexts across the world. Aiming to move the analysis of the history of violence away from a narrow focus on isolated regions like the Middle East and North Africa, Khalili has appealed to scholars to produce broader analyses which 'bridge [the] archipelagos of scholarship' on the subject of violence.[14] This book takes up this call by analysing the counterinsurgency operations conducted in Algeria and Kenya. Fabian Klose's *Human Rights in the Shadow of Colonial Violence* has gone a long way to provide an excellent example of such a comparison for these two colonial conflicts.[15] But while Klose has shown how the French and British colonial powers actively sought to limit the application of the nascent human rights regime to their colonial subjects in these two conflicts, this book focuses attention on a profession that is commonly assumed to be agents of beneficence and healing. Moreover, by focusing explicitly on colonial medicine and doctors, it provides fresh perspectives on a largely underexplored aspect of counterinsurgency violence. The aim, ultimately, is not only to provide new insights into the ways that some doctors can support acts of extreme violence, but also to offer a nuanced and empirically strong explanation of the reasons why they might be led to do so.

Historical background

Before addressing the anatomy of this book in more detail, it is worth exploring the recent historical events and changes in the historiography of colonial violence that enabled it to come together. Even during the Algerian War, victims of violence and critics of the war more generally published various accounts about atrocities playing out in North Africa. However, with the passage of time, other testimonies have come to light, as participants in the conflict have, as Mildred Mortimer notes, 'begun to unburden themselves of guarded secrets'.[16] Similarly, memoirs from various Kenyans were published soon after the events which explained life behind the barbed wire of Britain's detention camps. As such, the world has had knowledge of these bloody contexts for multiple decades. Even so, the roles played by the doctors in both accounts remain underexplored. Indeed, the contribution of medicine to the violence of these two colonial wars more generally has largely fallen outside the scope of existing studies. This may be because, until recently, historians lacked the necessary documentary evidence to make sense of what appeared to be comparatively minor features of two otherwise sensational stories about wider abuses. However, recent high-profile scandals related to the legacy of these two colonial wars, as well as a distinct evolution in the historiography of colonial violence more generally, have brought to light previously unknown archives for historical research. This section focuses on these developments and the impact they have had on our understanding of violence during the Kenya and Algerian emergencies. This provides a crucial background for assessing the place of the current study in relation to this literature and how an investigation into the role of medicine can provide new perspectives on the application of violence in these conflicts.

It has long been known that excessive violence such as torture was used by French and British forces during the Algerian War and the Mau Mau uprising, respectively. Until recently, however, it was not clear to what extent such violence had been exceptional or how aware the respective colonial governments had been of its use. The British approach to counterinsurgency operations in Kenya, as well as other locations, has often been perceived as less heavy-handed and violent than that of other colonial powers. In fact, until the late

1990s, Britain's methods for suppressing African insurgents were hailed as exemplary; they represented a more civilised and peaceful approach to non-conventional warfare in the postwar period which utilised 'minimum force' to appeal to the loyalties and sensibilities of colonial subjects.[17] This success is often contrasted with France's failed counter-revolutionary tactics in Indochina and Algeria, which were known to be more violent. As such, the Algerian War has had a longer and more explicit association with the practice of torture than its East African counterpart.

There are a number of explanations for this. Firstly, ever since the early days of the Algerian War, reports of torture, such as Henri Alleg's 1958 book *La Question*, have generated international outrage at France's tactics in North Africa.[18] Secondly, as David Anderson has noted, the British have always been 'coy' about digging into the unsettling features of their colonial past.[19] Torture has long been identified as a double-edged and destructive weapon in any war – one which can have serious corrosive effects on the prestige and reputation of the states which practise it. As such, allegations of its use by British colonial forces were allowed to disappear for many decades.[20] Thirdly, and more significantly, torture in Algeria has received wider academic and public attention because of events that took place at the end of the 1990s. The court trial of Maurice Papon in 1997–98 for crimes against humanity committed during the Second World War brought wide attention to police violence against Algerian protestors in Paris, in 1961.[21] The trial raised questions about France's past activities during the war and turned attention towards the availability of police and military archives for historical work. In addition, in 2001, Louisette Ighilahriz, a former Front de libération nationale (FLN) militant, published her memoir detailing the appalling treatment she had received at the hands of the notorious 10th Parachute Division while being detained over a ten-week period in 1957.[22] Her account implicated prominent military officers who served in the Battle of Algiers as being personally involved, and triggered a large public debate about torture. Ighilahriz's account corroborated details from the earlier memoir of General Jacques Massu, who had personally overseen the use of torture at the time when Ighilahriz and Alleg were being detained.[23] In the same year that Ighilahriz published her memoir, Paul Aussaresses produced his unrepentant account, which not only confessed to using torture and murdering FLN nationalists in Algeria, but also actively praised the results of such activities.[24] Thus, what started with Papon's trial quickly turned into a new social and political-cultural attitude in France, one that sought to understand the role of torture in its colonial past.

In Britain, the situation changed between 2009 and 2012, when the High Court ruled against the Foreign and Commonwealth Office (FCO) after five elderly Kenyan claimants filed suits against their former colonial rulers. These Mau Mau veterans alleged that, while being held by British security forces during the Kenya Emergency, they had been subjected to torture and various other abuses in the British detention and screening camps. This case, as Caroline Elkins has observed, '[stirred] the strategic amnesia of the British colonial government', leading to the disclosure of thousands of new end-of-empire documents that had previously been hidden away in a high-security facility in Hanslope Park, near Milton Keynes.[25] The Hanslope Disclosure, or Migrated Archives as it is often referred to, contains 8,000 files pertaining to thirty-seven former colonies and revealing detailed evidence of the extent to which excessive violence was used during the British counterinsurgency efforts. For Elkins, who served alongside David Anderson and Huw Bennett as a historical expert witness for the trial, the fact that these files 'had been spirited away [from Kenya] at the time of decolonization' was evidence of a wider British plan to bury the secrets of its torturous past.[26] She argues, compellingly, that the circumstances surrounding the disappearance of these files are themselves a story worth telling, especially as, in addition to illuminating the extent of violence taking place in the camps, they reveal the degree to which the colonial state in London – including but not limited to the Colonial Office – was complicit in condoning and covering it up.[27]

It is these recently disclosed sets of documents released by the French and British governments, along with other official (especially for the Kenya case) and unofficial records and other published materials, which form the core of the present study.[28] Scholars who have already accessed these archives have highlighted several important themes for understanding the ways in which torture and related violence were exercised in these wars. Firstly, research has demonstrated that the practice was not just common among the colonial police, military and other members of the colonial security forces during the wars, its practice also took different forms in each context which changed over time. For instance, Raphaëlle Branche has shown that, rather than being an isolated phenomenon practised by a few fanatical French soldiers, torture was in fact an instrumental part of the military's approach to population control in Algeria. As she says, it was a 'weapon of war, a violence used by design' to defeat a revolutionary enemy.[29] For torture's apologists, both during the Algerian War and more recently, this was a key argument to justify its use: torture, they contend, was a vital method for obtaining operational intelligence in a new type of conflict, one taking place within heavily populated urban centres riddled with 'terrorist' networks.[30] Central to this logic, Branche has shown, is the assumption that those undergoing interrogation had something to confess and were therefore guilty. Torture thus became a kind of preliminary punishment that eliminated the recourse to legal proceedings, which, the military complained, were too slow and too lenient.[31] By utilising such justifications, soldiers armed themselves with a utilitarian imperative to act brutally towards an individual in order to save the lives of the many.

In addition to being seen as a precision tool for extracting intelligence, torture was also a weapon of domination. As Branche notes, 'much more than a method of obtaining information, torture was a warning to all', and rumour served the military's aims by propagating the terror among the population.[32] If its use occasionally killed a detainee, then the same death communicated the power of France to the Algerians. This made torture an expression of political domination.[33] To appreciate how significant this is, it is necessary to understand its use not only as an act of excess in a chaotic war but as part of the wider system of repression within the colonial context which allowed such practices to emerge in the first place.[34] This is a particularly important point that has since been stressed by other scholars: the military's use of illegal violence in Algeria, not just torture, formed part of a long history of repression that can be traced back to the earliest days of France's occupation of the territory.[35]

In order to create these environments of repressive violence, the colonial governments manipulated and misused various institutions to support their rule. The law, Sylvie Thénault has shown, was a vital tool in France's military strategy, since it produced legally 'exceptional' conditions in which violence could take place.[36] Similar to the 'state of exception' described by the philosopher Giorgio Agamben, Thénault has revealed the extent to which the French legal system was inverted and weaponised against the nationalists to create environments where extreme violence – torture, rape, disappearances and summary executions – became permissible.[37] This was achieved through the use of key emergency laws issued in Paris which transferred the control of the civil courts in the North African colony to the military tribunals.[38] The introduction of these emergency powers by the political authorities allowed the military to conceive of and wage a war that twisted justice into a form of judicial repression within the Algerian courts and sanctioned the semi-legal practice of internment and the illegal practice of torture.[39] Importantly, Thénault has shown how magistrates became accessories to these exceptional circumstances and aided in perpetuating the misappropriation of their professional institutions. Through inaction and a passivity born out of 'fear of resisting the army by acting against torture, disappearances or summary executions', the French magistrates in Algeria showed remarkable solidarity with the military's aims.[40]

Just as the history of colonial violence had deep roots in the early stages of France's conquest of the North African territory, so too were the conditions of the emergency immersed in a colonial legal exception that dated back to the colony's earliest days.[41] French policy towards its colonial subjects was one of deep inequality where the access to legal and political office and representation was always skewed in the Europeans' favour. The colonial character of justice in Algeria was therefore a manifestation of French sovereignty on a conquered territory and people. The Muslims were by default French subjects who were denied the rights associated with French citizenship. They existed outside the 'normal' rule of law of metropolitan France.[42] By the time war broke out after 1 November 1954, the long colonial past, an 'exceptional regime' in an 'exceptional environment', was inherited by the military.[43] The French authorities sought to control the Algerian population and to sift rebels and their supporters from the wider population through the use of an extensive system of concentration camps. This was brought about by Article 6 of the emergency law of 3 April 1955, which allowed the 'Minister of the Interior in all cases and, in Algeria, the Governor General' to 'pronounce the assignment of residence in a territorial division or a specified locality of any person' residing within the territory whose activities might be deemed 'dangerous for public safety and security' of the territory.[44] However, the same article continued to state that 'Under no circumstances may the assignment of residence result in the creation of camps for the detention of the persons referred to in the preceding paragraph'. Despite this, the first camps in Algeria were opened in May 1955 as part of the law's allowance for placing suspects under house arrest.[45] Over the course of the conflict, over two million Algerians were relocated into what were called *camps de regroupement*, which formed a prominent part of the Plan de Constantine reforms launched by President Charles de Gaulle after his return to power in 1958.[46] While these camps were officially intended to protect the rural Algerian population while also helping to disrupt the nationalist underground networks, they were often the locations of extraordinary violence. Alongside these regroupment camps were detention camps designed for purely military purposes. The military established networks of *centres de tri et transit* (CTTs), which were legalised in 1957, to screen and categorise detainees. The fates of the detainee varied, depending on how they were categorised.[47] After 1958, there were also the military internment camps where selected detainees were subjected to 're-education' in order to turn them to the French cause.[48]

The situation in Kenya was not dissimilar; the excessive, punitive and retaliatory nature of the violence perpetrated by both sides of the Mau Mau uprising had its roots in the longer history of the British settler colony. The so-called 'pacification' of the territory had been achieved through savage campaigns of destruction by British military forces in the late nineteenth century.[49] Corporal punishment was a pervasive feature of interracial relations in pre-Emergency Kenya, where the European settlers, police forces and even school teachers beat the Africans in order to enforce a racial hierarchy in the country.[50] Any anticolonial resistance throughout the years of occupation was similarly met by collective punishment, imprisonment, executions and terror.[51] Although all these forms of force were unleashed upon Mau Mau and suspected Mau Mau supporters during the Emergency, it would be a mistake to conceive of colonial violence as unchanging. Indeed, when it comes to understanding how violence played out in the Emergency itself, David Anderson has usefully shown that there were two relatively distinct phases. The first took place between October 1952 and the end of 1955, when the emphasis was on the gathering of tactical intelligence to identify the enemy.[52] This was of prime importance for waging a successful counterinsurgency campaign, just as it was in Algeria. As Colonel J. M. Forster noted in 1957, the 'identification of terrorists and an early appreciation of their methods and habits is essential for the efficient conduct of operations'.[53] However, as time went on, the practice of screening evolved into a coercive exercise designed to extract confessions from detainees and to punish them for their defiant ways. By the end of the emergency, specific forms of torture had become systematised within the British detention centres and were being used to break the will of hard-core Mau Mau.[54]

In Kenya, the British authorities framed their use of emergency powers in relation to the British Emergency Powers (Defence) Act of 1939, a statute that gave the government unrestricted power to detain individuals deemed dangerous to the state during a time of war.[55] Yet they also drew inspiration from the Malayan Emergency Regulations ordinance of 1948, which had been used to suppress a communist insurrection in that colony a few years earlier. In contrast to the Act of 1939, these regulations empowered the state to detain suspected insurgents indefinitely and allowed for detention to continue even after the colonial state of emergency had expired.[56] Given that Mau Mau was interpreted as a form of 'collective African atavistic insanity', the British authorities devised the 'rehabilitation programme' to 'treat' this perceived ideological sickness. Once arrested, detainees were meant to make their way through the 'pipeline', a series of detention camps, transit camps, work schemes and relocation settlements that were built by the British colonial authorities to isolate, discipline, punish and ultimately 'rehabilitate' supposed Mau Mau followers.[57] Originally, the rehabilitation programme was conceived as a humanitarian project by a limited number of the more liberal-minded colonial officers who hoped to offer social and economic benefits to the Kikuyu who confessed to having taken Mau Mau oaths.[58] The British campaign for the 'hearts and minds' of their Kenyan subjects thus reinforced the idea of Britain's 'civilising mission', what Caroline Elkins refers to as its 'raison d'être for colonizing the Kikuyu people'.[59] Yet Elkins has shown that the rehabilitation camps became spaces of torture, punishment and death, as liberal ideals gave way to what she regarded as 'eliminationist' racism that ran riot. By her reckoning, the British had detained '1.5 million people, or nearly the entire Kikuyu population' who were subsequently 'physically and psychologically' beaten into submission.[60]

Later works by Daniel Branch and A. R. Baggallay show that, far from being an institutionalised plot to wage a racial war, the history of violence and torture in the detention camps is more detailed and complex. Branch, who explores the history of imprisonment in colonial Kenya in the years between 1930 and 1952, explains how poor funding had always meant that Kenyan prisons were understaffed and were sites of disease and violence. As such, there was a reliance on untrained officers who exercised a punitive approach to imprisonment. Although finances were set up to help expand these camps during the Emergency years, the underlying logic running them had not changed – they were still cramped, understaffed and prone to disease and violence. As such, I would argue, there is no evidence to suggest the Emergency, set up to combat the Mau Mau, introduced a new desire to eliminate the Kikuyu people – violence here is part of a longer history of colonial abuse and neglect.[61] Both Baggallay's and Branch's work demonstrates that the decline in efforts to meet the original rehabilitation programme had a more textured history than Elkins had originally suggested.

Indeed, a closer look at the provisions set aside for the rehabilitation programme indicates that the escalation in violence and increased reliance on torture were also influenced by changes in available finances and demands from the government. Baggallay argues that the British government had originally planned to embrace the liberal rehabilitation programme, but after the success of Operation Anvil in 1954 – an effort to eliminate Mau Mau from Nairobi – the detention camps swelled with suspects. In order to operate effectively, the rehabilitation programme would have required additional funds, but the Ministry of Finance actually reduced their budget and, instead, increased that available to 'Internal Security and Defence', including prison officers.[62] The department responsible for rehabilitation was thus stretched too thin and could not afford to provide the requisite training for its staff. Instead, Thomas Askwith, the head of the Community Development Department in Kenya, was forced to employ members of the Prison Department who had a long history of using violence, as Branch has demonstrated.[63] Moreover, after 1955, the introduction of release targets eroded any hope for rehabilitation and resulted in the transformation of camps into sites of torture – any action was deemed acceptable if it led to confession, the prerequisite for release.[64]

Given that a large portion of this study takes place within the confines of detention centres, Elkins's and Thénault's works on the British and French camps, respectively, are particularly useful. While Thénault's assessments have been careful and measured, Elkins's earlier work has caused more controversy as a result of her belief that 'there was in late colonial Kenya a murderous campaign to eliminate Kikuyu people, a campaign that left tens of thousands, perhaps hundreds of thousands, dead'.[65] By evoking 'genocide', Elkins simplified the meaning of torture and colonial violence, turning them into rhetorical tools for producing a 'black-and-white' representation of the Emergency. Less consideration has been paid to the wider historical context or the variables that motivated individual actors or groups to get involved in the repression activities at different stages of the conflict. More recently, however, Elkins has conceded that the situation was more complicated than she originally assumed and has even cautioned us against 'an overtly state-dominated understanding of mass violence'.[66] Instead, we need to ask questions about 'who organized the violence' in order to understand how weak states and their actors responded to violent insurgents.[67] With the release of the Migrated Archives, historians have started to ask important questions about those who participated in abuse, their personal culpability and how the torture and abuse was organised.[68]

Taken together, these studies of violence and torture in Algeria and Kenya have demonstrated the extent to which such practices were embedded within the two countries' colonial situations. They have addressed questions related to the evolution of violence within specific contexts, while also assessing the ways in which institutions, especially the colonial legal systems, created the local conditions of exception that allowed torture and related atrocities to be carried out by colonial security forces. Yet few of these studies have considered the role of other institutions and professions in supporting the exercise of state repressive force during emergency conditions. Given that doctors were almost ubiquitously present when instances of torture took place, the dearth of scholarship on the role of medicine during the Kenyan and Algerian emergencies is especially surprising and, indeed, unsatisfactory.[69] It is, after all, not coincidental that, in *The Gulag Archipelago*, Alexandr Solzhenitsyn referred to the doctor in the Soviet concentration camps as the torturer's 'right-hand man'.[70] This book thus represents the first focused analysis of medical practitioners who were involved in the use of torture in these two contexts.

Doctors, medicine and violence

The idea that medicine as a healing art could be regarded as an extension of colonial authority and power is not new. When Michel Foucault first articulated the ways in which clinical knowledge and medical practice came to shape the rise of Western modernity, he inspired generations of scholars to assess and map the formation of biopolitical knowledge and its implications in various settings.[71] For Foucault, medicine and medical institutions, such as hospital and asylums, functioned as tools of control whereby doctors and their technical knowledge helped discipline society through the organisation and isolation of their bodies, especially those deemed politically or socially undesirable.[72] Although Foucault focused on European contexts, his ideas have nevertheless been applied to the subject of empire whereby Western medicine and science were used to define non-Western bodies as political subjects while pathologising their laws, religions and structures of governance. As David Arnold has written, colonial rule 'built up an enormous battery of texts and discursive practices that concerned themselves with the physical being of the colonized'. Through this, he argued, the colonised body became a 'site for the construction of [colonialism's] own authority, legitimacy, and control'.[73]

However, it would be a mistake to suggest that Foucault's ideas can be transported onto the colonial world wholesale. There are, as Megan Vaughan has demonstrated, 'real differences between the nature of the colonial power/knowledge regime and that described by Foucault'.[74] Vaughan articulates several important objections to Foucault's claims when it comes to overseas territories. For one thing, she argues, colonial states were 'hardly "modern states" for much of their short existence', which meant they relied on 'repressive' power rather than the 'productive' power Foucault identified in European examples. Secondly, because the colonised individual was nearly always regarded as 'Otherly' by the colonial authorities, there was no need for the type of widescale incarceration in asylums that Foucault saw as fundamental tools for isolating the 'mad' and unproductive elements of society (more on this later). Finally, and significantly for this current work, there was the fact that Africans, and other colonial populations by extension, were seldom seen as 'individuals'. According to Foucault, an outcome of biopolitical power was the formation of individual 'subjects' as well as 'objects', but, as she notes, 'in colonial medical discourse and practice [the colonised] were conceptualized … as members of groups'.[75]

Yet while historians have shown how colonial medicine could be exercised as a means for expanding imperial control, there has been remarkable silence over its involvement in obviously violent situations, such as the emergencies addressed here. Indeed, in 2008, Richard Keller explicitly noted that the 'complicity of medicine in the structural violence of the colonial situation reveals a range of iatrogenic forms of suffering and a setting in which medicine cannot be construed without also accounting for its operation as a force of oppression'.[76] Within this context, the clinic itself was a space where the colonial conflict could play out, and it was the bodies of the indigenous populations that were the focus of this conflict. As such, the encounter between doctor and patient, where the doctor was a representative of the colonial oppressor and the patient an indigenous subject, could become an opportunity for the latter to exercise resistance and political defiance. Yet I would argue that even Keller has not gone far enough: rather than simply looking at the structural contributions medicine made to the exercise of colonial violence, what about such instances where doctors participated in explicitly violent acts themselves, acts that were exercised upon the very bodies of the colonial subject?

This point was made by Frantz Fanon, the Martinique-born psychiatrist and anticolonial writer, when he drew on his experience as a psychiatrist working at the Blida Psychiatric Hospital in Algeria, during the emergency. Fanon's work is well known to postcolonial critics and some historians of colonial medicine.[77] For the former, he is the founding father of the field of postcolonial studies, but for the latter, he has had limited application outside the history of colonial psychiatry.[78] This is unfortunate, given that his work is rich in material for studying African colonial medicine during the period of decolonisation. What Fanon offers, unlike other theorists such as Agamben, is an account of the lived experience of colonial subjects facing the everyday reality of colonial violence and their methods of resistance. More importantly for this book's purposes, Fanon is one of the few contemporary thinkers who attempted to wrestle with the entanglements of medicine and the colonial system and its impact on both the indigenous population and the make-up of the colonists' society. This is a point that is regularly underplayed or altogether forgotten by postcolonial writers, who fail to account for Fanon's role as an historical actor in the Algerian War or, indeed, his position as a psychiatrist schooled in the medical knowledge and skills of the 'oppressor'.[79] His interpretations of the impacts the colonial encounter had on both the coloniser and the colonised were indebted to his educational background and his experience as a black subject of colonialism working as a doctor in the colonial setting of Algeria. This should be stressed: Fanon's medical career, as recent studies by Keller and Filippo Menozzi have argued, was the linchpin that connected his work on racial identity to his later work as an anticolonial thinker and revolutionary.[80] It was his experience as a psychiatrist that exposed him to the injustices of colonialism and its effects on the personalities of the colonised.

However, this too should be problematised. Fanon became a vocal supporter of the Algerian nationalists and eventually threw his lot in with the FLN. As such, his anticolonial writing comes to us as testament to his outrage, disappointment and anger against the colonial authorities, which will have certainly influenced the way he constructed his cases. Both of his most famous publications, *A Dying Colonialism* and *The Wretched of the Earth*, contain specific instances where medical practitioners, his colleagues working in Algeria, abused their power, took advantage of the Algerians or actively abused their status as doctors in order to assist the police or military during the war.[81] In fact he even directly implicates doctors in torture operations. Yet Fanon does not always provide names or details that can be used to verify his claims. The identities of both the victims of abuse and its perpetrators are missing while the reader is faced with anecdotal evidence of serious breaches in ethical conduct and professionalism. The lack of tangible evidence accompanying Fanon's work may give reason for caution but it does not make it useless. In fact, it provides an opportunity to test Fanon's claims for historical accuracy. By comparing the accounts contained in his publications with other sources related to the Algerian War, it becomes possible not only to gain a greater appreciation for Fanon's work, but also to assess its applicability to other African contexts, such as the Kenya Emergency.

While a significant body of research has covered the subject of colonial medicine, tropical hygiene policy and scientific practice across the British and French empires,[82] somewhat less attention has been paid to colonial doctors and healthcare providers as a distinct social group within these colonial settings.[83] More bafflingly, the little social historical research that is relevant to these two contexts has adopted a comparatively limited chronological span. For instance, Charlotte Ann Chopin has recently shown how the French doctors in Algeria were representatives of the Third Republic in the colony, while also fitting in as local settlers among the other European communities. Rather than being simple agents of empire, Chopin argues, these doctors embodied the ideals and attitudes of a distinct form of 'whiteness' among the settlers.[84] Her analysis highlights specific tensions within the French medical culture in Algeria that arose from this dual identity as government employees and members of the settler societies, but her study stops at 1911.

Similarly, in the British context, Anna Crozier has provided one of the few histories of the British Colonial Medical Service (CMS) in East Africa.[85] Rather than examining the policies and practices of medicine in this region, Crozier's account tracks the evolution of this underexplored branch of the Colonial Services, its recruiting processes and culture and the experience of individual Medical Officers working in Kenya, Uganda and Tanganyika during the twentieth century. While Crozier's work provides excellent contextual detail for understanding the characters and attitudes of those selected by the Colonial Services to work in their overseas territories, her focus tapers off at the start of the Second World War. Although she provides a brief overview of the years leading up to independence, it forms a short coda to her concluding chapter. More recently, the same author has also produced an edited volume which seeks to shine greater light on the various medical practitioners and healthcare providers who competed and occasionally collaborated in East Africa in the first half of the twentieth century.[86] This collection of essays does add greater texture and diversity to the previous account, but it still fails to cover the postwar years.

This is a startling omission given that, as members of the colonial order, doctors would have embodied what Ann Laura Stoler referred to as 'imperial formations' upon which the legal, institutional and cultural bases of colonial discrimination were built.[87] These were shared presumptions and cultural norms that were commonplace in the late nineteenth and twentieth centuries which justified coercion and discrimination, as Stoler states, through ideas of 'imperial guardianship, trusteeship, delayed autonomy, temporary intervention, conditional tutelage, military takeover in the name of humanitarian works, violent intervention in the name of human rights, and security measures in the name of peace'.[88]

Over the last three decades, there have been multiple reports and studies into doctors involved in torture regimes and human rights violations in the various contexts mentioned above. The problem is that few of these studies, if any, have been conducted by historians; rather, the authors tend to be medical practitioners or involved in medical-related organisations. While much of this work shows little consideration for the wider historical contexts surrounding these instances of state-sponsored violence, it nevertheless provides a useful framework to guide an investigation into such abuses with this perspective. The overriding emphasis within this work has been to understand *how* doctors have contributed to regimes that torture while also seeking measures, regulations, codes of conduct and other solutions to prevent future participation.

There are a number of useful points identified by these studies when taken as a whole. Importantly, this body of work has shown that while many types of medical practitioners can get involved in human rights violations, those most likely to assist in torture are those responsible for examining and caring for prisoners.[89] Within detention camps, doctors appear to perform several important tasks that are common across these disparate contexts. These activities can be understood as either passive or active forms of collusion and include: evaluating the victim's capacity to withstand torture; providing medical treatment to victims if complications occur;

falsifying autopsy reports or providing false diagnoses in order to hide the evidence of torture; violating the professional confidence of the doctor–patient relationship by providing medical information to security staff; actively participating in the interrogation itself, especially through the use of so-called 'truth drugs'; and finally, failing to respond to the signs of torture and to take wounds and complaints seriously, and generally remaining silent in ways that allow the practice to continue.[90]

While this list of methods of collusion might be useful for comparing and contrasting the ways that doctors took part in violence in the Algerian War or the Kenya Emergency, these studies tend to favour psychological explanations for *why* doctors colluded in the first place, which is less helpful. In particular, the concepts of 'doubling' and 'atrocity-producing situations', which were created by the American psychiatrist Robert Jay Lifton, have featured heavily within this literature.[91] Lifton himself has used these concepts, whereby otherwise 'moral' and 'ethical' individuals become supporters or perpetrators of cruel conduct, to explain why American physicians took part in the abusive environments of the recent War on Terror, especially in Abu Ghraib, in Iraq.[92] Although these explanations remain popular among medical practitioners seeking to account for medical involvement in atrocities, they are nevertheless epistemologically limited for historical research. They are too generalised, deterministic and place too much emphasis on the corrupting influence of institutions and the state. They also reveal little about the specific factors that may lead a given individual at a given time and place to take part in violence; nor do they provide an explanation for the extent of this violence and how such activities are carried out. Ultimately, these perspectives play down the agency of those doctors who participated in atrocities while maintaining an image of the profession as otherwise ethical.

Alternatively, other scholars have adopted a similar structural-normative approach to produce more nuanced accounts of violence than Lifton, who has been accused of making grandiose claims and overstatements.[93] Through an examination of torture among Brazilian police, Huggins, Haritos-Fatouros and Zimbardo have explained the perpetration of violence as a result of a slow and gradual normative process whereby individuals become acclimatised to such acts over time.[94] Similarly, Christopher Browning's famous study of Polish Reserve Police Battalion 101 under Nazi occupation has shown how mass murder and routine, the exceptional and the normal, became fused during the everyday experience of these 'ordinary men'. Browning's approach is particularly useful for the present study as it is multi-layered; it allows for groups or subgroups at the centre of analysis to behave differently while also offering multi-causal explanations for why this may be the case.[95] Although he draws on psycho-sociological perspectives to guide his assessment, Browning is not rigidly bound to them, as he balances these perspectives with historical factors concerning individual beliefs, ideology and opportunity.

Unlike other sets of professionals involved in modern conflicts, doctors as a group are often associated with ethical standards which are *expected* to play some part in guiding their conduct. Yet these expectations, along with the development of modern medical codes of ethics, are themselves the products of complicated historical variables. Lifton's psychological explanations reveal little about the influence medical ethics exert on professional conduct in a given time and place. What types of pressures can come into play when a doctor participates in a conflict scenario where torture is rife? How do they understand such dilemmas and how do they negotiate them? It would be a mistake to simply assume that the Hippocratic Oath has always meant the same thing to everyone at all times,[96] or that doctors operating in different types of conflict always understand their roles and responsibilities in the same way. Indeed, have doctors always seen themselves as the protectors of human rights they are commonly believed to be today?[97]

It is only in recent years that historians have begun to turn their attention to these questions. Thus scholars have taken a closer look at how contemporary medical ethics regimes have come into existence, especially those related to human experimentation (especially within the Nazi concentration camps), the development of the Nuremburg Code and medical and scientific involvement in the research, development and testing of chemical and biological weapons during the Cold War.[98] Such studies have not only drawn attention to the relative ineffectiveness of ethical codes in governing medical and scientific research using human participants, they have also offered important perspectives for contemporary research ethics.[99] Nevertheless, the dilemmas surrounding human experimentation, especially in relation to national security considerations and wartime conditions, are only one area where established medical ethics can become strained; medical participation in interrogation is, of course, another. When it comes to the subject of medical ethics and doctors' participation in torture, scholarly interest in bioethics has tended to favour the subject of professional loyalty itself.

The use of so-called 'enhanced interrogation techniques' by British and American forces in Iraq and Afghanistan in the 2000s drew attention to the thorny problems posed by medical complicity in violent conflicts.[100] The concept of the 'dual-loyalty dilemma', sometimes referred to as the 'dual-obligation dilemma' or 'mixed agency', has become a common feature within bioethical discussion on this topic. This can be understood as a conflict between clinical professional duties to the patient, on the one hand, and, on the other, obligations, expressed or implied, real or perceived, to the interests of a third party, such as an employer, an insurer, the state or the military.[101] For instance, military physicians have medical obligations to those in medical need and are required to exercise beneficence and non-malfeasance, both of which form the foundation of modern medical ethics, to needy combatants on either side of the conflict and not to undertake any activity that might (intentionally) make anyone medically worse off.[102] Yet, at the same time, these professionals may have competing obligations to their regiment and the state, applying contrary pressures to their conduct.[103] These pressures, it is assumed, can lead some military physicians to use medical knowledge and skill for purposes other than healing – for instance, for conducting illegal human experimentation (as in the case of Nazi doctors during the Second World War); for designing and building such lethal weapons as biological or chemical weapons; or, as in the context of the present research, for assisting with torture and abusive interrogation.[104]

The dual-loyalty dilemma, especially within the military context, has continued to pose intractable challenges. While it is beyond the scope of this book to examine the range of potential options raised by these authors for current conflict scenarios, the examination of professional loyalty in relation to medical ethics and conduct is interesting from a historical perspective. This is especially so in the cases of Algeria and Kenya, where the nature of revolutionary warfare in settler colonies presented alternative challenges to the types of 'conventional' struggles these scholars have assessed. The contention is that, during irregular conflicts, such as those experienced during the Kenyan and Algerian emergencies of the 1950s, the situation becomes even more complex: under these conditions, civilian doctors can be drawn into the conflict and put into positions where they are required to behave or operate in ways that challenge the understanding of their professional and ethical obligations. This is not to say that the emergencies introduced an entirely new set of circumstances that radically changed the attitudes, behaviours or loyalties of these professionals per se. On the contrary, it seems that the emergencies merely polarised older, more deeply entrenched prejudices and allegiances, prompting some to act on them in ways that varied in degree, not in type, from pre-emergency conditions. Rather than simply witnessing a binary strain between the professional loyalties of the doctors, on the one hand, and the demands of the state and military, on the other, these two complicated contexts reveal a whole range of competing factors that might have influenced how physicians understood their obligations and interpreted their roles.

The road ahead

The analysis in this book is shaped by one overarching question: to what extent and in what ways did colonial doctors contribute to the practice of torture during the Algerian and Kenyan wars of decolonisation? To address it, I make use of a range of sources, both official and published materials, drawn from British, French and Kenyan archives, to assess when and how doctors participated in the colonial counterinsurgency efforts, especially within the detention centres.[105]

In many instances, the events being discussed here featured in the work of other historians who have examined allegations and cases of torture and abuse, but the doctors within these assessments have either only been mentioned in passing or else have been entirely overlooked. As such, care has been taken to situate the findings with reference to the secondary literature in order to show how a re-examination of some well-known cases can yield new perspectives when approached from this angle. However, this book's empirical bases pose a number of challenges that must be understood at this stage.

Given the depth of official denial and cover-up that took place during the Kenya Emergency, it is likely that we are still missing crucial information about alleged atrocities and the individuals involved, the availability of the Migrated Archives notwithstanding. The situation is not dissimilar in Algeria. The French government went to great lengths to conceal the official records regarding the use of torture. As Thénault and Branche have noted, 'the best way to keep a practice secret is to leave no trace of it'.[106] But while the French government and military tried to stymie the spread of information about their clandestine and illegal practices in Algeria, multiple participants on both sides of the conflict have recently published memoirs which add greater contextual detail to the official record. Of course, memoirs and the act of recalling events from the distant past present their own challenges for historical analysis. But when handled with due caution, these documents, some of which have been produced by former doctors, can still be used to substantiate areas where the official evidence is thin. In contrast, although there have been a number of memoirs published by police and military officers who fought against Mau Mau insurgents, the same cannot be said about their medical counterparts. This constitutes a frustrating absence in the historical record for this struggle. As mentioned above, in the years following decolonisation, a number of British medical officers published nostalgic accounts of their days in the East African colony, but when it comes to the Emergency, their accounts largely fall silent. Although the official records at TNA permit many doctors to be placed in direct proximity to the types of violence discussed in this study, these practitioners themselves have had little to say on the matter, either to explain the situation, to deny their participation or to denounce others. Where possible, I have therefore tried to draw attention to the gaps in evidence, as an omission can sometimes be just as telling as a direct admission.[107] Nevertheless, there are portions of the following analysis that draw on sparse and sometimes patchy material; where appropriate, any potential limitations to the interpretations have been acknowledged in the text while efforts have been made to provide alternatives if possible.

Regardless of these gaps, the material presented in this book makes it possible to argue that not only were French and British doctors involved in the torture and violence perpetrated by colonial security forces in Algeria and Kenya, they were also often central to their justification, systemisation and maintenance. Although it is not always possible to identify the extent to which a given practitioner was aware of the whole system of repression in which they operated, it is clear that when torture took place within these colonies, medicine and its professionals were frequently present in one form or another. Yet it would be a mistake to assume that the presence of these professionals in and around the torture chamber amounted to any real reliance on sophisticated scientific interrogation techniques within either state. In this sense, the findings of this book contribute to recent scholarship which debunks and challenges ideas about effective 'scientific' methods for gaining the truth through the application of pain and suffering.[108] More often than not, when doctors participated in torture, it was to monitor the health of victims or to help cover up or deny evidence of its application. Even in extreme cases such as the use of truth serums in Algeria, the existing evidence is clear that such methods were ineffective and unreliable tools of persuasion.

The role of the doctors discussed in this work and the reasons why each individual became entangled in counterinsurgency violence are predictably complicated and multifaceted. By contrasting and comparing both contexts within each chapter, this study seeks to untie several such explanations. The benefit of this type of approach is that it avoids drawing what Heather Jones refers to as 'partisan interpretations' of the perpetration of violence in both contexts.[109] This is because a comparative approach assumes there are key variables that influence the ways in which doctors participated in these programmes that are unique or common to these contexts. These include the ways Britain and France governed their respective colonies, the ways medicine was established within each setting and the place of different types of medical professionals who provided care for different groups of people. In order to explore these themes, I start by situating French and British colonial medicine as it was practised in Algeria and Kenya, along with its doctors, within the longer history of the colonies in North and East Africa. This is the primary function of Chapter 1. By exploring the ways these professionals were embedded in the social, economic and political milieu of the colonial situation, it is also possible to map out the rise of African and Muslim nationalism in each colony and how doctors, as a privileged set of historical actors, may have contributed to local grievances and complaints.

Once violence broke out in both colonies, the governments found themselves facing what they regarded as a new type of warfare inspired or directly managed by Communist subversion. As such, it is not possible to grasp the logic governing the colonial authorities' responses to these threats to colonial rule without accounting for their place in the broader history of the Cold War. With this in mind, Chapter 2 addresses initial colonial appraisals of the nationalist movements. This is particularly interesting as, in both cases, colonial authorities utilised the expertise of a range of experts of the mind, including sociologists, anthropologists and psychiatrists, not only to explain the nationalists' mindsets, but also to prescribe appropriate treatment for their perceived psychological conditions. These experts drew on old, established and fundamentally local racial perspectives about the ostensibly irrational and violent tendencies inherent in African populations. These, I shall show, were then married with contemporary anxieties about brainwashing and vulnerable minds. Rather than interpreting the nationalists' recourse to violence as a response to long-held grievances or as the tactical outcome of guerrillas fighting an asymmetrical war, British and French authorities chose to regard them as displays of innate savagery and religious fundamentalism.

Chapter 3 moves the analysis into the detention camps themselves and demonstrates how colonial doctors and medicine performed a range of activities and provided services behind the barbed wire that have hitherto been overlooked in the existing historiography. Indeed, this chapter shows that not only were many detention camps in both Algeria and Kenya fitted with rudimentary medical provisions and facilities, sometimes there were doctors living on site who held daily clinical hours and treated patients for a variety of conditions. Nevertheless, many detention camps were extremely unsanitary locations where a number of deficiency and contagious diseases were endemic. In some cases, the colonial security forces actually regarded the poor conditions as part of the punishment process and believed that disease and starvation were easier ways to eliminate more recalcitrant members of the detainee populations. In this context, ideas about abuse expand to include indirect forms of suffering caused by such conditions. Although doctors may not have shared in these ideas, when news of the appalling sanitary and health conditions of certain camps reached wider public audiences, especially in the case of Kenya, it was these medical officers who provided evidence and statements that helped mitigate embarrassment for the government. The chapter also explores the nature of the clinical encounter within these facilities, an encounter that was often a complicated experience for detainees who would sometimes see camp doctors as functionaries of colonial oppression. Indeed, doctors regularly offered expert interpretation of detainee behaviour and complaints that translated what could be seen as acts of detainee resistance, into further evidence of the patient's psychological instability, something that helped justify the camp's continued existence.

It should be stated here that Chapters 4 and 5 contain material that some readers may find challenging or disturbing, as the focus of the analysis moves onto the ways that doctors employed by the state assisted with and responded to the use of torture in the detention centres. In particular, Chapter 4 examines the development of new international codes of medical ethics in the immediate postwar period to show how the language enshrined within these instruments was often too imprecise and vague to be of practical use for doctors faced with the challenges associated with interrogation and torture. When it came to justifying the use of state-sponsored and systematised torture techniques, the military and colonial authorities appealed to doctors to provide a humanitarian and scientific veneer to the administration of pain. Whether it involved them directly endorsing specific techniques or simply monitoring the health of detainees before and after its application, the colonial authorities required medical assistance. In other instances doctors became directly involved in the interrogation process. The use of truth drugs on terrorist suspects in Algeria remains an important distinction between these two conflicts, as there is little evidence to suggest that British doctors were prepared to use such methods against Mau Mau.

While military doctors in Algeria may have played a more active role in the interrogation and torture of detainees, this does not mean their British counterparts were any less instrumental in similar activities in Kenya. In particular, the Medical Officers working in the detention centres appear to have either turned a blind eye to the signs of torture within these camps or else conducted their clinical duties in order to maintain the bodies of those undergoing torture. In fact, doctors responded to the realities of torture in various ways; this is the topic of Chapter 5. Although such reactions could be rationalised in several ways, often the result was that doctors remained silent in the face of such abuse. This silence and potential indifference to suffering went a long way to maintaining the efficiency of Kenya's preferred torture technique, the now notorious 'dilution technique' designed by the British security forces to quickly overwhelm and break new detainees. In a few rare cases, news of excessive abuse reached wider audiences in the metropoles, generating public outcry. In order to quell concerns or to help cover up evidence of torture, doctors could act in various ways that played into the hands of the colonial authorities. By manipulating reports, doctors concealed the true causes of death. In other cases, a rigid adherence to professional neutrality, which neither confirmed nor denied evidence of torture, allowed other government agents to fill in the explanatory gap with their own narrative. Interestingly, in both countries, there were high-profile scandals related to the victims of torture and other abuses that foreshadowed the end of the conflicts. In Algeria, public interest in the trial of Djamila Boupacha, a young Algerian nationalist who attempted to bring rape and torture charges against the French military, revealed not only the types of barbarous treatment that Algerians experienced while in detention, but also the lengths to which military doctors were prepared to go to hide and downplay signs of abuse. In Kenya, the deaths of eleven detainees at Hola Camp brought the realities of British conduct in the detention camps to the British public, a scandal that had a direct impact on ending British rule in that colony. Here too, it will be shown, the doctors involved with the camp hospital, and the subsequent inquest into the deaths, played a number of roles in supporting the government's efforts to conceal the true extent of violence.

Notes

1 For the Compton Report, see Edmond Compton, *Report of the Enquiry into Allegations Against the Security Forces of Physical Brutality in Northern Ireland Arising out of Events on the 9th August, 1971*

(London: Her Majesty's Stationery Office, 1971). For the *Parker Report*, see Hubert Lister Parker, *Report of the Committee of Privy Counsellors Appointed to Consider Authorised Procedures for the Interrogation of Persons Suspected of Terrorism* (London: Her Majesty's Stationery Office, 1972).

2 *Parker Report*, Majority Report, paragraph 34.

3 *Parker Report*, Majority Report, paragraph 41.

4 This issue was raised by the representatives of the BMA in a statement to the WMA in February 1975. See 'Statement by the British Medical Association Upon the Medical Aspects of Interrogation and of Artificial Feeding of Prisoners', 1975 held by the WMA archives.

5 The current version of the Declaration of Tokyo can be seen here: www.wma.net/policies-post/wma-declaration-of-tokyo-guidelines-for-physicians-concerning-torture-and-other-cruel-inhuman-or-degrading-treatment-or-punishment-in-relation-to-detention-and-imprisonment/ [Accessed 18 November 2022].

6 Anonymous, 'Cruel treatment', *British Medical Journal*, 9 August 1975.

7 William Refshauge, 'Statement from the Secretary General to the 29th World Medical Assembly', 1975, held by the WMA archives.

8 See Sidney Bloch and Peter Reddaway, *Soviet Psychiatric Abuse: The Shadow Over World Psychiatry* (London: Gollancz, 1984); M. G. Bloche, 'Uruguay's military physicians: cogs in a system of state terror', *JAMA* 255 (1986), pp. 2788–2793; Mark Hurst, *British Human Rights Organizations and Soviet Dissent 1965–1985* (London and New York: Bloomsbury, 2016); E. Stover, *The Open Secret: Torture and the Medical Profession in Chile* (Washington, DC: American Association for the Advancement of Science, 1987); T. A. Brennan and R. Kirscher, 'Medical ethics and human rights violations: the Iraqi occupation of Kuwait and its aftermath', *Annals of Internal Medicine* 117 (1992), pp. 78–82; Mary Rayner, *Turning a Blind Eye: Medical Accountability for Torture in South Africa* (Washington, DC: American Association for the Advancement of Science, 1987); Steven H. Miles, *Oath Betrayed: Torture, Medical Complicity and the War on Terror* (New York: Random House, 2006).

9 Today, doctors are often recognised as the enforcers and monitors of the international human rights regime; their participation in acts of organised and systematised violence is therefore seen as inherently wrong or concerning. The roles within this capacity of protecting human rights is enshrined within the four Geneva Conventions of 1949 and the two Additional Protocols of 1977, as well as the WMA's Tokyo Declaration, 1975.

10 In 2004, members of the US army and the CIA used torture and other cruel and inhumane acts such as rape and even murder on detainees being held at the Abu Ghraib prison in Iraq. Although military doctors did not participate directly in the abuse, significant questions were asked as to where they were and why they did not try to stop it. More recently, in 2014, the *New York Times* and, later, Human Rights Watch called for two American psychologists, John Bruce Jessen and James Elmer Mitchell, to be investigated and tried for their development of a set of 'enhanced interrogation techniques' which were used by the CIA to interrogate detainees in Afghanistan. In 2017, the lawsuit against these two scientists was settled out of court. Since then, in 2018, the American Civil Liberties Union managed to win the release of a ninety-page account of the involvement of the CIA's Medical Services in torture, which demonstrates the extent to which military physicians willingly and actively took part in American torture activities in Iraq and Afghanistan.

11 David Anderson, *Histories of the Hanged: The Dirty War in Kenya and the End of Empire* (New York and London: W. W. Norton & Company, 2005); Caroline Elkins, *Britain's Gulag: The Brutal End of Empire in Kenya* (London: Jonathan Cape, 2005).

12 Raphaëlle Branche, *La Torture et l'armée pendant la guerre d'Algérie: 1954–1962* (Paris: Gallimard, 2001).

13 David Anderson, 'British abuse and torture in Kenya's counter-insurgency, 1952–1960', *Small Wars & Insurgencies* 23 (2012), pp. 700–719; and Caroline Elkins, 'Looking beyond Mau Mau: archiving violence in the era of decolonization', *The American Historical Review* 120 (2015), pp. 852–868.

14 Laleh Khalili, 'Thinking about violence', *International Journal of Middle East Studies* 45 (2013), pp. 791–792.

15 Fabian Klose, *Human Rights in the Shadow of Colonial Violence: The Wars of Independence in Kenya and Algeria*, trans. Dona Geyer (Philadelphia: University of Pennsylvania Press, 2013).

16 Mildred Mortimer, 'Tortured bodies, resilient souls: Algeria's women combatants depicted by Danièle Djamila Amrane-Minne, Louisette Ighilahriz, and Assia Djebar', *Research in African Literatures* 43 (2012), p. 107.

17 For instance, Robert Thompson's 1966 book *Defeating Communist Insurgency* (London: Chatto & Windus, 1966) is recognised as one of the influential sources that promoted a special British approach to winning insurgency wars. More recently, scholars like Thomas Mockaitis have published a number of studies that praise the successes of British counterinsurgency campaigns in Malaya, Cyprus and Northern Ireland. Although Mockaitis acknowledges that the

situation in Kenya was not always as 'clean' as in other conflicts, any use of excessive violence – in his view – was the work of untrained police personnel at the local level and was confined to the start of the emergency. See Thomas R. Mockaitis, 'The origins of British counter-insurgency', *Small Wars & Insurgencies* 1 (1990), p. 223.

18 During the Algerian War itself, several high-profile cases were reported to French and international audiences which made detailed allegations of the use of torture by French forces. In particular, the cases of Henri Alleg, Maurice Audin, Djamila Bouhired and Djamila Boupacha were reported in the French press, bringing the realities of the military's conduct to the metropole. In addition, during and soon after the war, a number of historians began publishing accounts of the struggle which kept the subject of torture within French memory.

19 Anderson, *Histories of the Hanged*, pp. 292–293.

20 Anderson, *Histories of the Hanged*, p. 293.

21 Joshua Cole, 'Massacres and their historians: recent histories of state violence in France and Algeria in the twentieth century', *French Politics, Culture & Society* 28 (2010), pp. 106–107.

22 Louisette Ighilahriz, *Algérienne. Récit recueilli par Anne Nivat* (Paris: Fayard/Calmann-Lévy, 2001).

23 Jacques Massu, *La Vraie Bataille d'Alger* (Paris: Plon, 1971).

24 Neil Macmaster, 'The torture controversy (1998–2002): towards a "new history" of the Algerian war?', *Modern & Contemporary France*, 10 (2002), p. 450. See also Paul Aussaresses, *The Battle of the Casbah: Terrorism and Counter-Terrorism in Algeria, 1955–1957*, trans. Robert L. Miller (New York: Enigma Books, 2004).

25 Elkins, 'Looking beyond Mau Mau', p. 857.

26 Elkins, 'Looking beyond Mau Mau', p. 857.

27 Elkins, 'Looking beyond Mau Mau', p. 860.

28 Official records include, but are not limited to, publications by the British government such as F. D. Corfield, *Historical Survey of the Origins and Growth of Mau Mau* (London: Her Majesty's Stationery Office, 1960) and United Kingdom Parliament, *Report of the Kenya Land Commission* (London: Her Majesty's Stationery Office, 1933).

29 Branche, *La Torture et l'armée pendant la guerre d'Algérie*, p. 27.

30 Raphaëlle Branche, 'Torture of terrorists? Use of torture in a "war against terrorism": justifications, methods and effects: the case of France in Algeria, 1954–1962', *International Review of the Red Cross* 89 (2007), p. 549.

31 Branche, 'Torture of terrorists?', p. 549.

32 Branche, *La Torture et l'armée pendant la guerre d'Algérie*, p. 590.

33 Branche, *La Torture et l'armée pendant la guerre d'Algérie*, p. 591.

34 Branche, *La Torture et l'armée pendant la guerre d'Algérie*, p. 29.

35 Olivier Le Cour Grandmaison, *Coloniser. Exterminer. Sur la guerre et l'Etat colonial* (Paris: Fayard, 2005); Sylvie Thénault, *Violence ordinaire dans l'Algérie colonial. Camps, internements, assignations à résidence* (Paris: Odile Jacob, 2012).
36 Sylvie Thénault, *Une drôle de justice. Les magistrats dans la guerre* (Paris: Découverte, 2001).
37 Giorgio Agamben, *Homo Sacer: Sovereign Power and Bare Life*, trans. Daniel Heller-Roazen (Stanford: Stanford University Press, 1998); Sylvie Thénault, *Une drôle de justice.*
38 The state of emergency was first voted on 3 April 1955 and later extended on 22 August 1955.
39 Thénault, *Une drôle de justice*, p. 9.
40 Thénault, *Une drôle de justice*, p. 160.
41 Thénault, *Une drôle de justice*, pp. 15–28.
42 Thénault, *Une drôle de justice*, pp. 18–22.
43 Thénault, *Une drôle de justice*, p. 22.
44 Article 6 of loi 55–385 du 3 avril 1955 instituant un état d'urgence et en déclarant l'application en Algérie.
45 Sylvie Thénault, 'L'Internement en France pendant la guerre d'indépendance algérienne', *Recueil Alexandries* 15 (2008). reseau-terra.eu/article917.html
46 Sibylle Scheipers, 'The use of camps in colonial warfare', *The Journal of Imperial and Commonwealth History* 43 (2015), p. 689.
47 The categories included 'to be released'; the 'unwanted', who would be detained for longer in either the CTT or in a civilian-run camp called a *centre d'hébergement*; and finally, the 'criminals', who were to undergo trial under common law. See Raphaëlle Branche, 'The French in Algeria: can there be a prisoner of war in a "domestic" operation?', in Sibylle Scheipers (ed.), *Prisoners in War* (Oxford: Oxford University Press, 2010), pp. 178–179.
48 Sylvie Thénault, 'Personnel et internes dans les camps français de la guerre d'Algérie. Entre stéréotypes coloniaux et combat pour l'indépendance', *Politix* 1 (2005), p. 67.
49 Klose, *Human Rights in the Shadow of Colonial Violence*, p. 61.
50 Paul Ocobock, 'Spare the rod, spoil the colony: corporal punishment, colonial violence, and generational authority in Kenya, 1897–1952', *The International Journal of African Historical Studies* 45 (2012), pp. 29–56.
51 Elkins, *Britain's Gulag*, p. 55.
52 Anderson, 'British abuse and torture in Kenya's counter-insurgency'.
53 TNA WO 291/1670, p. 74. J. M. Forster, Operational Research Unit Far East, *A Comparative Study of the Emergencies in Malaya and Kenya*, Report No. 1/1957.

54 Anderson, 'British abuse and torture in Kenya's counter-insurgency', p. 701.
55 Stephen Morton, *States of Emergency: Colonialism, Literature and Law* (Liverpool: Liverpool University Press, 2013), p. 125.
56 Morton, *States of Emergency*, p. 125.
57 Throughout this book I will use both 'the Mau Mau' and 'Mau Mau' without the definitive article. The former refers to the political movement itself, while the latter captures something of the pervasive and abstract ideology the colonial authorities imagined the movement to be. As will be discussed in subsequent chapters, the Mau Mau rebellion came to represent and embody a variety of anxieties and distorted beliefs held by the settlers and the administration.
58 Elkins, *Britain's Gulag*, p. 101.
59 Elkins, *Britain's Gulag*, p. 100.
60 Elkins, *Britain's Gulag*, pp. xii–xiii.
61 Daniel Branch, 'Imprisonment and colonialism in Kenya, *c.* 1930–1952: escaping the carceral archipelago', *The International Journal of African Historical Studies* 38 (2005), p. 263.
62 A. R. Baggallay, 'Myths of Mau Mau expanded: rehabilitation in Kenya's detention camps, 1954–60', *Journal of Eastern African Studies* 5 (2011), p. 560.
63 Branch, 'Imprisonment and colonialism in Kenya', p. 243.
64 Baggallay, 'Myths of Mau Mau expanded', p. 568.
65 Elkins, *Britain's Gulag*, p. xiv.
66 Elkins, 'Looking beyond Mau Mau', p. 868.
67 Elkins, 'Looking beyond Mau Mau', p. 868.
68 Anderson, 'British abuse and torture in Kenya's counter-insurgency', p. 700.
69 Elaine Scarry, *The Body in Pain: The Making and Unmaking of the World* (Oxford: Oxford University Press, 1985), p. 42.
70 Alexandr Solzhenitsyn, *The Gulag Archipelago, 1918–1956: An Experiment in Literary Investigation*, trans. Thomas P. Whitney (New York: Harper & Row, 1974), p. 208.
71 Michel Foucault, *Birth of the Clinical Gaze: An Archaeology of Medical Perception*, trans. A. M. Sheridan-Smith (New York: Vintage, 1973). See also Michel Foucault, *Madness and Civilization: A History of Insanity in the Age of Reason*, trans. Richard Howard (London and New York: Routledge, 1989); and Michel Foucault, *Discipline and Punish: The Birth of the Prison*, trans. A. M. Sheridan (London: Penguin Books, 1977).
72 Foucault's work has inspired many scholars, including Ann Laura Stoler, *Race and the Education of Desire: Foucault's History of Sexuality and the Colonial Order of Things* (Durham and London:

Duke University Press, 1995); Jacques Donzelot, *The Policing of Families*, trans. Robert Hurley (New York: Pantheon, 1979); Paul Rabinow, *French Modern: Norms and Forms of the Social Environment* (Cambridge, MA: MIT Press, 1998). For a broader look at the history of colonial medicine, see Gerald W. Hartwig and Karl D. Paterson, *Disease in African History: An Introductory Survey and Case Studies* (Durham: Duke University Press, 1978); Michael Worboys, 'Science and British Colonial Imperialism: 1895–1940' (Unpublished DPhil thesis, University of Sussex, 1979); Daniel R. Headrick, *The Tools of Empire: Technology and European Expansion in the Nineteenth Century* (Oxford: Oxford University Press, 1981); Roy Macleod and Milton Lewis (eds), *Disease, Medicine and Empire: Perspectives on Western Medicine and the Experience of European Expansion* (London: Routledge, 1988); and Alfred W. Crosby, *Ecological Imperialism: The Biological Expansion of Europe 900–1900* (Cambridge: Cambridge University Press, 1993).

73 David Arnold, *Colonizing the Body: State Medicine and Epidemic Disease in Nineteenth-Century India* (Berkeley: University of California Press, 1993), p. 8.

74 Megan Vaughan, *Curing Their Ills: Colonial Power and African Illness* (Stanford and Cambridge: Stanford University Press, 1991), p. 10.

75 Vaughan, *Curing Their Ills*, p. 11.

76 Richard C. Keller, *Colonial Madness* (Chicago and London: Chicago University Press, 2008), p. 161.

77 In particular, see Frantz Fanon, *A Dying Colonialism*, trans. Haakon Chevalier (New York: Grave Press, 1965); and Fanon, *The Wretched of the Earth*, trans. Constance Farrington (London: Penguin Books, 2001).

78 Richard C. Keller, 'Clinician and revolutionary: Frantz Fanon, biography, and the history of colonial medicine', *Bulletin of the History of Medicine* 81 (2007), p. 825.

79 Keller, 'Clinician and revolutionary', p. 825.

80 Keller, 'Clinician and revolutionary', p. 826; and Filippo Menozzi, 'Fanon's letter: between psychiatry and anticolonial commitment', *Interventions* 17 (2015), pp. 360–377.

81 For example, in *A Dying Colonialism*, Fanon includes a description of how a medical practitioner would 'very often [assume] an aspect of systematized piracy', which included injecting patients with 'twice-distilled water' and charging them for penicillin or vitamin B12. He explained how, in rural settings, doctors would 'boast of taking X-rays with the aid of a vacuum cleaner' and on market days, would offer patients a variety of 'salt serum' injections sold at varying prices.

The doctor, Fanon assures us, knew that the Algerian would 'almost always choose the most expensive injections'. See Fanon, *A Dying Colonialism*, p. 133.

82 Influential work on the history of colonial medicine includes, but is in no way limited to: Ann Beck, 'Medical administration and medical research in developing countries: remarks on their history in colonial East Africa', *Bulletin of the History of Medicine* 46 (1972), pp. 349–358; Shula Marks, 'What is colonial about colonial medicine? And what has happened to imperialism and health?', *Social History of Medicine* 10 (1997), pp. 205–219; William Gallois, *The Administration of Sickness: Medicine and Ethics in Nineteenth-Century Algeria* (Basingstoke: Palgrave Macmillan, 2008); Mark Harrison, *Medicine in an Age of Commerce and Empire* (Oxford: Oxford University Press, 2010); Pratik Chakrabarti, *Medicine & Empire, 1600–1960* (Basingstoke: Palgrave Macmillan, 2014); Olivier Le Cour Grandmaison, *L'Empire des hygiénistes. Faire vivre aux colonies* (Paris: Fayard, 2014).

83 Some notable work on this subject does include, for example, Vaughan, *Curing Their Ills*; Mary P. Sutphen and Bridie Andrews (eds), *Medicine and Colonial Identity* (London and New York: Routledge, 2003); Warwick Anderson, *The Cultivation of Whiteness: Science, Health & Racial Destiny in Australia* (Melbourne: Melbourne University Press, 2005); and Charlotte Ann Chopin, 'Embodying "the new white race": colonial doctors and settler society in Algeria, 1878–1911', *Journal for the Social History of Medicine* 29 (2015), pp. 1–20.

84 Chopin, 'Embodying "the new white race"', pp. 1–20.

85 See Anna Crozier, *Practising Colonial Medicine: The Colonial Medical Services in British East Africa* (London: I. B. Tauris, 2005).

86 Anna Greenwood (ed.), *Beyond the State: The Colonial Medical Services in British Africa* (Manchester: Manchester University Press, 2016).

87 Ann Laura Stoler, 'Imperial debris: reflections on ruins and ruination', *Cultural Anthropology* 23 (2008), pp. 193–194.

88 Stoler, 'Imperial debris', p. 193.

89 British Medical Association, *Medicine Betrayed: The Participation of Doctors in Human Rights Abuses* (London: Zed Books, 1992), p. 40.

90 This list, which I compiled from a number of summaries of medical involvement in torture, is not exhaustive. See Stover, *The Open Secret: Torture and the Medical Profession in Chile*; Laurel Baldwin-Ragaven, Jeanelle de Gruchy and Leslie London (eds), *An Ambulance of the Wrong Colour: Health Professionals, Human Rights and Ethics in South Africa* (Cape Town: University of Cape Town Press, 1999),

pp. 91–112; and Darius Rejali, *Torture and Democracy* (Princeton and Oxford: Princeton University Press, 2009), pp. 398–399.

91 In part three of *The Nazi Doctors*, Lifton explained the concept of 'doubling' to account for the psychological mechanism that allowed German doctors to undertake appalling breaches of medical ethics, such as assisting in the euthanasia programmes. Doubling, as Lifton sees it, is 'an active psychological process, a means of *adaptation to extremity* [...] The adaption requires a dissolving of "psychic glue" as an alternative to a radical breakdown of the self'. Alternatively, and more specifically for doctors involved in torture, Lifton proposed the 'atrocity-producing situation' to account for why individuals become complicit in violence. Lifton describes the atrocity-producing situation as 'one so structured, psychologically and militarily, that ordinary people can readily engage in atrocities'. This mechanism for producing complicit physicians, Lifton argues, takes place through gradual acclimatising to violence and abuse by way of a 'sequence of socialization'. For 'doubling', see Robert Jay Lifton, *The Nazi Doctors: Medical Killing and the Psychology of Genocide* (New York: Basic Books, 2000), p. 422; and for a clear explanation of 'atrocity-producing situation' in relation to doctors involved in torture, see Robert Jay Lifton, 'Doctors and torture', *The New England Journal of Medicine* 351 (2004), pp. 415–416.

92 Lifton, 'Doctors and torture', p. 416.

93 Ben Shephard, *A War of Nerves* (London: Jonathan Cape, 2000), p. 361.

94 Matha K. Huggins, Mika Haritos-Fatouros and Philip G. Zimbardo, *Violence Workers: Police Torturers and Murderers Reconstruct Brazilian Atrocities* (Berkeley: University of California Press, 2002).

95 Christopher R. Browning, *Ordinary Men: Reserve Police Battalion 101 and the Final Solution in Poland* (New York: HarperCollins, 1998), pp. 191–223.

96 Vivian Nutton, 'Beyond the Hippocratic Oath', in Andrew Wear, Johanna Geyer-Kordesh and Roger French (eds), *Doctors and Ethics: The Earlier Historical Setting of Professional Ethics* (Amsterdam and Atlanta, GA: Rodopi, 1993), pp. 10–37. See also Carsten Timmermann, 'A model for the new physician: Hippocrates in inter-war Germany', in David Cantor (ed.), *Reinventing Hippocrates* (Aldershot: Ashgate, 2002), pp. 302–324.

97 Rejali identifies doctors as the front line in the identification of torture, as they have 'a specialized set of skills to diagnose the use of' some techniques. See Rejali, *Torture and Democracy*, p. 16.

98 George J. Annas and Michael A. Grodin (eds), *The Nazi Doctors and the Nuremberg Code: Human Rights in Human Experimentation* (New York and Oxford: Oxford University Press, 1992); Jay Katz, 'The consent principle of the Nuremberg Code: its significance then and now', in Annas and Grodin (eds), *The Nazi Doctors and the Nuremberg Code*, pp. 227–239; Jay Katz, 'The Nuremburg Code and the Nuremberg Trial: a reappraisal', *JAMA* 276 (1996), pp. 1662–1666; Jay Katz, 'Human sacrifice and human experimentation: reflections at Nuremberg', *Yale Journal of International Law* 22 (1997), pp. 401–418; U. Tröler and S. Reiter-Theil (eds), *Ethics Codes in Medicine* (Farnham: Ashgate, 1998); Andreas Frewer and Markus Rothhaar, 'Medicine, human rights and ethics: paths to universal rights', *Medical Health Care Philosophy* 13 (2010), pp. 247–249; Volker Roelcke and Giovanni Maio (eds), *Twentieth Century Ethics of Human Subjects Research: Historical Perspectives on Values, Practices, and Regulations* (Stuttgart: Franz Steiner Verlag, 2004); Ulf Schmidt, *Justice at Nuremburg: Leo Alexander and the Nazi Doctors' Trial* (Basingstoke: Palgrave Macmillan, 2004); Wolfgang U. Eckart (ed.), *Man, Medicine, and the State: The Human Body as an Object of Government Sponsored Medical Research in the 20th Century* (Stuttgart: Franz Steiner Verlag, 2006); Ulf Schmidt, 'Medical ethics and human experimentation at Porton Down: informed consent in Britain's biological and chemical warfare experiments', in Ulf Schmidt and Andreas Frewer (eds), *History and Theory of Human Experimentation: The Declaration of Helsinki and Modern Medical Ethics* (Stuttgart: Steiner, 2007), pp. 283–313; Ulf Schmidt, *Secret Science: A Century of Poison Warfare and Human Experiments* (Oxford: Oxford University Press, 2015).

99 Schmidt, *Secret Science*, pp. 9–11.

100 Fritz Allhoff, 'Physician involvement in hostile interrogations', *Cambridge Quarterly of Healthcare Ethics* 15 (2006), pp. 392–402.

101 Leslie London, Leonard S. Rubenstein, Laurel Baldwin-Ragaven and Adriaan Van Es, 'Dual loyalty among military health professionals: human rights and ethics in times of armed conflict', *Cambridge Quarterly of Healthcare Ethics* 15 (2006), p. 391.

102 Fritz Allhoff, 'Introduction', in Fritz Allhoff (ed.), *Physicians at War: The Dual-Loyalties Challenge* (Springer, 2008), p. 5.

103 It is worth noting that dual loyalty is not just limited to military physicians. As Fritz Allhoff has noted, there are cases where modern physicians outside the armed forces also have responsibilities beyond those to their patients. These include forensic psychiatry, occupational

health and public health. See Allhoff, 'Physician involvement in hostile interrogations'.

104 Allhoff, 'Introduction', pp. 5–7.

105 Due to the size restrictions, I have not been able to provide the original French text in all instances. I have therefore relied on my own translation of these documents which I have had checked by native speakers. I am therefore confident that the translations I offer here are suitable for this work.

106 Sylvie Thénault and Raphaëlle Branche, 'Le Secret sur la torture pendant la guerre d'Algérie', *Matériaux pour l'histoire de notre temps* 58 (2000), p. 57.

107 For example, in the now famous trial of David Irving who, in addition to falsifying and distorting evidence about Hitler's involvement in the Final Solution, also carefully omitted evidence of his awareness and approval of the *Reichskristallnacht*. See Richard J. Evans, *Telling Lies About Hitler: The Holocaust, History and the David Irving Trial* (London and New York: Verso, 2002), pp. 213–215.

108 See Rejali, *Torture and Democracy*; and Erik Linstrum, *Ruling Minds: Psychology in the British Empire* (Cambridge, MA and London: Harvard University Press, 2016), pp. 175–188.

109 Heather Jones, *Violence Against Prisoners of War in the First World War: Britain, France and Germany, 1914–1920* (Cambridge: Cambridge University Press, 2011), p. 8.

1

First blood

On 24 January 1953, the white settler community in Kenya was shocked by the murder of Roger and Adeline Esmee Ruck (referred to as Esmee), their six-year-old son, Michael, and a farm worker called Muthura Nagahu. These deaths, which took place on their farm in North Kinangop, near the Aberdare Forest, were to be a definitive moment for the state of emergency that had been in effect since October 1952. The Ruck family, as David Anderson noted, represented everything that Kenya's European settlers held dear.[1] The family were young, sociable and popular, and both Roger and Esmee were active in the colonial community: Roger was a member of the Kenya Police Reserves (KPR), while Esmee was a qualified doctor who ran a clinic on their farm, where she treated African squatters from the whole neighbourhood.[2] To many, the fact that the Kenyan insurgents had slaughtered such a respectable family proved that Mau Mau was little more than a savage group of 'terrorists'. While the family's murder generated great concern within the Kenyan and British press, the medical community were particularly shaken by the death of one of their own.

Less than a week after the Ruck murders, the Kenya Branch of the British Medical Association (BMA) held their annual general conference in Nairobi. Those present at the meeting felt that the wider medical community should be acquainted with what Dr Robert Howitt Wiseman, the Honourable Secretary of the Kenya Branch, described as 'the wanton attacks which have been made and of the continuing threat to life in Kenya'.[3] Wiseman, writing in the *BMJ* in February 1953, asserted that dangerous 'gangs' of Mau Mau exercised 'no discrimination in the choice of victims [...] unless it [was] to choose those who [were] elderly or who [were] held in especial esteem by Africans whom they [had] befriended'. That doctors seemed to be potential targets is implied by Wiseman, but it is further supported by the fact that Dr Ruck was not the only practitioner to be attacked by Mau Mau. Indeed, Wiseman pointed out that Dr Dorothy Meiklejohn and her husband, Commander I. H. Meiklejohn, had also been attacked on their property in Thomson Falls, Rift Valley, in November 1952. Although Dr Meiklejohn survived with extensive wounds, her husband was less fortunate.[4] Then, on 15 May 1954, Dr C. H. R. Pentreath, a retired ophthalmic specialist, was 'senselessly attacked by Mau Mau terrorists' while walking to buy cigarettes from a nearby inn. He died from his injuries four days later.[5]

The murder of doctors by Mau Mau may at first appear to be evidence of the desperate tactics employed by the Kenyan nationalists. Both the Ruck family and the Meiklejohns lived on isolated farms outside the relative protection of larger towns or cities. In fact, the Meiklejohn property was so remote that Dr Meiklejohn had to drive seven or eight miles to reach the police station following her attack.[6] These settlers may have appeared more vulnerable and therefore less likely to pose a threat to Mau Mau gangs, who, in the early stages of the conflict, would raid settler properties to secure food, medication and weaponry.[7] Yet the explanation that these attacks were purely opportunistic fails to account for their apparent brutality. The extent of the mutilations could represent deeper resentments.

Just as doctors appeared among the early victims of the Kenyan insurgency, European doctors were also targeted by the Algerian FLN. For example, on 14 November 1954, thirteen days after the Algerian War had started, a band of about forty 'outlaws' attacked Pasteur, a small Algerian village in the north of the country named after the famous French microbiologist. The violence broke out near the home of Dr Vezon, who, after seeing his wife to safety, returned to the scene in the company of a rural guard called Bouakar Ahmed. They then encountered and confronted a 'bandit' hiding in the shadows who shot at Dr Vezon and the guard. While Ahmed was killed, Dr Vezon was wounded but still able to fire his own weapon, killing the assailant.[8] Then, on 5 January 1956, Dr Jacques Vanier, a volunteer with the military's *sections administratives spécialisées* (SAS), designed to provide free healthcare to the rural population during the Algerian War, was ambushed and killed in Bouzina while en route to assist an allegedly injured Muslim woman.[9]

Dr Vanier was not the only doctor associated with the military to be directly targeted during the war.[10] Civilian doctors were also targeted. On 15 November 1956, a Dr Nackach was murdered by rebels while leaving his home in Vallee to treat a sick Muslim patient. On 8 January 1957, in Alma, a town near Algiers, a Dr Ettighoffer, who was also the vice-president of the Confédération des vignerons des trois départements algériens [Confederation of Algerian Vinegrowers], was attacked by 'outlaws' while surveying his property with his manager. Both men were seriously injured but not killed.[11] Finally, on 28 February 1957, *Le Monde* reported the death of Dr Jouane, the General Councillor of Guelma, in north-eastern Algeria, who was killed by a 'terrorist' as he left the home of a Muslim woman he had been treating. According to the article, Dr Jouane's death 'provoked strong emotion' among the locals, as he was held in 'general esteem'.[12]

This evidence suggests that, during the respective emergencies in 1950s Kenya and Algeria, members of the medical profession found themselves to be the direct targets of rebel violence. Yet while the number of doctors involved in these attacks is too small to claim that the rebels undertook a targeted programme against medical professionals, that does not mean they cannot offer valuable insights into the wider colonial situation. To date, little historical attention has been given to these attacks, yet that does not mean historians are unaware of the symbolic significance of such events. Jonathan G. Katz and Ellen Amster, respectively, have examined a different context to show how the death of a colonial doctor can provide valuable insights into the interplay between colonial politics, science and local communities.[13] The case study focuses on the murder of a doctor of the French government, Emile Mauchamp, who was beaten to death by a mob outside his clinic in the city of Marrakech, Morocco, in March 1907. According to contemporary French reports, Mauchamp was a victim of 'clash of civilizations'; his murder was interpreted as a violent rejection of Western science by an 'irrational' Islamic society. It was apparently a symbol of their hostility, barbarism and backwardness. However, Katz and Amster have shown that, in reality, this was not the case. If anything, the death of a European doctor offered France an excuse to justify colonial occupation of Morocco.[14]

More importantly for understanding the situation in Kenya and Algeria, Mauchamp's death and the rumours circulated about it provide insights into the ways in which the Moroccan community 'conceptualize both foreign threat and the Moroccan polity'.[15] Rather than snubbing Western science, as traditional explanations suggested, the Muslim community integrated French technology and science and gave it local social meaning. The Moroccans were therefore less concerned with Mauchamp's status as a doctor and more worried about the political influence he had over the sultan, whose court Mauchamp had access to. The rumours concerning Mauchamp's death revealed fears that he was an agent of French imperial penetration, a poisoner of Moroccans and an organiser of a French invasion.[16]

Similarly, the attacks in Kenya and Algeria were presented in ways that emphasised the rebel's sheer brutality. The aforementioned Wiseman, of the *BMJ*, described the Ruck family murder as an expression of Mau Mau's indiscriminate violence. The fact that Esmee Ruck was a doctor is repeatedly stressed in the memoirs of Europeans involved in the Kenya Emergency; the nature of her charitable work was contrasted against the extremely violent circumstances surrounding her death.[17] In the Algerian cases, *Le Monde* presented the attacks as distinct, stand-alone segments of larger reports. The separation of these cases from other victims mentioned in the same articles implies there was something particularly significant or symbolically depraved about their murders. Yet, as with contemporary explanations for the death of Dr Mauchamp in Morocco, these accounts do not consider alternative explanations for why these individuals were killed. Repeatedly, there is a feeling of shock and confusion over how the terrorists could reject the civilisation that the colonial powers were offering them. However, for Frantz Fanon, there were plenty of reasons for this phenomenon.

When it came to doctors being murdered or targeted by FLN forces, Fanon believed it was because they had betrayed their ethical positions, the very core of what it was to be a healer. As he stated in *A Dying Colonialism*, colonial doctors had excluded themselves from 'the protective circle that the principles and the values of the medical profession have woven around [them]'.[18] This was something that was 'never [...] clearly understood by world opinion'.[19] The violent deaths of doctors in Algeria stood out as being irregular and disturbing for Europeans, even when compared to the 'cruellest wars', where it was traditional for 'the medical corps to be left unscathed'.[20] Fanon continues to assure us that the 'Algerian political men', the FLN and their supporters, were 'quite aware of the existence of the laws of war. They [knew] the complexity of the problem and the dramatic situation of the European population'.[21] Killing a doctor was therefore a conscious decision, one made with a full understanding of its significance. Colonial doctors had, for the FLN and Fanon at least, shed their commitment to the patient and given their loyalty to the authorities and to their own sectional interests.

Although it is not clear which 'principles and values' Fanon is referring to here, his critique of colonial medicine is useful for identifying three ways in which colonial doctors could be seen as contributing to the atmosphere of repression and violence in Algeria. Firstly, medicine and its practitioners were often viewed as being closely associated with the French authorities and the exercise of power. Doctors as well as engineers, school teachers, the police and rural constables were all seen as representatives of colonial power, extensions of colonial oppression in the eyes of the colonised. They made even routine activities, like the compulsory visit by the doctor to the *douar* – small rural indigenous villages – seem suspicious.[22] Doctors were simply too closely associated with colonial rule. Secondly, there was also the problem of their social standing within the colonial order itself. According to Fanon, '[b]ehind "the doctor who heals the wounds of humanity" appears the man, a member of a dominant society and enjoying in Algeria the benefits of an incomparably higher standard of living than that of [their] metropolitan colleagues'.[23] This was largely because, in centres of colonisation, the doctor was more often than not a landowner as well. 'It is exceptional', Fanon tells us, 'to see in Algeria, a colony which attracts settlers, a doctor who does not take up farming, who does not become attached to the soil'.[24] Finally, there was the social and political standing of these individuals within the colonial administration and settler communities. The flexibility of colonial society meant the type of divisions between professions that existed in the metropoles were less pronounced or else absent entirely. Professionals such as medical practitioners, lawyers and engineers could also benefit from agricultural pursuits to supplement their incomes and provide a legacy for their children. By owning land in these overseas territories, doctors became politically invested in maintaining the colonial order. They therefore often took up prominent positions within the local administration and settler communities where they became, Fanon claimed, 'leaders of colonialist movements'.[25]

As is made clear by some of the aforementioned examples, a number of the doctors targeted by the rebels in Kenya and Algeria were closely associated with colonial security forces. In fact, the focus on Dr Ruck's professional status actually obscures that of her husband, who, unlike Esmee, was known to be 'less kindly' towards the Kenyans.[26] As a member of the KPR, Roger would have been associated with an institution renowned for its heavy-handed and repressive approach to law enforcement, especially in the eyes of Kenyans. Similarly, Dr Meiklejohn was married to a retired military commander. In Algeria, multiple doctors who worked with the military were assassinated during 1956. In addition, several of the attacks took place on the private farmland of the doctors in question, especially in Kenya. The ownership of this property, as will be discussed in detail below, was a contentious issue for both colonised Kenyans and Algerians. By owning land and hiring local workers for cheap labour, these doctors may have become synonymous with the types of inequalities the rebels sought to address, especially with relation to the apparent wealth that came with land ownership. Finally, it is clear from the obituaries concerning doctors in Kenya that many of them held important ties to the administration and wider settler communities. In Algeria, too, Dr Jouane was not only a practising physician but also a local General Councillor.[27]

Far from being isolated occurrences with little value, the deaths of doctors in Kenya and Algeria highlight points of interests concerning the wider story of how the respective rebellions came to pass. Individually, these accounts may appear insignificant and unrelated; however, it can be argued that, if taken together, they expose deeper connections between the colonial situation and the wider grievances that produced the respective rebellions in each context. The question is, however, how did these situations and conditions take root in the first place? How did doctors come to inhabit such prominent and contentious positions within the colonies, and how did this contribute to the growing resentment that surrounded them?

Algeria: conquest, medicine and subjugation

When it came to conquering overseas territories, medicine played a fundamental role in the French military's wider aims. Not only did doctors administer to the army's needs, they also served a broader political purpose. As Hubert Lyautey, the French conqueror of Morocco admitted as late as 1933, '[t]he physician, if he understands his role, is the primary and the most effective of our agents of penetration and pacification'.[28] For the French, Western medicine and the perceived benefits it offered indigenous populations represented the core impetus for its so-called *mission civilisatrice*, its justification for colonial occupation.[29] The healing of locals was thought to demonstrate the superiority of European civilisation and could provide 'backwards' peoples with a means for progress. This is not to say medicine was solely a vehicle for colonial ideology, as recent studies have shown.[30] But its association with the military conquest of Algeria and its support for the European population came at the expense of Algerians and their needs.[31] In fact, the administration of medicine in the colony during the nineteenth and early twentieth century helped establish and reinforce some of the more significant political divides between the colonial state and the indigenous populations.

The conquest of Algeria was a particularly bloody struggle which started in 1830, when General Thomas Robert Bugeaud, marquis of la Piconnerie, undertook a military expedition to help prop up the Bourbon throne and to satisfy the financial interests of the merchants in Marseille.[32] With a fleet of 635 French ships loaded with 34,184 soldiers, Bugeaud occupied the seaports of Algiers, Oran and Bône. Over the next forty years, French forces conducted an increasingly cruel and repressive conquest of the Algerian population at large, not just Arabs but also Kabyles and other Tamazight peoples, by way of 'scorched earth' tactics which saw whole towns, cities and even the culture fall victim to extraordinary violence.[33] It has been estimated that during the conquest the size of the Algerian population dropped from about three million to two million.[34] Contemporaneously, in order to consolidate control of the territory, the French initiated an intensive settlement policy which sought to marginalise the Arab population by increasing the number of Europeans in the country.[35]

It was as a result of this increase in the number of European settlers that a connection between medicine and the colonial conquest first came about, since medical expertise was used to promote the health of the fledgling settler communities. In the 1830s and 1840s, Bugeaud placed medicine and the need for an ambitious healthcare system at the centre of debates surrounding the future of the colony. This was not without good reason. Thousands of settlers routinely died from the cholera or malaria epidemics that plagued the cities and wiped out a number of new villages. In 1835, for instance, cholera killed 12,000 people in Algiers and 14,000 in Constantine (these figures included indigenous Algerians).[36] The policies envisaged by Bugeaud and others were thus vigorously debated in the colony and in Paris, highlighting deep tensions between the two.[37] Even at this early stage, the provision of medical care was informed by political differences between, on the one hand, the interest of the military and settler society in Algeria and, on the other, the expectations of decision makers in France. These tensions would continue to exist throughout the colonial period right up to the emergency of the 1950s. Yet the expectations and desires of the military and the settlers in Algeria were themselves frequently at odds. Algeria came to be governed by a so-called *mixte* system, which combined civil and military powers. In terms of the organisation and administration of medicine, a highly incoherent system emerged where military, civil and commercial medical practitioners often competed for clients and expressed conflicting views on how medicine should operate in the colony.[38] From an outside perspective, such as that of a local Algerian, it would have been difficult to differentiate between these various practitioners and therefore between military and civilian medicine.

During the 1850s, the French government established the Service médical de colonisation (SMC) following the long period of conquest. The SMC existed to assist the Second Empire in its consolidation of French control in its North African territories. It supplied treatment to the registered needy while relaying disease statistics to the central administration.[39] As the conquered territory expanded, the SMC passed from military to civil jurisdiction in 1861. Through a series of decrees, a grade system was established for doctors which confirmed their positions as 'agents of special services', essentially civil servants with some professional autonomy. The SMC then remained under the control of the General Government of Algeria, even after administrative responsibility for the colony was transferred to the French Home Office in 1870.[40] However, the military also continued to have a significant medical presence in the colony. On 7 January 1890, a decree issued by the office of the State Secretary of the Colonies established a Colonial Health Advisory Council, a Colonial Health Corps (Corps de santé colonial, a company of French colonial doctors) and provided for hospitals services in every French colony and protectorate.[41] The establishment of this corps further blurred the lines between military and civilian medical affairs and meant that doctors across the range of service providers were forced to compete with one another for clients.[42] Over the next six decades, the administration of medicine in Algeria would be beset by two constantly reoccurring themes: firstly, both the military and civilian medical communities (SMC doctors and commercial practitioners) would struggle for dominance of a system that was consistently underfunded and mismanaged by successive French governments;[43] secondly, the benefits of such healthcare as was available were enjoyed by a very small proportion of society, namely the European settler communities.

For the most part, SMC doctors resisted the need to practise medicine in rural zones. As Clark has shown, those who did were referred to as *toubib du bled*, a sort of 'backwater doctor'.[44] Each physician attempted to cultivate a private practice but also received a stipend from state coffers for performing a statutory number of free public consultations; a monthly inspection of schoolchildren and sex workers; food and water quality inspections; and various administrative functions. But working in the rural communities, which could be separated by vast expanses of unpaved mule tracks, was a daunting and unattractive prospect for many.[45] While this was not a rewarding job in the eyes of the doctor, this type of clinical encounter was, as mentioned above, a site of suspicion for the Algerians who saw the collection of nosological data as a form of state surveillance and control. This was because the doctor's presence in the *douar* was often preceded by the police authorities who gathered the population for the visit.[46] Given the strong ties between medicine and the police, as well as the infrequency of doctors' visits, it is easy to see why rural Algerians may not have been convinced by the agents of France's *mission civilisatrice*. A programme to deal with this situation was initiated in 1904, when Muslim youths began to be trained as auxiliaries to provide medical outreach to Muslim villages in the *douar*. These auxiliaries assisted colonial physicians and provided hygiene education to local people. Their efforts were valuable in combining the biomedical ideas of the Europeans with autochthonous notions, forming a hybrid system of medicine and care.[47] Yet the overall impact of this effort was limited. Indeed, those living away from the larger urban centres may never have encountered state medical services such as doctor's consultations, vaccination and drug distribution at all, though they would have certainly been affected by the state's sanitary policy.[48]

Generally speaking, the imperial powers had little interest in improving the health of colonial populations over the long term. Whereas medical research centres, such as the network of Pasteur Institutes established across the French empire, sought to classify and quantify tropical infections, their fixation on microorganisms in the first half of the twentieth century meant they were preoccupied with fighting 'isolated phenomena' rather than intervening to address the general socio-economic conditions that produced them.[49] It was only when key aspects of colonial management came under threat that a concerted effort to intervene occurred. That is to say that, as Sunil S. Amrith explains, 'colonial states only mobilized their medical policy at moments of crisis and emergency, and particularly in response to epidemic disease'.[50] Despite the introduction of basic public health measures, such as smallpox vaccinations, water purification and quarantine measures, the infant mortality rate in Algeria remained at 160 per 1,000 live births at the start of the Second World War.[51] So while medicine was one of the pillars of the French civilising mission in Algeria, the indigenous populations were often excluded from its benefits.

As with Britain, France had been party to the ten International Sanitary Conferences which first took place in Paris in 1851 and then concluded in 1938.[52] The Conferences attempted to create health codes governing the human body in order to limit the spread of disease throughout the world. Following the end of the First Word War, France also joined the League of Nations Health Organization (LNHO), which represented a second attempt at formulating global health policy and introducing a common vocabulary about hygiene.[53] The postwar belief in scientific advances and the practical achievements in disease prevention instilled into this community a belief that research and internationally organised preventative measures could eliminate many diseases and socio-economic causes of ill health. This culminated in a collective effort to improve the health of all humans. Yet these international initiatives had limited impact on daily life in the colonies. Any targeted programmes for specific diseases, such as malaria and sleeping sickness, did not tackle the social root causes and structural inequalities that produced disease and ill health in the colonies.[54] As Randall Packard asserted, 'despite a great deal of rhetoric around the health of the empire, little change occurred in the direction or definition of health in the tropics between the [world] wars. Health remained defined as the absence of disease and the control of disease continued to be viewed in narrow technical terms'.[55]

Instead of regarding the locals as individuals to be treated and enhanced by Western bioscience, many Europeans regarded them as harbingers of infection to be controlled and even eliminated. For example, in April 1921, the mayor of Cherchell, a town along the Mediterranean coast, wrote to the Prefect to complain about the threat to health posed by migrants travelling from the interior. The migrants, the mayor explained, 'brought with them the threat of typhus [...] to a settlement which had until then been spared'. Evoking language that presented the town as being under siege, the mayor added that 'the only means we had of defending ourselves against this invasion was to guard all the gates into the town'.[56] The Prefect responded by coordinating with the mayor of Algiers to impose travel restrictions on migrants by introducing a ticket system so that only the uninfected could travel on to the capital. This, William Gallois has suggested, was a calculated move on the Prefect's part as the latter knew that the mayor of Algiers objected to charitable assistance that drew on the city's budget for 'beggars who needed to be purged from Algiers'.[57] Rather than feel any obligation towards the sick, colonial officials made a distinction between the lives worth protecting, those of the white settler 'public', and those to be segregated and excluded from the healthy society of the European cities, the Muslim.[58]

Here, a deep divide between the settler communities, on the one hand, and the poor indigenous populations, on the other, comes to the surface. Throughout the period of colonial occupation, the Muslim population, especially the rural communities, were regarded as vectors of disease. Such beliefs had deep roots within Western medical circles, who regarded the poor and non-European races as inferior and, more often than not, natural sources of infection that posed a threat to security.[59] French medicine conceived of the Muslims as wholly Other, and produced theoretical foundations for justifying European dominance and a range of racial inequalities in the colonies.[60]

L'Algérie, c'est la France

Since the conquest, the Muslim population had been relegated to an underclass status defined on racial grounds. The white settler population, known as the *colons* or *pieds-noirs*, dominated every facet of life. As the former FLN member and historian, Mohammed Harbi, explained:

> Racial affiliation was the line of demarcation among people. The privileged were, regardless of all class differences, the Europeans, even the workers among them. They all understood themselves as French, as the occupiers of Algeria, and as victorious conquerors. The vanquished were to pay tribute to them in one way or another.[61]

When Algeria became an extension of France in October 1871, the Ministry of the Interior took responsibility for the country and its indigenous population. However, for the Arabs, little changed. Although they were de facto French subjects, they were without representation and enjoyed few civil rights.[62] Even Algerians who became doctors, for example, could be regarded as tacitly joining the oppressor's camp while distancing themselves from the medical and traditional practices of their people.[63] They were at once divorced from their heritage while also not quite 'French' enough to fit in with the colonisers among whom they worked. On a legal level, Muslims were not subject to French law; instead, they were regulated under the Code de l'indigénat, a penal code whose harsh provisions were only applicable to 'subjects', which was first established in 1874 and subsequently modified in 1876, 1877, and 1881.[64]

Excluded from the provisions of French law and politically disenfranchised, Algerian Muslims were also marginalised in terms of land ownership – something they shared with the East Africans in Kenya. As the first country conquered by the French in the nineteenth century, Algeria was made a colony for settlers. Its constitutional status as an extension of the metropole made it 'France-outside of France', providing a superficial excuse for the French political class to affirm that '*l'Algérie, c'est la France*' [Algeria, it is France].[65] This sentiment was fiercely stressed by a politically active and vocal settler community, whose members hailed not just from France, but also Spain, Italy, Greece and Malta. Their influence was especially prominent along the coastline, in the large Europeanised city ports and the Mitidja – rich, flat farmland which the French had cultivated from swamp. This was fertile terrain that boasted all the benefits of the south of France. As Alistair Horne wrote, 'in a country that might be Languedoc, straight eucalyptus-shaded roads led through a prosperous and tidy succession of cereal and citrus farms, drenched with orange-blossom scent in May, and vast vineyards, owned by *pieds-noirs* and operated by Muslim labour'.[66] This land, some of the most fertile in Algeria, had been seized by Europeans following the imposition of the Warnier Law of 1873. This law, introduced by Auguste Warnier, the representative of the settlers in the French parliament, transformed the process of buying and selling land by imposing private, rather than tribal, ownership.[67]

The principles of free trade imposed by the French were meant to lead to progress and civilisation for the Algerian Muslims, which would lead to greater assimilation and *francisation*. In reality, the act legalised a veritable land grab whereby the best and most fertile land was bought from the locals.[68] This process typified the general history of the Algerian colony. Few Muslims in rural Algeria had a notion of private ownership, and none understood the French concept of legally binding property contracts, in particular the way in which contracts had to be signed by a surnamed individual.[69] Opportunities for fraud, as Martin Evans notes, were plentiful, and the result was that between 1880 and 1908 as many as 451,000 hectares of land were purchased by Europeans at little cost.[70] A process of dispossession that had been in place since the French arrived in Algeria in 1830s was rapidly accelerated. By 1870, settlers had acquired 481,000 hectares supplemented by an additional 687,000 hectares which were annexed in retaliation for the 1871 Muslim uprising. This additional land was granted directly to the settlers by the state.[71] Through this dispossession, Bugeaud's plan to consolidate the subjugation of the populace and to strengthen French rule was realised.

The conversion of the land into a profitable entity was part of a global economic phenomenon; the same process could be seen in French Tunisia and Morocco, or the British territories of Rhodesia, South Africa and, as will be argued below, in Kenya.[72] This transformation became the foundation stone of French Algeria. The settlers had a right to remain in the country because the land had been acquired legally. Moreover, the cash crops they produced, notably cork, alfalfa and wine grapes, were sold competitively in foreign markets, while the Muslim population struggled to even feed their own families. Wine production was potentially one of the more contentious industries in Algeria for the North Africans. While accounting for half of Algeria's exports to France and, as a result, granting considerable power to the wine lobby, it hardly helped the economic predicaments of the Muslim population, as it provided little steady work, produced a crop that could not nourish a starving family and was ultimately offensive to the Islamic religion.[73] Within this context, it is easy to see why Dr Ettighoffer may have become a target for FLN hostility. Dr Ettighoffer was not only a trained medical practitioner, he was also the Vice-President of the Confédération des vignerons des trois départements algériens.[74] It seems that the attacks against colonial doctors were not completely random or arbitrary, but linked to wider colonial policies of repression, humiliation and (religious) disrespect, especially when concerning the growing of wine grapes.

Algeria was, until the 1960s, one of the world's largest wine exporters, and by a wide margin.[75] Although the height of the industry in Algeria was reached during the 1930s, wine production continued to prosper until the period of decolonisation, save for a sharp decline during the Second World War. Following the war, the production of Algerian wine doubled from nine million hectolitres in 1945 to eighteen million by 1953. Algerian wine producers were therefore in a prodigious position, but the crucial point here is that the benefits of this industry rested almost entirely in the hands of the *pieds-noirs*. This small, but socially dominant minority owned 97 per cent of Algerian vineyards and produced 99 per cent of the wine.[76]

The private purchase of the best land by the Europeans created two unequal agricultural systems that led to the collapse of Muslim rural society. Not only was their land less fertile, they also lacked the agricultural technologies and techniques available to the settlers.[77] The result was an unstable system that regularly tipped into famine conditions, notably in 1905, 1908, 1912 and 1937, the 'year of great hunger'.[78] Under such circumstances, children, so Albert Camus claimed, were often seen fighting with dogs for scraps of food.[79] Reflecting on this situation, Jean-Paul Sartre asked pointedly: 'Will we ask the Algerians to thank our country for allowing their children to be born into poverty, to live as slaves and to die of hunger?'[80] The only possibility for many Muslims was to sell their properties or face destitution. Hundreds of thousands of young rural labourers found themselves in need of work and became increasingly antagonistic towards the European population.[81] Large numbers flocked to the cities and towns, or to the Mitidja, where the settlers' prosperous vineyards needed cheap labour. By 1930, 428,000 Muslims were employed by large farming enterprises, but the country was deeply divided between the successful Europeans and the downtrodden Muslim population who felt they had been robbed of their land and forced into subjugation.[82] The cities experienced their own migration boom at the same time.[83]

The land question caused embittered resentment in Algeria and gave birth to a form of 'agrarian patriotism' from the 1920s onwards. Landowners increasingly found themselves to be at odds with their workers.[84] Overall, discontent over landownership, the repressive nature of the colonial regime and its racial discrimination led to various strikes, acts of defiance and ultimately nationalism throughout the first half of the century. Although many of these grievances were shared by other colonial peoples, not least in Kenya, there was one feature of the Algerian context which makes it stand out. That is, a significant number of the prominent nationalist leaders had some form of medical training. Although there were certainly other intellectuals and professional men among the politically active Algerians, such as layers and imams, the number of doctors, especially among the moderates, is interesting. This is a point briefly acknowledged by Horne in a footnote to *A Savage War of Peace* where he said: 'It will be noted that many of the nationalist intellectuals [...] were doctors, pharmacists or lawyers'.[85] For

Horne, this was because these professions offered fewer barriers to advancement for educated Muslims. Although Fanon had more complicated views on this,[86] it nevertheless demonstrates that colonial medicine was not simply a tool of oppression and repression. In fact, it was more Janus-faced: in some instances, it contributed to the general atmosphere of alienation in the colony while also providing, in isolated cases at least, a means for social liberation. In some cases, French education provided some Algerian doctors with greater social standing within their communities when it came to championing nationalists' causes.

At the start of the twentieth century, after years of silence from resistance movements, a new generation of Algerian youths found their voices. These individuals, known as the Young Algerians, were French-educated and often from privileged backgrounds. They formed associations and mutual aid societies that promoted the idea of greater assimilation of the North Africans into French society.[87] One of the more prominent members of this group was Dr Belkacem Benthami Ould Hamida, a French citizen who eventually became a professor of ophthalmology.[88] Benthami, who was elected to the Algiers Municipal Council in 1908, ran the most important Young Algerian delegations in Paris and was recognised as the leader of this early political movement. In 1926, Benthami became the first president of the Fédération des élus indigènes [the Federation of Elected Natives], which adopted a programme for greater incorporation with France, until he was unseated in 1930.[89] The Fédération was then split into three departmental groups, the most dominant of which was in Constantine. The leaders of this branch of the reorganised Fédération were themselves both trained in medical-related subjects. The first, Dr Mohammed Saleh Bendjelloul, held a medical degree from the University of Algiers and served as a public health service physician in 1924.[90] His political views were slightly more radical than Benthami's, as he championed equal rights as well as assimilation for the Young Algerians.[91] While Bendjelloul was the most visible and powerful leader of the Fédération, he is not as well remembered as the second leader, Ferhat Abbas, who remains one of the most significant moderate nationalist politicians of modern Algeria. Abbas was born in Affirs, a small village in the eastern region of Djidjelli, in 1899. His privileged background allowed him to climb the social ladder and to qualify as a pharmacist at Algiers University.

In 1931, he established his own pharmacy in Sétif, which served as a personal 'fiefdom', with a population of roughly 30,000, two-thirds of whom were Muslim.[92] Then, in 1933, Abbas was elected to the General Council of the Constantinois, and, in 1936, he joined the Municipal Council of Sétif and the Délégations financières in 1936.[93]

For Abbas, as for the other moderates, education was a key source for ensuring a fairer, more integrated Algeria. This was in contrast to more radical nationalists such as those from the Ulama d'Algérie, a religious organisation which grew out of the Koran schools and which was avowedly anti-Western.[94] Assimilation of any form was to be rejected by the Ulama, who wanted to unite Arabs and Berbers, without discrimination, in a formal Islamic community built around Koranic laws. The Ulama slogan was 'Islam is our religion, Algeria our country, Arabic our language'.[95] There was also the radical views of individuals like Ahmed Messali Hadj, founder the Paris Etoile nord-africaine, which became the first Algerian party in 1926 and clearly advocated Algerian independence. Messali and his followers were frequently in conflict with the French administrative authorities and the judiciary, which forced him to continue his campaigns underground. In 1937, Messali established the political party, the Parti du peuple algérien (PPA) after the Etoile was disbanded. With independence as its primary aim and a well-structured propaganda campaign to circulate its agenda, the PPA gained considerable influence across Algeria. Yet moderates like Abbas continued to push for assimilation rather than independence. In 1938, Abbas founded the Parti de l'Union Populaire Algérienne pour la conquête de droits de l'homme et du citoyen, which refused to accept a future divorced from France.[96]

The situation, however, changed significantly during the Second World War as conditions in Algeria deteriorated. Food shortages due to crop failures and rationing from 1940 to 1942 and an outbreak of typhus radicalised many nationalists. In addition, the educated bourgeoisie took inspiration from the news broadcast on the radio and, in particular, the principles enshrined in the Atlantic Charter by President Roosevelt and Prime Minister Winston Churchill in 1941.[97] Increasingly, the attitudes of moderate nationalists were hardened as they came to realise that assimilation was meaningless; independence from France was the only reasonable future for the colony. Eventually, Algerian nationalism, which had been diverse and divided prior to the conflict, was unified in 1943 by Abbas when he drew up the *Manifeste du peuple algérien*. The text, which decried the Algerian condition, called for, among other demands, an end to colonisation and exploitation, equality for all regardless of race and religion, the recognition of the Arabic language, and compulsory education for children of both sexes.[98] Algeria was to be a unified, autonomous and democratic state which would be recognised and protected by a federal relationship with France.[99] Keen to recruit indigenous people for the war effort, General Henri Giraud and the then General Governor of Algeria, Marcel Peyrouton, initially accepted the *Manifeste* as a working hypothesis and encouraged the Muslims to make a list of realisable proposals. However, this was largely interpreted as time saving measure which forced Abbas to produce the *Additif au Manifeste*, a more radical document that espoused national self-determination and independence.[100]

Eager to outmanoeuvre the nationalists, the government under General Charles de Gaulle and his deputy, General George Catroux, who governed Algeria, promulgated the Ordinance of 7 March 1944 which granted French citizenship without requiring Muslims to renounce their heritage and submitted the indigenous population to the rules of French common law. Article 3 of the Ordinance allowed the new citizens to be 'registered on the same electoral lists as non-Muslim citizens' and allowed them to participate 'in the same polls'.[101] In addition, in the years following the end of the Second World War, France and Britain both attempted to overcome some of the long-standing health and labour conditions for the colonial subjects. This was, as Jennifer Johnson noted, only undertaken because Empire 'presented a potential solution to the crisis in Capitalism'.[102] The war had left both colonial powers in urgent need of resources to fuel their economic recovery. Throughout the war itself, the colonial territories had provided essential raw material and foodstuffs, yet their true potential remained unrealised.[103] As such, rather than move towards decolonisation in the postwar period, the colonial powers recommitted themselves to restoring the colonial status quo to their prewar hegemonic positions. Both Britain and France focused their attention on introducing planned economies for the colonies. Africa, in particular, became a prized asset at a time when the future of the colonies in Asia was more contentious. Money poured into infrastructure such as roads and railways, as well as social welfare, hospitals and education. At this point, the idea that the state played a role as agent for the promotion of the welfare of its inhabitants was introduced to the colonies with increased medical services.[104] In particular, attention was paid to improving health and nutrition for the Algerians, but, as with earlier targeted medical campaigns surrounding infectious disease, the colonial authorities did not address the social roots of inequality.

For the nationalists, all these efforts were too little too late. Firstly, Abbas, the Messalists and most of the ulama rejected de Gaulle's 1944 proposals. Abbas responded by creating the association Amis du manifeste et de la liberté on 14 March 1944, through which he intended to create a national front extended to the ulamas and the clandestine supporters of Messali Hadj.[105] Algerian nationalism was now more radical, more separatist and increasingly hostile towards colonial rule at the end of the Second World War. Yet as demonstrated by the postwar recolonisation efforts, the French had little intention of abandoning Algeria. If necessary, they would resort to extreme violence to protect it.

In May 1945, dissident violence broke out in Sétif during demonstrations and resulted in the deaths of twenty-one Europeans. The insurrection movement spread over the following days to the countryside and to cities such as Bône, Guelma and Batna. Several French victims were subsequently mutilated and displayed.[106] Yet while this violent nationalist outburst was shocking for the Europeans in Algeria, France's retaliatory repression was, as Bernard Droz and Evelyne Lever note, 'pitiless and often blind'.[107] It will never be clear just how many Algerians were killed by France's retribution, but the FLN propaganda suggested over 40,000 people were killed.[108] If these figures are questionable, then the limited 1,500 admitted by the French administration seems just as suspicious. The reality is probably four or five times higher than this, but either way, the Sétif massacre served as the spark that ignited the fires of revolution for the Algerian nationalists. On the night of 31 October into the morning of 1 November 1954, a radical group of insurrectionists called the Comité révolutionnaire d'unité et d'action (CRUA) led coordinated guerrilla strikes across six military districts (*wilayas*). Although casualties were low, the psychological impact was huge.[109] The CRUA later reformed itself into the FLN and organised a national liberation army called the Armée de libération nationale (ALN).[110] The Algerian War of Independence had started.

Yet while the war would come to engulf all members of colonial society on both sides of the conflict, as will be shown in subsequent chapters, the FLN were keen to also wage an organised and effective propaganda campaign which struck at the heart of the occupying power's failures. This campaign, too, demonstrates the extent to which France's inability or reluctance to address entrenched health and social inequalities was a significant political issue for the Muslims. As the war started, the FLN took note of the language surrounding healthcare, international development and modernity which was being promoted by the colonial powers in the postwar period and used it to create their own alternative healthcare system. The ultimate expression of this effort was the formation of the Croissant-Rouge algérien in 1957, the FLN's vehicle for disseminating medical aid and healthcare to both, so their pamphlets claimed, 'combatants and civilians' during the war.[111] The Croissant-Rouge was a valuable propaganda device, as it allowed the FLN to demonstrate their humanitarian aspirations and to appeal for international aid in their struggle. This came in direct contrast to the ways in which the French security forces and some doctors corrupted medicine during the war and used it as a weapon against the rebels, as will be demonstrated later in this work.

Jennifer Johnson has recently argued that by establishing national healthcare institutions, like the Croissant-Rouge, the FLN were presenting themselves as a 'proto-state' that could provide better care than the colonial authorities.[112] Although this was a political move performed by other anticolonial groups in the British and French empires during the Cold War, it nevertheless demonstrates the extent to which healthcare provisions and medicine were political matters for the rebels.[113] This is an important point that distinguishes the nationalist campaigns of the FLN from those of Mau Mau in Kenya. While the FLN successfully launched a viable programme for delivering healthcare to the Muslim population and drew international support to their efforts, the Kenyan nationalists did not. In fact, it seems the senior members of the political dissidents in East Africa still hoped for a limited number of British doctors to continue to immigrate to the country, even after they won their independence. This desire for medical migrants contrasted with a general call for the cessation of European migrants more generally, which suggests that the nationalists did not have an effective plan for medical provisions.[114] The FLN's ability to produce the Croissant-Rouge therefore marks a significant point of contrast between the two contexts and shows how important medicine and its administration were for the rebels. By the time hostilities erupted in the colony, the French had become all too aware of this fact.

In 1955, the Governor General of Algeria, Jacques Soustelle, created the military-run *sections administratives spécialisées* (SAS) to perform security and welfare work in mostly rural areas – places where colonial doctors had largely failed to minister to the sick throughout the colonial period.[115] The SAS was therefore largely a propaganda organisation: their purpose was simultaneously to provide medical care in rural settings and to convince the rural communities of the benefits of the French presence in Algeria. Johnson has convincingly argued that the SAS was established to woo the hearts and minds of the Algerian inhabitants away from the FLN's attempts to foster humanitarian support and to cast themselves as better providers of healthcare and welfare. The French authorities believed that the SAS could promote a more humane version of empire by offering greater healthcare for those previously neglected portions of Muslim society.[116] By doing so, they acknowledged not only the level of inequality that had characterised much of the period of colonial occupation but also the close association between healthcare and military objectives.[117] It is this final point which helps to explain the number of French doctors who were killed by the FLN in 1956, as mentioned in the first section. These individuals, especially Dr Vanier, were providing healthcare through the SAS as part of a wider military strategy. It is therefore clear that the FLN's attacks on some doctors was not random. While the French press described the provision of this care as an act of humanitarianism, the FLN recognised it as another French tactic in the war. In fact, as early as 1961, a group of young French conscripts denounced the darker side of the SAS when they wrote in *Esprit*:

> the soldier turned schoolmaster, the S.A.S. officer, even the doctor of the Free Medical Service are not just teachers, administrators, and doctors; they are military personnel and are never allowed to forget it. In this war, which is overturning all our values, they are not

> primarily serving the Muslim children, or the sick of the village; they are serving a cause; they are one more weapon in the battle. The army only supports the S.A.S. system because it plays this dual role.[118]

Under the state of emergency, the military would use their control of the civilian medical services as a means for policing the Muslim population. Following their defeat at the hands of the nationalists in the protracted war in Indochina (1946–54), the French army had little time to dissect or make sense of what had happened before they were plunged into the Algerian War. The loss of their influence in the east left them embarrassed and terrified that Algeria, the last colony of significance, would also be lost to nationalist fervour. The French army, especially the paratrooper divisions, therefore carried out extreme levels of violence and waged a terror campaign against the FLN that included the use of torture, extrajudicial executions, assassinations and disappearances. A more detailed analysis of these aspects of the war will take place in later chapters, but at this stage it is important to note that the extent of the military's involvement in the conflict is a crucial factor that distinguishes the Algerian War from the Kenyan Emergency. In the context of the former, the civilian administration found itself constantly tussling with the military for control, especially as the army had a propensity for excessive and ill-judged interventions in politics and dissident behaviour that resulted in a failed military coup in April 1961.[119] The result was that medicine, in the eyes of the politically active on both sides of the conflict, was a weapon to be harnessed against the enemy. As in the early years of the colony, medicine was once again being controlled by the military – a development which goes a long way towards explaining why so many medical practitioners undertook activities that supported torture and violent interrogation. Although many civilian doctors also took part in forms of terrorism and violence, the military's control of Algeria during the war meant that the medical-assisted violence in this territory followed a distinct course from Kenya.

Doctors or soldiers of God?

In the early stages of colonial settlement in Kenya, medicine was, unlike its French counterpart, closely aligned with trade rather than military occupation. This is arguably because British officials were not really interested in the territory for its own sake; it was a link in the overall British Mediterranean and central African policy.[120] This should not be taken to imply that the British military were less aggressive than their French counterparts, however.[121] In 1888, the Imperial British East Africa Company (IBEAC) was issued a royal charter to trade in, and administer, the region. The Company brought with it administrators, commercial managers and the first government doctors to attend to the medical needs of the British residence. Prior to this, there had been little medical presence in the region, save for a few pioneering doctors attached to expedition parties and missionary physicians.[122] Doctors worked for the IBEAC until it was officially disbanded in 1895, when the territory of Kenya became a British protectorate and settler colony, whereupon they were absorbed into government service. Although the IBEAC quickly realised they were unable to establish trade in the hinterland without British military and financial support, the military only played a role in the administration until the first decade of the twentieth century, after which its influence was greatly diminished.[123] During these early years, the distinction between military and civilian roles was blurred, especially when it came to practising medicine. Military doctors had often been the first to establish the foundations of a medical infrastructure, but once the protectorate fell under civil management, these individuals usually transferred to civilian posts.[124] This is in marked contrast to the situation in Algeria, where military and civilian administrators continued to struggle for dominance throughout the colony's history.

Another distinction of note has to do with how the British administered their overseas territories more generally. It was assumed that British colonies should be largely self-supporting and funded by taxes drawn from the indigenous populations.[125] As such, the Colonial Services in each territory were afforded a certain degree of independence from central authority in London. Even though the Secretary of State for the Colonies and the Colonial Office had ultimate responsibility, individual colonial governors exercised a great deal of power.[126] This autonomy was also reflected in the CMS, which, employing nearly a third of all Colonial Staff in 1900, was the second-biggest personnel branch of the British Empire.[127] Although often referred to as a single body, the CMS was run as a distinct administrative organisation in each country, often with its own terms and conditions of service.[128] The Medical Department was one of the major departments of each colony and like others, such as the Treasury, the Legal Department and the Public Works Department, was headed by a member of the profession concerned – the head of the Medical Department was therefore always a civilian doctor. Unlike in Algeria, where it was mostly military doctors who would be involved in the counterinsurgency tactics employed against the FLN, it would be members of this CMS who had the most prominent role to play in the detention camps where the majority of Mau Mau detainees were held.

The CMS was, like other departments within the colonial administration, underfunded and low on personnel. This remained a constant challenge for the administration of medicine in East Africa and would have implications in the Kenyan detention camps during the Emergency.[129] The healthcare that the Medical Services could provide for the nascent settler community was thus limited, especially in the early days of British rule. Similar to the medical services in Algeria, colonial medicine in Kenya was principally aimed at protecting the lives of settlers, traders and the members of administration from the infectious diseases that threatened their interests.[130] The welfare and provision of healthcare for the African population lay outside their purview until after the First World War, unless disease prevalence among their communities posed a threat to the health of the British.[131] For example, in 1902, an epidemic of plague broke out in Nairobi. In order to stop it spreading to the European community, several doctors took it upon themselves to burn down the local Indian bazaar, with seemingly little consideration for the consequences.[132] In the end, a Dr Spurier was brought in from Zanzibar to take over the medical measures and to stop the sporadic burnings, despite those responsible for these extreme measures being thanked by the Secretary of State in England.[133] Consequently, as with Algeria, the benefits of Western medicine were largely reserved for the white settlers living in the colony.[134] If care was extended to the indigenous peoples, it was only when they presented a threat to the health of the nascent settler communities.

Moreover, due to financial restraints, the CMS in Africa rarely acted entirely autonomously. In fact, resources and expertise from other locally based health agencies were often pooled together, formally or informally, even if their interests did not always agree with one another.[135] In particular, running alongside the official administration of medicine in East Africa was the work performed by medical missionaries of various denominations.[136] These services, unlike those offered by the CMS in the early days of the colonies, were directed at the indigenous population. Although missionaries were not part of the CMS per se, the work of the two institutions was, as Markku Hokkanen states, deeply 'intertwined, with each benefitting from the other's cooperative co-existence'.[137] In essence, the colonial government was required to contribute very little to the civilising mission being carried out by various Christian denominations in East Africa. This is not to suggest that missionary societies and the CMS had an easy relationship, nor that the former were the handmaids of the latter. Indeed, recent scholarship has shown that although there were many instances of collaboration between the colonial authorities and various missionary societies across Africa, disagreements between the two were common, especially when related to administrative policy.[138] As Michael Jennings states, medical missionaries did function as 'agents of empire' to a certain extent, 'but in ways more complex and nuanced than is often presented [...]. Ultimately, missionaries were agents of their mission first and foremost'.[139] For many Africans living outside the urban and administrative centres, however, the distinction between the two was meaningless: missionary medicine was not an alternative form of Western medicine, it *was* Western medicine.[140] Where interests were shared, the two supported one another. In some cases, the level of collaboration between missionary doctors and the CMS was so intense that doctors with the Church Missionary Society[141] negotiated dual roles as missionaries and colonial medical officers up to the period before the 1940s.[142]

Yet the missionaries' ultimate aim differed from that of the colonial authorities. Missionaries emphasised the gospel of healing as an essential aspect of their work among the Africans. Their medical care was supplied alongside their greater aim: the Africans' spiritual salvation. As David Hardiman notes, the 'sickness' of the African, for Evangelicals, reflected both 'moral and physical contamination'. As such, 'any Godly person who understood the rudimentary principles of hygiene and sanitation was in a position to bring health to the "native" by cleansing their bodies with soap and their minds with the Gospel'.[143] Healing was an important tool for conversion, and so missionary medicine had a dual purpose for which the objective of healing bodies was subservient to saving souls.[144] This was a contentious problem for many of these 'hyphenated-hybrids', as Dr Chesterman called them, who felt torn by the dual nature of their role.[145] In fact, there was a long-running debate among missionary doctors regarding the extent to which they should capitalise on the opportunity to evangelise at the bedside. Some, like the famous missionary doctor Albert Cook, had the conversion of souls as their priority, and maintained that medical work would water down evangelisation, leading to superficial conversions only.[146] However, in times of epidemics and given the scarcity of available personnel and resources, it was not unusual for missionary doctors working in remote locations to find their time for spiritual commitments compromised by the sheer number of patients. As Dr Frank Lake of the Church Missionary Society for the Christian Medical College in Vellore, southern India, queried in 1949:

> How do we do it? Do we close the dispensary when we have seen the first six hundred patients? Do we say to the next two hundred, who because of greater infirmity took longer to crawl the weary road to the hospital: Sorry no more to-day; the priorities of the Kingdom of God must be served?[147]

Lake's question was raised as part an address he gave at a conference of the British Missionary Societies which was subsequently reproduced and circulated among the Kenya CMS staff. In answer to this question, Dr Lake ultimately echoed Cook. Lake suggested missionaries follow the example set by Christ in the 'Synoptic accounts of our Lord's healing miracles', and asked: 'What do our acts of physical healing achieve?' It was foolish, he argued, to believe that a physical cure would result in a patient entering 'within the sphere of spiritual redemption'.[148] Secular medicine emphasised obligations to all patients, but missionaries, Lake stressed, had to limit their clinical duties if they were to effectively deliver on their spiritual ones. It is not clear as to how members of the Kenyan Church Missionary Society responded to Lake's views. Reverend W. Scott Dickson, the General Secretary of the Church Missionary Society, asked readers to 'not assume [that] I agree with the paper', but it seems they were at least indicative of debates that run throughout the colonial period, as Megan Vaughan notes.[149]

There are a few points of interest here. Firstly, as mentioned above, missionaries were among the first to introduce Western medical practices to Kenya and many other countries that would become part of the British and French empires.[150] Indeed, in many instances, missionary hospitals and dispensaries were set up decades before colonial governments accepted any general responsibility for African health.[151] Medicine in East Africa was thus associated with Christianity from the outset. It was the missionaries who pioneered biomedical science in these colonies, who established rural hospitals and clinics, trained personnel and introduced 'Western' midwifery and childcare practices to the Africans.[152] It was not until the years following the First World War, as with the French example, that the CMS started to provide some healthcare to the indigenous population in East Africa and therefore limit their unofficial cooperation with missionary doctors. This provided a significant amount of political strength to the missionaries who administered healthcare to the Africans. In fact, it highlights a crucial factor in the rise of nationalism in Kenya: for the Africans the link between the missionaries' Christian zeal and their medical aid could be extremely contentious, especially when they interfered with their traditional customs.

The emphasis on Christian spirituality was often fundamental and sometimes unyielding. In this world view, if illness was the result of sin, then the roots of that sin, in many cases, were the evils of traditional society.[153] African indigenous religious beliefs were viewed as unacceptable, primitive, uncivilised and as potential sources for infection. The missionaries took particular exception to the practices of witchcraft, ancestor worship, modes of dress, African dances, polygamy and burial practices.[154] In some instances in Kenya, the services provided by missionary schools and hospitals could only be accessed by the Africans such as the Kikuyu – Kenya's largest ethnic group, which made up the vast majority of Mau Mau – if they renounced their own traditional beliefs and 'pagan' customs.[155]

One of these traditional customs that caused political controversy for the medical community and the colony more generally was the Kikuyu's practice of female circumcision, or clitoridectomy. As a Dr John W. Arthur explained in 1942, 'the missionaries, many of whom are medical men, and nurses have spoken of "the sexual mutilation of women" as being a more correct term than "circumcision" '.[156] Dr Arthur explained that, from a medical perspective, the operation had 'physical and psychological' effects on 'girls in puberty' and could lead to excessive bleeding and even death. Yet, according to Arthur, the 'most disastrous results of the operation occur[ed] at times of childbirth, especially with primiparae'. This meant that labour was often delayed and the mother or child, or even both, could die 'from the unfavourable conditions of the operation'.[157] In the early part of the twentieth century, some missionary hospitals working with the Kikuyu had banned the practice for their converts. 'As the result of a strong stand taken by some of the missions working among the Kikuyu from 1916 on', Arthur tells us, 'many Christian girls are now saved from this operation, and thus in certain areas the custom is becoming a thing of the past'.[158] The reference to 'Christian girls' in this passage is interesting as, up to this point, Arthur had made no reference to the Kikuyu's religious beliefs. Indeed, the correspondence says nothing else related to religion. One could be forgiven for assuming that Arthur's views on female circumcision were based purely on medical grounds, but this final line betrays a certain religious objection, one that almost seems to link Kikuyu's 'pagan' practice with dangers to health.

What Arthur fails to mention in his correspondence is that he himself played a direct role in a political clash that came about because of the ban on female circumcision in Kenya. Arthur had started his medical work in Kenya in 1909 and had been opposed to the practice from the start.[159] He and two colleagues, Dr Stanley Jones and Dr H. R. Philip, the Church of Scotland Mission doctor of Tumu Tumu province, had also been 'vigorous' campaigners against the practice on religious, medical and humanitarian grounds.[160] During the late 1920s, several missions, including the Church of Scotland Mission, the Africa Inland Mission and the Gospel Missionary Society, applied pressure on colonial officials in Nairobi to change their approach of indirect rule. Typically, the British colonial authorities allowed local chiefs or what were known as Local Native Councils to exercise authority over the Africans and their customs.[161] In this situation, however, the officials in Nairobi urged local African authorities to regulate and restrict female circumcision. In 1929, Dr Arthur, who was the 'feisty' head of the Church of Scotland Mission, along with his European staff had insisted that all their African employees, primary teachers, as well as church elders and members sign an oath renouncing the custom of female circumcision. He even insisted that the Africans swear that they were not members of the Kikuyu Central Association (KCA) – a radical African political organisation that came to prominence in Kikuyuland in the early 1930s.[162]

According to Anne Beck, Dr Arthur had always had a pro-African attitude and a history of trying to protect African land rights and access to education from more hardline settlers like Lord Delamere.[163] However, the political repercussions of his anti-female circumcision stance were far larger than Arthur had anticipated. As Donald Schilling notes, 'Seventeen of the bush school teachers refused to sign and were dismissed; the church at Kikuyu lost nine-tenths of its members, including eighteen of fifty elders; and the mission's bush schools, assigned teachers who had taken the oath, were boycotted and shut down'.[164] Other missions that took a similar stance also found their flocks depleted in their thousands. The Kikuyu founded their own churches that permitted the practice, in response. On 11 December 1929, the Kikuyu's practice of female circumcision became a hotly debated subject in Parliament back in London.[165] The policy embarrassed more moderate missions while straining relations between government officials and the missionaries opposed to circumcision. This single cultural issue ended up mobilising Kikuyu peasants for the first time and, in doing so, provided the KCA with a mass political basis that would contribute to a growing sense of nationalism among the politically minded Kikuyu.

The controversy caused by missionary doctors like Dr Arthur and his colleagues demonstrates the delicate situation medical missionaries working in the colonies faced. Although the fundamental principles underlining the ban on clitoridectomies were grounded in humanitarian and medical terms, the missionaries' continual desire to stamp out all unchristian indigenous practices nevertheless contributed to the Kikuyu's negative response. Arthur's medical responsibilities were tainted by his missionary zeal in the eyes of the Kenyans, causing them to transmute into political issues. Indeed, while on an evangelical tour of central Kenya, where he was preaching on the 'evils' of clitoridectomy prior to the ban in 1929, Arthur reportedly accused the KCA of being agitators and despoilers of 'God's work'. He even reportedly thumped the pulpit in anger, causing concern among the other European missionaries who were present.[166] Arthur's controversy thus highlights an interesting alternative to the type of dual-loyalty dilemma discussed so far. Rather than being torn between his commitments to the healing profession and the military, as is the case in other contexts, Arthur was caught between his professional role and his religious beliefs. This is an area worth wider investigation, but for now it is important to note that the divide created by the circumcision topic served as a point of orientation for the nationalists in Kenya.

The KCA, who aimed for a progressive spread of education and training for Africans, were also determined to preserve tribal customs, which included female circumcision. Jomo Kenyatta, the future president of Kenya, felt strongly about the retention of circumcision itself and the rites that accompanied it.[167] For him and for many other Kikuyu, the practice was part of the essence of Kikuyu life. A Kikuyu girl who refused to undergo the operation could not marry a Kikuyu husband; and this meant, as Anderson argued, that there would be no exchange of bridewealth – livestock and goods given to the family of the bride by the family of the groom. This exchange served as a social glue that bound families to one another in relations of obligation and reciprocity.[168] A challenge to this tradition was a direct challenge to the survival of the Kikuyu society. The repeated demands that were issued by Kikuyu politicians in defence of circumcision demonstrated, in their eyes, the realities of Britain's 'civilising mission'. The colonial government responded to the KCA with unequivocal hostility, labelling it a dangerous and subversive organisation that was unrepresentative of the Kikuyu majority.[169] Arthur's ban was therefore further evidence in the minds of the KCA that colonial authority, religion and the limited medical aid the Africans received were all part of a system that would erode traditional values; the price for 'progress' in this instance was too steep.

The clitoridectomy controversy allowed the KCA to gain significant strength.[170] In the 1930s, they turned their attention to one of the most significant grievances of the Kikuyu, the struggle for land that, they believed, had been stolen by white settlers. The politics that played out over the next decade would shape the rise of Mau Mau in the 1950s. The issue of land was central to the politically active Kikuyu's list of grievances and ultimate demands.

Land, nationalism and the rise of Mau Mau

Since the arrival of the first European settlers in 1902, land in Kenya had been divided by race, just as it had been in South Africa. In 1915, the Crown Land Ordinance recognised 'native rights' in lands reserved for their use, and in 1926 the British consolidated this division by creating African Reserves for each of Kenya's 'tribes', leaving the highlands, what would be known as the 'White Highlands', for the Europeans.[171] The White Highlands had absorbed large chunks of land in Kiambu and Murang'a, as well as areas further north, around Nyeri and Nanyki, and great tracts of land in the Rift Valley, and far to the west on the plateaus beyond.[172] Prior to the arrival of the Europeans, most of these lands were grazed by the Masai, while the richest part, little more than 1 per cent of the area, had belonged to the Kikuyu. Once the settlers took possession of them, however, the only Africans allowed on the land were the squatters employed as labourers by the Europeans. Settlers saw this land as rightfully theirs as they had, as John Lonsdale says, claimed it 'by virtue of treaty and achievement; it was their own sure footing in uncertain times'.[173] For two generations, these Europeans had been tending to and taming the land; their young had prosperous futures tied to its soil and their dead had been buried within it.

The same was true for the medical community. Since the early days of European settlement in Kenya, some doctors were attracted to the colony for the financial opportunities it offered. For example, in 1896, Henry Albert Bödeker arrived in Kenya seeking to make his fortune from private practice before eventually joining the Colonial Service in 1899.[174] However, the land offered the greatest opportunities for securing a living, even for medical practitioners. In 1919, following the First World War, the pro-European War Council in Kenya established the Soldier Settlement Scheme, with support from Governor Sir Edward Northey. The scheme enabled veterans to claim land as British settlers, even if they lacked capital to develop their holdings.[175] Yet one feature of this scheme solidified the connection between the land issue and the medical community in a way that was more defined than in North Africa: an amendment to the scheme made by Northey himself saw ex-service doctors being offered free farms to encourage them to attend to the newly arriving soldier settlers.[176] The provisions of this medical scheme were designed to keep the doctors on their farms for as long as possible. If the farms were sold to anyone other than a doctor in the first five years after allotment, the full stand premia on the land had to be paid. Thereafter, the stand premia were reduced to a fifth for each year the doctor remained on the farm, and after ten years the land became free.[177] Although the number of doctors who benefitted from this scheme was relatively low – twenty-five doctors, four nurses and a dentist – those who did gain land seem to have received a substantial amount.[178] For instance, the family of Lieutenant-Colonel C. A. Cunningham, the only doctor in the district of Laikipia, in central Kenya, gained 10,255 acres through the Soldier Settler Scheme.[179]

Although the scheme offered ex-service doctors a chance at securing a livelihood in Kenya, it still had significant drawbacks. One of the most frustrating seemed to be that these doctors were often tied to land in extremely isolated locations with few resources at their disposal. Competition for clients was tight, and settler doctors often had to compete with Government Medical Officers for civil service patients, some of the few in Kenya who could be relied on to pay their bills.[180] Overall, the medical settlers attempted to avoid proceeding to the soldier settlement districts. For example, Dr Pentreath, one of the victims of Mau Mau mentioned above, engaged in a series of five attempted exchanges of land in order to both secure a farm and reside close to Nairobi so he could maintain an eye practice he had established. Flexibility was needed, and the Government exercised it where possible. Dr M. C. Wetherell, a local medical settler who had been assigned a farm in the Kipkarren area, was also appointed as District Surgeon for Eldoret and allowed to use his practice there to count as occupation of his farm. Cunningham was permitted an extension of his then 1,760 acre farm in response to local demand for a doctor, in order that he might work it as an economic unit.

If a steady flow of patients was insufficient to maintain a 'colonial' lifestyle, then doctors were forced to either subsidise their incomes by cultivating the land or else return to Britain.[181] As such, those who remained in Kenya were tied to the land as a necessity for survival. This meant they would be responsible for maintaining the health of the European community, and to a lesser extent the Africans, in their allotted district as well as tending to their own agricultural enterprises. The hardship of this role was not necessarily without reward. Indeed, the need for qualified doctors meant that those who took up positions in the settler districts became invaluable members of the community and could rise in the ranks of the local hierarchy. On these extensive farms, doctors were not only benefiting from the soil at the expense of the Kikuyu, they were also among the settlers who exploited their labour.

This is where the significance of the farming scheme with respect to the Mau Mau uprising starts to take shape. Following the end of the First World War, colonial authorities began to consider vital reforms in their management of African communities. Missionaries, colonial officials in East Africa and reformers in the metropole supported efforts to improve the standard of education available to Africans. The idea was that an expansion of education should be principally directed at increasing the number of Africans with technical qualifications. But, crucially, this limited goal of advancement for the indigenous population met strong resistance. As Beck notes, 'European settlers felt that their need for African unskilled labor should be given priority over any other consideration'.[182] African advancement was a secondary consideration when it came to protecting the interests of the settler community. The Soldier Settler Scheme added pressure to this problem as the need for more African labour came at a time when African wages were already being depressed by the new settlements.[183]

Rather than offer wage incentives, European employers and colonial authorities relied on coercion to recruit African labour, which was mostly drawn from the Kikuyu population. This was achieved in four ways. Firstly, the Africans were forced into reserves (through the 1915 Crown Lands Ordinance), which were defined rural areas, much like the homelands in South Africa.[184] Each ethnic group had their own separate reserve. This practice of divide and rule was also a cornerstone of the colonial government's labour policy. With insufficient land in their reserves, many Africans had little choice but to migrate to the Europeans' farms in search of work. Increased taxation on their huts also pressured Africans to migrate in search of employment, but the government regulated this too. It forced all African men by law to carry a pass, or *kipande*, that recorded a worker's fingerprint, name, employment history, ethnicity and current employer's signature. Finally, when the Europeans and authorities realised that African farmers were more successful than the largely inexperienced settlers, further regulations were imposed that forbade Africans from growing the major cash crops – coffee, tea and sisal.[185]

By the 1920s, the British presence in Kenya was secure. Whereas colonists in other territories, most obviously Australia, had to live or die by the labour of their own hands, those in Kenya could count on the sweat of African peasants to maintain agricultural development.[186] Doctors brought to Kenya under the Soldier Settlement Scheme would have presumably benefitted from this cheap labour as well, along with other settler doctors drawn to Kenya for its opportunities. This, it can be argued, helps explain why doctors featured so prominently among the first causalities of the Mau Mau uprising. It was not necessarily their medical titles that made them targets, though it should be apparent by now that, from the perspective of the Africans, such qualifications were unlikely to be associated with benevolence and non-malfeasance. Instead, because of their links to the land, these doctors contributed directly to one of the most contentious political issues in the colony and would have undoubtedly appeared as representatives of the wider settler communities who had marginalised the Africans.

Many Africans, especially the Kikuyu, still claimed ownership of the land they were forced to cultivate for the European settlers. With the passage of time, and the steady increase in African population, pressure on the African reserves became apparent. By the 1930s, both the moderate nationalists, the KCA, and the conservative chiefs who maintained close loyalty to the British authorities, agreed on the extent of the land problem. Chief Koinange was particularly vocal in drawing attention to the issue and successfully persuaded the British government to inaugurate the Kenya Land Commission in 1932.[187] The hope was that the Commission would be 'above suspicion' and, according to Lord Sanderson speaking in Parliament on 4 May 1932, should have 'secure[d] the complete confidence of the African population'.[188] However, this was never realised. Prior to the Commission's arrival in Kenya, the KCA and the chiefs set about obtaining evidence of land claims from the African population. A questionnaire was prepared and circulated by the KCA and filled in with help from the chiefs. A Kikuyu Land Board Association was created by the KCA to gather additional evidence, collate land claims and find witnesses to give testament to the Commission. In total, the land claimed by the Kikuyu amounted to about 60,000 acres. But when the Commission reported its recommendations in 1934, the Kikuyu were to be greatly disappointed.[189] Far from taking African grievances seriously, the Commission decided to confirm the status quo, merely offering Africans, by way of consolation, lands of substandard quality in areas in which the Europeans had no interest. This infertile and less accessible land amounted to only a fraction of that lost to the Africans – an increase of about 3 per cent to 'the native reserves' and an additional 21,000 acres as 'Native Lands'.[190]

The report felt that a 'great disservice' would be done to the country if the British were to 'compromise future development by locking up rigidly in tribal compartments land not yet required by the tribes, because we apprehend that at some uncertain date in the future it might be required'.[191] That is, the contested land was better off being used by Europeans for productive agriculture than squandered while waiting for Africans to develop it themselves. The outcome of the Commission's recommendations hit the Kikuyu particularly hard and effectively removed all hope of ever recovering their loss, but it also hardened attitudes. As Anderson notes, '[t]he Land Commission report was the stone upon which moderate African politics was broken'.[192] For the Kikuyu, the real struggle for land had just begun and more militant nationalism found expression in the everyday effort to resist the colonial authorities from implementing the Commission's recommendations. Over the next twenty years the seeds of rebellion continued to grow as the African population increased in size and pressures on their limited land holdings prompted further resentment towards the tightening grip of the settler community. Kikuyu militancy and a full uprising eventually erupted in the late 1940s and early 1950s in what would be known as the Mau Mau uprising.

On 20 October 1952, following the assassination of Chief Waruhiu by Mau Mau commandos earlier that month, Governor Baring declared a state of emergency in the colony.[193] Through the use of various emergency regulations, the colonial authorities were vested with far-reaching powers which enabled them to arrest and detain Mau Mau suspects without court orders and to suspend civil rights.[194] Unlike in Algeria, however, the emergency regulations did not provide for martial law to be enacted in Kenya. As such, the military played a more limited role in Kenya than they did in Algeria. Their presence was initially enhanced by way of five regiments of the King's African Rifles (KAR) and the Lancashire Fusiliers for what was a relatively short military campaign that was concluded by 1955.[195] The military's initial response was to undertake the mass arrest of 180 leading African political figures, including Kenyatta, who were suspected of being the ringleaders of Mau Mau. Operation Jock Scott, as this initiative was named, sought to sever the heads of the movement from its body through a pre-emptive strike. Unlike the French in Algeria, who were caught unaware by the FLN's coordinated attacks in 1954, the British authorities attempted to outmanoeuvre the nationalists before they could act. But rather than weaken the nationalist sentiment, Britain's opening strategy merely radicalised Mau Mau militants under the command of individuals like Dedan Kimathi and Stanley Mathenge, who waged a guerrilla war in the Kenyan jungles. If Mau Mau's violence had been inspired by the conditions created by the state of emergency, as Carl Rosberg and John Nottingham have surmised, then Klose is certainly correct in arguing that 'the planned preventive strike of the emergency thus achieved the exact opposite of its intended purpose'.[196]

When violence broke out, members of the Kenyan medical community were eager to offer their own explanations for its causes. According to Dr Wiseman, who wrote to the *BMJ* following the death of Dr Ruck, it was overpopulation and the shortage of food for the Africans that had led to the rebellion. Wiseman notes that in 1947–48, the Kenya Branch put forward the case for a Royal Commission to investigate the 'population problem'.[197] The Kenya representatives at the Annual Meeting at Cambridge in 1948 pleaded for support for the proposal and subsequently the Council of the BMA recommended it to the Colonial Office. However, as Wiseman pointed out, 'the Government then in office [...] declined to recommend the appointment of a Commission'. The consequences of this were dire: 'some African "intelligentsia" have been encouraged to believe that their prosperity lay in expelling the British and seizing political power by force'.[198]

Absent from this explanation of the rise of Mau Mau was any reference to the land grievances raised by the politically active Kikuyu. Wiseman does draw attention to land-based issues, but only with reference to comments made by 'casual visitors to the Colony', that is, the views of European travellers, not the African inhabitants themselves. He writes that these visitors 'are impressed by the disparity between the productive farmlands of European settlements and the soil-eroded areas of certain native reserves'. Wiseman, however, is quick to state that 'no competent authority has ever advocated that the solution of the food problems of the Africans lay in interfering with the successful farming of the former'.[199] Wiseman's statement echoes the aforementioned views of the Land Commission: the fertile farmlands of the White Highlands were better off in European hands, since Africans would not be able to use them effectively. This was the most important point of Wiseman's correspondence and, by extension, the views of Kenya Branch of the BMA. Under no circumstances were the metropolitan colleagues of the Kenya medical profession to attempt to interfere with the situation in Kenya:

> The Kenya Branch is anxious that the profession should become acquainted with these facts, lest in a desire to help the Africans of Kenya some of its members might misinterpret events and hinder a return to orderly progress on which alone the health of all communities, but especially that of the African depends.[200]

It is clear from this extract that the 'return to ordinary progress' and 'the health of all communities' meant a return to pre-Emergency conditions where Europeans had held unquestioned supremacy. Wiseman's views betray the type of attitude towards the plight of the African population that Fanon drew attention to. Colonial medicine in Kenya revealed itself to be closely aligned with the economic interests of the settler population. African health was contingent on the Europeans maintaining their land rights.

In light of all of this, it is easy to see how landowners like the Rucks could become targets for hostilities when the Kikuyu's frustrations finally turned violent. The CMS in Kenya, along with the assistance of prominent missionary doctors, had directly contributed to the political, economic and social conditions that eventually festered into outright resentment and aggression.

Conclusion

Doctors working in the colonies were not always viewed as simple healers or providers of medical care. The contention of this chapter has been that that, in both countries, doctors were so deeply embedded in the colonial order that they could be seen as representatives of the types of offences and grievances associated with European occupation in the eyes of the indigenous populations. This is because, in the colonies at least, these professionals were often involved in activities, or ways of life, that were similar to those of other settlers and that saw them benefiting in ways that excluded the indigenous populations. For some locals, the doctor was a potentially corrupt individual whose loyalties to patients had been subverted by their commitments to other institutions or their own self-interest. Practising medicine in the colonies, it seems, could be a highly political activity which rarely had the interests of the indigenous populations at heart. In order to examine this split-loyalty phenomenon and the factors that contributed to it, this chapter also critically engaged with the work of Frantz Fanon and, specifically, the claims he made concerning colonial doctors. Essentially, it is possible to identify a number of factors that appeared to cause the split in doctors' loyalties across both contexts, splits which contributed to the lists of grievances held by the respective nationalist groups.

Firstly, the administration of medicine in Algeria and Kenya helped to establish and maintain an atmosphere of alienation and exclusion whereby African and Muslim communities were reduced to an underclass status. This was partially achieved through the medical community's close connection with the colonial authorities, especially the military and security forces in both contexts. This connection, however, was particularly strong in Algeria, where medicine had played a fundamental role in supporting the military conquest of the territory in the nineteenth century. In this case, while the colony ceased to be controlled by the army towards the end of that century, the military nevertheless maintained a strong presence within the colonial order up until the Algerian War when they took control once again.

Although the military had less of a role to play in the management of Kenya, the medical system was no more coherent, especially for the indigenous population. The financial limitations on the CMS in East Africa resulted in medical missionaries of various denominations providing the majority of health services for the Africans. The work of medical missionaries provided healthcare to the Kikuyu and other Africans under the condition that they renounce their traditional beliefs and practices. Ultimately, the disquiet this caused in Kikuyu society led to their first mass political revolt, something that fed directly into the formation of Mau Mau in the 1940s and 1950s. This is an important distinction between the Algerian and Kenyan situations. The controversy surrounding clitoridectomy, which was framed on medical grounds though it was equally a moral question for the Christian missionaries, represented a rare moment where the acts of a doctor had real, tangible impacts on the political situation in the colony.

The question of land rights and ownership forms an important issue for both countries, though it arguably became a more central political grievance for the Kikuyu in Kenya. There is, at present, more evidence for the intimate connection between the Kikuyu's land claims and the land holdings of colonial doctors in this context. As in Algeria, British colonial authorities in Kenya enabled European settlers to claim ownership of the more fertile farming lands in the colony, the White Highlands. The loss of this land became a central issue for the KCA in the 1930s and 1940s and would be the main political rallying point for Mau Mau.

Notes

1 David Anderson, *History of the Hanged*, pp. 93–94.

2 Esmee Ruck actually practised medicine under her maiden name, Esmee de Smidt. See Anonymous, 'Search for murderers of British family', *Manchester Guardian*, 26 January 1953; and Anonymous, 'Obituary', *British Medical Journal*, 28 February 1953, p. 513.

3 Robert Howitt Wiseman, 'Mau Mau', *British Medical Journal*, 7 March 1953, p. 65.

4 Anonymous, 'SURVIVOR'S STORY OF MAU MAU RAID: Seven Kikuyu Charged with Murder', *Manchester Guardian*, 23 January 1953.

5 Anonymous, 'Obituary', *British Medical Journal*, 29 May 1954, 1270–1271.

6 Anonymous, 'SURVIVOR'S STORY OF MAU MAU RAID'.
7 Anderson, *Histories of the Hanged*, p. 94.
8 Anonymous, 'QUARANTE BANDITS EN ARMES ont attaqué le petit village de Pasteur', *Le Monde*, 17 November 1954. www.lemonde.fr/archives/article/1954/11/17/quarante-bandits-en-armes-ont-attaque-le-petit-village-de-pasteur_2026138_1819218.html> [Accessed 17 November 2017].
9 Anonymous, 'LES MEDECINS MILITAIRES et l'assistance médicale gratuite en Algérie', *Le Monde*, 28 August 1957. www.lemonde.fr/archives/article/1957/08/28/les-medecins-militaires-et-l-assistance-medicale-gratuite-en-algerie_2326178_1819218.html> [Accessed 17 November 2017].
10 On 29 March 1956, a medical officer, Lieutenant Guillemont was kidnapped and killed by FLN forces in Djidjelli; on the same day, a medical auxiliary called Maurice Feignon was captured and tortured by rebels. On 11 June 1956, a Lieutenant Petit, an administrative officer at the military hospital of Sétif, was shot and killed while, a day later, a medical officer called Captain Fauvy was killed in Djidjelli as well. These deaths have since been collected together within the websites of French right-wing organisations as evidence of France's apparent betrayal of her European subjects in the colony as well as the loyalists who sought to continue colonial rule in the territory. Even today, the death of doctors at the hands of the FLN is portrayed by these ultras as a sign of the barbarism among the FLN.
11 Anonymous, 'DES REBELLES HARCELENT SOUK-AHRAS', *Le Monde*, 9 January 1957. www.lemonde.fr/archives/article/1957/01/09/des-rebelles-harcelent-souk-ahras_2329536_1819218.html> [Accessed 17 November 2017].
12 Anonymous, 'Une patrouille ouvre le feu dans la Casbah d'Alger CINQ MORTS, TRENTE-SEPT BLESSES, *Le Monde*, 28 February 1958. www.lemonde.fr/archives/article/1957/02/28/une-patrouille-ouvre-le-feu-dans-la-casbah-d-alger-cinq-morts-trente-sept-blesses_3134093_1819218.html> [Accessed 19 March 2018].
13 See Jonathan G. Katz, *Murder in Marrakesh: Emile Mauchamp and the French Colonial Adventure* (Bloomington and Indianapolis: Indiana University Press, 2006); and Ellen Amster, 'The many deaths of Dr Emile Mauchamp: medicine, technology, and popular politics in pre-Protectorate Morocco, 1877–1912', *International Journal of Middle East Studies* 36 (2004), pp. 409–428.
14 Katz, *Murder in Marrakesh*, p. 2.
15 Amster, 'The many deaths of Dr Emile Mauchamp', p. 423.
16 Amster, 'The many deaths of Dr Emile Mauchamp', pp. 418–422.

17 For instance, see Michael Blundell, *So Rough a Wind* (London: Weidenfeld and Nicolson, 1964), p. 123; Peter Hewitt, *Kenya Cowboy: A Police Officer's Account of the Mau Mau Emergency in Kenya* (London: Avon Books, 1999), p. 55.
18 Fanon, *A Dying Colonialism*, p. 135.
19 Fanon, *A Dying Colonialism*, p. 135.
20 Fanon, *A Dying Colonialism*, p. 135.
21 Fanon, *A Dying Colonialism*, p. 135.
22 Fanon, *A Dying Colonialism*, p. 121.
23 Fanon, *A Dying Colonialism*, p. 133.
24 Fanon, *A Dying Colonialism*, p. 133.
25 Fanon, *A Dying Colonialism*, p. 134.
26 Peter Hewitt, a former member of the KPR, like Roger Ruck, explained that Roger had a reputation for being less friendly towards Africans, especially after the death of Eric Bowyer, another settler murdered shortly before the Rucks. Roger was also known to be a man of 'strong views', which, as David Anderson has noted, is 'settler shorthand for conservative and outspoken'. Such qualities may well have contributed towards the Mau Mau's decision to target him and his family on that fateful night. See Hewitt, *Kenya Cowboy*, p. 55; and Anderson, *Histories of the Hanged*, p. 93.
27 Anderson, *Histories of the Hanged*, p. 134.
28 As quoted in Richard C. Keller, 'Madness and colonization: psychiatry in the British and French Empires, 1800–1962', *Journal for Social History* 35 (2001), p. 297.
29 William Gallois, 'Local responses to French medical imperialism in late nineteenth-century Algeria', *Social History of Medicine*, 20 (2007), p. 315. More generally, see Mathew Burrows, '*Mission civilisatrice*': French cultural policy in the Middle East, 1860–1914', *The Historical Journal* 29 (1986), pp. 109–135.
30 In particular, recent work has sought to reassess the level of agency and resistance exercised by colonised peoples. In the Algerian context, see Hannah-Louise Clark, 'Expressing entitlement in colonial Algeria: villages, medical doctors, and the state in the early 20th century', *International Journal of Middle East Studies 48* (2016), pp. 445–472. For more general account of the changes in historiography around colonial medicine, see Chakrabarti, *Medicine & Empire*; and Keir Waddington, *An Introduction to the Social History of Medicine* (Basingstoke: Palgrave Macmillan, 2011), p. 278.
31 Clark's recent study shows that, in reality, few French doctors were willing to practice medicine in rural zones. Their absence was lamented by small rural villages and towns who requested medical

visits from colonial doctors even after the military had been involved in repressive activity in the local area.

32 Robert Aldrich, *Greater France: A History of French Overseas Expansion* (Basingstoke: Macmillan Press, 1996), pp. 26–27.

33 For a detailed assessment of France's occupation strategy and the destructive methods used to eliminate Arab opponents (as well as civilians), see Le Cour Grandmaison, *Coloniser. Exterminer*, pp. 7–22. See also pp. 138–140 for details on the French massacre of over 500 Arabs in 1845 in the grotto of Dahra.

34 Le Cour Grandmaison, *Coloniser. Exterminer*, p. 188.

35 Klose, *Human Rights in the Shadow of Colonial Violence*, p. 79.

36 Aldrich, *Greater France*, p. 144.

37 Aldrich, *Greater France*, p. 144.

38 Gallois, *The Administration of Sickness*, p. 63.

39 Chopin, 'Embodying "the new white race" ', p. 6.

40 Chopin, 'Embodying "the new white race" ', p. 6.

41 Laurence Monnais, 'Which medications did they trust? The role of French colonialism in Vietnamese attitudes towards pharmaceuticals, 1858–1939', Paper presented at Princeton Workshop in the history of science, 'Science across Cultures – Historical and Philosophical Perspectives', Princeton University, 24 October 2003, p. 2.

42 Philippe Bonnichon, Pierre Geny and Jean Nemo, *Présences françaises outre-mer (XVIe–XXIe siècles). Science, religion et culture* (Paris: Editions Karthala, 2012), p. 224.

43 Gallois, *The Administration of Sickness*, p. 39.

44 Clark, 'Expressing entitlement in colonial Algeria', p. 447.

45 Clark, 'Expressing entitlement in colonial Algeria', pp. 448–449.

46 Fanon, *A Dying Colonialism*, p. 121.

47 Clark, 'Expressing entitlement in colonial Algeria', p. 455.

48 Clark, 'Expressing entitlement in colonial Algeria', p. 446.

49 Anne Marcovich, 'French colonial medicine and colonial rule: Algeria and Indochina', in Macleod and Lewis (eds), *Disease, Medicine and Empire*, p. 114. See also Marie-France Laberge, 'Les Instituts Pasteur du Maghreb. La recherche médicale dans le cadre de la politique coloniale', *Revue française d'histoire d'outre-mer* 74 (1987), pp. 27–42.

50 Sunil S. Amrith, *Decolonizing International Health: India and Southeast Asia, 1930–65* (Basingstoke: Palgrave Macmillan, 2006), p. 22.

51 However, rates of epidemic disease had started to fall in the first half of the century. Outbreaks of plague, cholera and typhus, which had decimated whole villages for much of the nineteenth century, became less frequent. The death rate from such infections fell to lower than

20 per 1,000 during the interwar years and then, after a small peak in the 1940s, to 17.5 per 1,000 by 1954. See John Ruedy, *Modern Algeria: The Origins and Development of a Nation* (Bloomington and Indianapolis: Indiana University Press, 2005), p. 120.

52 Norman Howard-Jones, *The Scientific Background of the International Sanitary Conferences 1851–1938* (Geneva: World Health Organization, 1975).

53 Martin David Dubin, 'The League of Nations Health Organization', in Charles Webster and Charles Rosenberg (eds), *International Health Organisations and Movements, 1918–1939* (Cambridge: Cambridge University Press, 1995), pp. 56–80.

54 Jennifer Johnson, *The Battle for Algeria: Sovereignty, Health Care, and Humanitarianism* (Philadelphia: University of Pennsylvania Press, 2016), p. 31.

55 Randall Packard, 'Visions of postwar health and development and their impact on public health interventions in the developing world', in Frederick Cooper and Randall Packard (eds), *International Development and the Social Sciences: Essays on the History and Politics of Knowledge* (Berkeley: University of California Press, 1997), p. 96.

56 Quoted in Gallois, *The Administration of Sickness*, p. 1.

57 Gallois, *The Administration of Sickness*, p. 1.

58 Gallois, *The Administration of Sickness*, p. 6.

59 Mark Harrison, 'Medicine and the management of modern warfare', *History of Science* 34 (1996), p. 395. For a wider discussion on the twentieth-century history of disease and its links to security issues, see Nicholas B. King, 'Security, disease, commerce: ideologies of postcolonial global health', *Social Studies of Science* 32 (2002), pp. 763–789.

60 Keller, *Colonial Madness*, p. 123.

61 Mohammed Harbi, 'Bauern und Revolution', pp. 127–128. Quoted in Klose, *Human Rights in the Shadow of Colonial Violence*, p. 79.

62 Muslims could become French citizens only if they rejected Islam and their cultural habits, served in the military and learnt the French language. Few Muslims accepted these conditions, and those who did were viewed with suspicion by both the communities they rejected and the racially prejudiced Europeans they joined. Aldrich, *Greater France*, p. 212. See also Fanon, *A Dying Colonialism*, pp. 40–41.

63 Fanon, *A Dying Colonialism*, p. 132.

64 Sanctionable crimes included, for example, meeting without authorisation; departure from the territory of the municipality without a travel permit; disrespectful acts; and offensive remarks towards an officer of authority even outside of his functions. Punishments included

individual fines and imprisonment, as well as collective punishment, corporal punishment, forced labour, and the confiscation of property. See Patrick Weil, 'Le Statut des musulmans en Algérie colonial', *Histoire de la justice* 16 (2005), p. 96; and Le Cour Grandmaison, *Coloniser. Exterminer*, p. 22.

65 Martin Shipway, 'Algeria and the 'official mind': the impact of North Africa on French colonial policy south of the Sahara, 1944–58', in Martin S. Alexander, Martin Evans and J. F. V. Keiger (eds), *The Algerian War and the French Army, 1954–62: Experiences, Images, Testimonies, 2002* (New York: Palgrave Macmillan, 2002), p. 61.

66 Alistair Horne, *A Savage War of Peace: Algeria 1954–1962* (New York: New York Review Books, 2006), pp. 45–46.

67 Article 1 of Warnier Law says: *l'establishment de la propriété immobilière en Algérie, sa conservation et sa transmission contractuelle des immeubles et droits immobiliers, quels que soient les propriétaires, sont régis par la loi française. En conséquence, sont abolis tous droits réels, servitudes ou causes de résolutions quelconques, fondes sur le doit musulman ou kabyle, qui seraient contraires à la loi française.*] See Eugène Robe, *La Propriété immobilière en Algérie, commentaire de la loi du 26 juillet 1873* (Algiers: Juillet St Lager, 1875), p. 5.

68 Mahfoud Bennoune, *The Making of Contemporary Algeria, 1830–1987* (Cambridge: Cambridge University Press, 2002), p. 46.

69 Martin Evans, *Algeria: France's Undeclared War* (Oxford: Oxford University Press, 2012), p. 23.

70 Evans, *Algeria*, p. 23.

71 Evans, *Algeria*, p. 23.

72 Evans, *Algeria*, p. 25.

73 Although the consumption of alcohol was frowned upon within Quranic traditions, that does not mean Muslims did not drink. This aspect of history, the relationship between colonial Muslims and the cultures of alcohol introduced by the French into Northern Africa has received increased attention in recent years and shows that the story is far more complicated than previously assumed. See Shahab Ahmed, *What Is Islam? The Importance of Being Islamic* (Princeton and Oxford: Princeton University Press, 2016), pp. 57–73.

74 I was unable to find much of substance about Dr Ettighoffer other than his role within the Confédération des vignerons des trois départements algériens and to confirm that he was a doctor of medicine working in Algiers in the 1920s. It is possible he had retired by the time he was made vice-president in the 1950s. See *L'Echo d'Alger. Journal républicain du matin*, 3 July 1922.

75 Giulia Meloni and Johan Swinnen, 'The rise and fall of the world's largest wine exporter – and its institutional legacy', *Journal of Wine Economists* 9 (2014), p. 3.
76 Meloni and Swinnen, 'The rise and fall of the world's largest wine exporter', p. 3.
77 This subsistence economy was fragile and collapsed under the demographic explosion that saw the population triple to six million in the period between 1871 and 1936. See Evans, *Algeria*, p. 35.
78 Evans, *Algeria*, p. 35.
79 Albert Camus, 'Misère de la Kabylie', in Camus, *Actuelles III. Chronique algérienne, 1939–1958* (Paris: Gallimard, 1958), p. 29.
80 Jean-Paul Sartre, *Colonialism and Neocolonialism*, trans. Azzedine Haddour, Steve Brewer and Terry McWilliams (London and New York: Routledge, 2001), pp. 37–38.
81 W. B. Cohen, 'The legacy of empire: the Algerian connection', *Journal of Contemporary History* 15 (1980), p. 110.
82 Evans, *Algeria*, p. 35.
83 Prior to the First World War, roughly 8.5 per cent of the Algerian population lived within these urban centres, but by 1954 this had swollen to 16.6 per cent. See Ruedy, *Modern Algeria*, p. 124.
84 Evans, *Algeria*, p. 36.
85 Horne, *A Savage War of Peace*, p. 40.
86 Fanon, as mentioned above, believed Algerians who trained in Western professions, especially medicine, found themselves marginalised or trapped in a point of suspicion between both their traditional communities and the settlers.
87 Lizabeth Zack, 'Early origins of Islamic activism in Algeria: the case of Khaled in post-World War I Algiers', *Journal of North African Studies* 11 (2006), p. 209.
88 Ruedy, *Modern Algeria*, p. 108.
89 Ruedy, *Modern Algeria*, p. 108.
90 Ruedy, *Modern Algeria*, p. 133.
91 Weil, 'Le Statut des Musulmans en Algérie coloniale', p. 107.
92 Evans, *Algeria*, p. 56.
93 Evans, *Algeria*, p. 56.
94 Klose, *Human Rights in the Shadow of Colonial Violence*, p. 81. See also Henri Grimal, *Decolonisation: The British, French, Dutch and Belgian Empires* (London and Henley: Routledge & Kegan Paul, 1978), p. 74.
95 Grimal, *Decolonisation*, p. 74.
96 Klose, *Human Rights in the Shadow of Colonial Violence*, p. 81.

97 In particular, the nationalists were struck by the principle within the Atlantic Charter which extolled self-determination for all peoples. See Klose, *Human Rights in the Shadow of Colonial Violence*, pp. 11–17; Francis Koerner, 'Le Mouvement nationaliste algérien (Nov. 1942–mai 1945)', *Revue d'histoire de la Deuxième Guerre mondiale* 93 (1974), p. 55.
98 Ruedy, *Modern Algeria*, pp. 146–147.
99 Grimal, *Decolonisation*, p. 118. See also Bernard Droz and Evelyne Lever, *Histoire de la guerre d'Algérie 1954–1962* (Paris: Editions du Seuil, 1991), p. 31.
100 Klose, *Human Rights in the Shadow of Colonial Violence*, p. 82.
101 Bénédicte Fortier, 'L'Indigène algérien. Du sujet au citoyen (1944–1947)', *Le Genre humain* 32 (1997), p. 56.
102 Johnson, *The Battle for Algeria*, p. 32.
103 Klose, *Human Rights in the Shadow of Colonial Violence,* p. 52.
104 Michael Crowder, 'The Second World War: prelude to decolonisation in Africa', in Michael Crowder (ed.), *The Cambridge History of Africa Volume 8: From c. 1940 to c. 1975* (Cambridge: Cambridge University Press, 1984), p. 46.
105 Droz and Lever, *Histoire de la guerre d'Algérie 1954–1962*, p. 31.
106 Anthony Clayton, *The Wars of French Decolonization* (London and New York: Longman, 1994), p. 30.
107 Droz and Lever, *Histoire de la guerre d'Algérie 1954–1962*, p. 32.
108 Droz and Lever, *Histoire de la guerre d'Algérie 1954–1962*, p. 32.
109 Klose, *Human Rights in the Shadow of Colonial Violence*, p. 84.
110 Grimal, *Decolonisation*, p. 293.
111 Jennifer Johnson Onyedum, '"Humanize the conflict": Algerian health care organizations and propaganda campaigns, 1954–62', *Journal of Middle East Studies* 44 (2012), p. 713.
112 Johnson, *The Battle for Algeria*, p. 4.
113 Johnson, *The Battle for Algeria*, pp. 2–5.
114 TNA FCO 141/5667/17/1. Letter of complaint from Mau Mau detainees addressed to Governor Baring, 17 November 1954.
115 Although these communities had contact with auxiliary medical practitioners, as Clark demonstrates, the general belief among the French at the start of the Emergency was that these inhabitants had never encountered European medicine, the core of the French 'civilising mission'. How then could they reject it? See Hannah-Louise Clark, 'Doctoring the *Bled*: Medical Auxiliaries and the Administration of Rural Life in Colonial Algeria, 1904–1954' (Unpublished dissertation, Princeton University, 2014), p. 11.

116 Jacques Frémeaux, 'Les SAS (sections administratives spécialisées)', *Guerres mondiales et conflits contemporains* 208 (2002), pp. 55–68.
117 Increasingly during the twentieth century the armed forces were required to supply healthcare and medical provisions to their soldiers, as Mark Harrison has shown. Yet the SAS's medical aid formed part of a broader propaganda campaign where offering healthcare to the indigenous populations was a weapon in the war against the rebels. For more on the connection between healthcare provisions and modern warfare, see Harrison, 'Medicine and the management of modern warfare'.
118 Quoted in Pierre Vidal-Naquet, *Torture: Cancer of Democracy*, trans. Barry Richard (Middlesex: Penguin Books, 1963), p. 45.
119 Martin S. Alexander, Martin Evans and J. F. V. Keiger, 'The "war without a name", the French Army and the Algerians: recovering experiences, images and testimonies', in Alexander, Evans and Keiger (eds), *The Algerian War and the French Army, 1954–62*, p. 9.
120 Ann Beck, *A History of the British Medical Administration of East Africa* (Cambridge, MA: Harvard University Press, 1970), p. 11.
121 Klose, *Human Rights in the Shadow of Colonial Violence*, p. 61.
122 Crozier, *Practising Colonial Medicine*, p. 5.
123 Beck, *A History of the British Medical Administration of East Africa*, p. 19.
124 Beck, *A History of the British Medical Administration of East Africa*, pp. 8–9.
125 Beck, *A History of the British Medical Administration of East Africa*, p. 14.
126 Crozier, *Practising Colonial Medicine*, pp. 2–3.
127 Crozier, *Practising Colonial Medicine*, p. 3.
128 Crozier, *Practising Colonial Medicine*, p. 9.
129 Indeed, even in 1958 the problem was debated in the House of Commons, where the systemic shortage of doctors in the colonies was causing considerable concern. See Hansard. House of Commons Debate, 'Doctors', Mr Blenkinsop MP, 17 June 1958, paragraphs 887–888.
130 Michael Worboys, 'Colonial medicine', in Roger Cooter and John V. Pickstone (eds), *Companion to Medicine in the Twentieth Century* (London: Routledge, 2003), p. 67; see also Michael A. Osborne, 'Acclimatizing the world: a history of the paradigmatic colonial science', *Osiris* 15 (2000), pp. 135–151.
131 The diseases that caused the most trouble for the CMS in Kenya were malaria, plague (bubonic and pneumonic), smallpox and sleeping sickness, which all had recurring epidemics in the years between 1900

and the start of the First World War. During this period, the colonial government spent a considerable amount of time experimenting with various measures to address the issue, but the impact was limited. See Beck, *A History of the British Medical Administration of East Africa*, pp. 24–25; Marc H. Dawson, 'Socioeconomic change and disease: smallpox in colonial Kenya, 1880–1920', in Steven Feierman (ed.), *The Social Basis of Health and Healing in Africa* (Berkeley and Oxford: University of California Press, 1992), pp. 90–91.

132 John Carman, *A Medical History of the Colony and Protectorate of Kenya: A Personal Memoir* (London: Rex Collings, 1976), p. 5.

133 Carman, *A Medical History of the Colony and Protectorate of Kenya*, pp. 5–6.

134 There was also a large Indian community in Kenya who played an important role in the early years of the colony, especially in relation to the construction of the railway line. Some of them even served as CMS doctors in the first years of the twentieth century. Interestingly, I have not encountered the names of any Indian doctors in the detention camps used by the British to hold those arrested during the Emergency. This is likely because, by the 1920s, there was a general effort within the CMS to limit the number of Indian doctors. See Anna Greenwood and Harshad Topiwala, 'The maintenance of hegemony: the short history of Indian doctors in the Colonial Medical Services, British East Africa', in Greenwood (ed.), *Beyond the State*, pp. 64–84.

135 Greenwood, 'Introduction', p. 2.

136 There was a missionary presence in Algeria during the period of French colonialism, especially during the second half of the nineteenth century. Different orders of missionary societies saw it as their responsibility not only to convert the North African Muslims to Christianity, in order to fend off the perceived rise of Islam in Africa, but also to fight the rise of secularism in France. Despite the important role Catholic missionaries played in Algeria, there is currently less evidence that medical missionaries had the same type of impact on the political situation in the colony as their East African counterparts in Kenya, which is why they have not received as much attention in the present work. For details on French missionary presence in the French empire, see Aldrich, *Greater France*, pp. 128–131.

137 Markku Hokkanen, 'The government medical service and British missions in colonial Malawi, *c.* 1911–1940: crucial collaboration, hidden conflicts', in Greenwood (ed.), *Beyond the State*, p. 40.

138 Hokkanen, 'The government medical service and British missions in colonial Malawi', pp. 55–57.

139 Michael Jennings, 'Healing bodies, salvation of souls': missionary medicine in colonial Tanganyika, 1870s–1939', *Journal of Religion in Africa* 38 (2008), p. 34.
140 Jennings, 'Healing bodies, salvation of souls', p. 28.
141 The Church Missionary Society is often abbreviated as CMS; however, in this book I will continue to refer to it in full so as to avoid confusion with the Colonial Medical Service.
142 Yolana Pringle, 'Crossing the divide: medical missionaries and government service in Uganda, 1897–1940', in Greenwood (ed.), *Beyond the State*, p. 19.
143 David Hardiman, 'Introduction', in David Hardiman (ed.), *Healing Bodies, Saving Souls: Medical Missions in Asia and Africa* (Amsterdam and New York: Clio, 2006), p. 5.
144 Jennings, 'Healing bodies, salvation of souls', p. 36.
145 Kenya National Archives (KNA) MSS/3/479/91. Quoted by Dr Frank Lake, 'An address delivered at the Conference of the Medical Advisory Board of the "Conference of British Missionary Societies"' reproduced in 'The Realignment of Medical Missions To-Day to Meet New Demands' and circulated among the Kenyan Church Missionary Society medical staff in 1949.
146 Vaughan, *Curing Their Ills*, p. 58.
147 KNA MSS/3/479/91. Dr Frank Lake, 'An address delivered at the Conference of the Medical Advisory Board'.
148 KNA MSS/3/479/91. Dr Frank Lake, 'An address delivered at the Conference of the Medical Advisory Board'.
149 Vaughan, *Curing Their Ills*, pp. 58–59.
150 Missionaries also played a role in the colonisation of Algeria, but as noted above, it was military medicine which had the most influence over the colony for most of its formative years.
151 Charles M. Good, 'Pioneer medical missions in colonial Africa', *Social Science and Medicine 32* (1991), p.1.
152 Vaughan, *Curing Their Ills,* p. 56.
153 Vaughan, *Curing Their Ills*, p. 57.
154 Anderson, *Histories of the Hanged*, p. 18.
155 Elkins, *Britain's Gulag*, p. 20.
156 John W. Arthur, '"Female circumcision" among the Kikuyu', *British Medical Journal*, 24 October 1942, p. 498.
157 Arthur, '"Female circumcision"', p. 498.
158 Arthur, '"Female Circumcision"', p. 498.
159 Beck, *A History of the British Medical Administration of East Africa*, p. 93.

160 Beck, *A History of the British Medical Administration of East Africa*, pp. 93–94.

161 Authorised in 1925 by an amendment to the Native Authority Ordinance, Local Native Councils were established in the more progressive districts of Kenya by 1952. They served as a 'safety valve' for acceptable African political expression and action. By bringing together competing political segments of the community in each district, the colonial government sought to reduce potentially dangerous frictions and at the same time undermine the purpose of the African protest organisation. See Donald G. Schilling, 'Local Native Councils and the politics of education in Kenya, 1925–1939', *The International Journal of African Historical Studies* 9 (1976), p. 221.

162 Beck, *A History of the British Medical Administration of East Africa*, p. 94.

163 Beck, *A History of the British Medical Administration of East Africa*, p. 96.

164 Schilling, 'Local Native Councils and the politics of education in Kenya, 1925–1939', p. 236.

165 Hansard. House of Commons Debate, 'Colonial Policy in Relation to coloured races', 11 December 1929, paragraphs 581–616.

166 Anderson, *Histories of the Hanged*, pp. 19–21.

167 Jomo Kenyatta, *Facing Mount Kenya* (London: Secker & Warburg, 1974), pp. 130–154.

168 Anderson, *Histories of the Hanged*, p. 19.

169 Elkins, *Britain's Gulag*, p. 21.

170 Daniel Branch, *Defeating Mau Mau, Creating Kenya: Counterinsurgency, Civil War, and Decolonisation* (Cambridge: Cambridge University Press, 2009), p. 31.

171 Anderson, *Histories of the Hanged*, p. 21.

172 Anderson, *Histories of the Hanged*, p. 21.

173 John Lonsdale, 'Mau Maus of the mind: making Mau Mau and remaking Kenya', *The Journal of African History* 31 (1990), p. 402.

174 Ann Crozier, 'The Colonial Medical Officer and Colonial Identity: Kenya, Uganda and Tanzania Before World War Two' (Doctoral thesis, University College London, 2005), p. 148.

175 Beck, *A History of the British Medical Administration of East Africa*, p. 74.

176 C. J. D. Duder, 'The Soldier Settlement Scheme of 1919 in Kenya' (Doctoral thesis, University of Victoria, 1978), p. 200.

177 Duder, 'The Soldier Settlement Scheme of 1919 in Kenya', p. 200.

178 C. J. D. Duder, '"Men of the officer class"': the participants in the 1919 Soldier Settlement Scheme in Kenya', in *African Affairs* 92 (1993), p. 77.

179 Duder, 'The Soldier Settlement Scheme of 1919 in Kenya', p. 612.
180 Duder, 'The Soldier Settlement Scheme of 1919 in Kenya', pp. 454–455.
181 Duder, 'The Soldier Settlement Scheme of 1919 in Kenya', p. 455.
182 Beck, *A History of the British Medical Administration of East Africa*, p. 74.
183 Beck, *A History of the British Medical Administration of East Africa*, p. 74.
184 Elkins, *Britain's Gulag*, p. 15.
185 Sisal is cultivated and naturalised in many countries. The fibres produced from its leaves are used to make rope, cord, twine and various other products. Elkins, *Britain's Gulag*, pp. 15–17.
186 Anderson, *Histories of the Hanged*, p. 81.
187 David Anderson, *Eroding the Commons: Politics of Ecology in Baringo, Kenya, 1895–1963* (Oxford: James Currey, 2002), pp. 126–135.
188 Hansard. House of Lords Debate, 'Kenya Land Commission', Lord Sanderson, 4 May 1932, paragraphs 307–308.
189 Anderson, *Histories of the Hanged*, p. 23.
190 O. F. Watkins, 'The Report of the Kenya Land Commission', *Journal of the Royal African Society* 33 (1933), p. 209.
191 United Kingdom Parliament, *Report of the Kenya Land Commission*, pp. 518–519.
192 Anderson, *Histories of the Hanged*, p. 23.
193 Anonymous, 'Mau Mau Shoot Africa's Churchill', *Daily Mail*, 8 October 1952.
194 Morton, *States of Emergency*, pp. 125–126.
195 Branch, *Defeating Mau Mau, Creating Kenya*, p. 49. See also Huw Bennett, 'The other side of the COIN: Minimum and exemplary force in British Army counterinsurgency in Kenya', *Small Wars and Insurgencies* 18 (2007), p. 648.
196 Carl Rosberg and John Nottingham, *The Myth of Mau Mau: Nationalism in Kenya* (London: Pall Mall Press, 1966), p. 277; Klose, *Human Rights in the Shadow of Colonial Violence*, p. 71.
197 Wiseman, 'Mau Mau', p. 65.
198 Wiseman, 'Mau Mau', p. 65.
199 Wiseman, 'Mau Mau', p. 65.
200 Wiseman, 'Mau Mau', p. 65.

2

Fragile hearts and vulnerable minds

For the British and French security forces, the conflicts in Kenya and Algeria represented struggles that were familiar while also being peculiar to the postwar world. On the one hand, 'guerrilla' wars, literally 'small wars', had long been waged between imperial authorities and various indigenous groups in their colonies.[1] Yet on the other, the paranoia produced by the start of the Cold War coloured the perception of these rebellions, making them appear distinctly *modern* in their eyes. As the guerrilla wars unfolded against the backdrop of this bipolar, geopolitical conflict, many officials in London and Paris detected communist interference, if not directly involved in the conflicts, then at least inspiring their manifestation. International Communism, they believed, would not be achieved through overt expansion, but by spreading dissent between nations, exploiting national and racial movements and backing them if necessary by the clandestine supply of arms and money.[2] For example, even as late as 1960, the British Colonial Office believed Jomo Kenyatta, whom they regarded as 'the architect' of Mau Mau, had learnt communist methods for promoting political agitation while visiting Russia in 1929–30 and again in 1933.[3] The French, on the other hand, believed Moscow was trying to build a 'solid communist core' by inspiring revolutions in North Africa and the Middle East with the hope of establishing pro-communist postcolonial states.[4] Yet it was the Chinese Revolution, led by Mao Tse-Tung, that had signalled the arrival of a new form of warfare that would, in the minds of British and French military theorists, come to define future wars.[5]

Mao's teachings highlighted the key objectives for waging a successful war of national liberation and could be used as a recipe for others. Chief among these objectives was the mobilisation of the masses. The very life of a successful guerrilla campaign rested on this support: '[the guerrilla] can neither exist nor flourish if it separates itself from [the masses'] sympathies and cooperation'.[6] Not only could this support provide food, shelter and other resources, it was also a source of new recruits, intelligence and shelter. Through popular support, so Mao's often quoted phrase goes, the guerrilla becomes 'a fish' that can swim in the water provided by the people. Where the conditions are right, these fish can thrive where their enemies drown.[7] This was the only means by which a revolutionary war could hope to engage in a prolonged guerrilla campaign against a technically advanced and seemingly overpowering enemy. Yet the question that vexed many counterinsurgency theorists was a simple one: how did Mao gain popular support from the masses? The answer they arrived at would become a defining feature of the Cold War as well as of counterinsurgency responses in the colonial wars: Mao, it was believed, had achieved mass indoctrination during the Chinese Revolution through mind-control programmes that 'brainwashed' the population into subservience.

Brainwashing is arguably the essence of cold warfare, even if it is a vague and, until recently, underexplored concept.[8] As Timothy Melley notes, the Cold War was 'a conflict of ideas and persuasion fought not on the battlefield but through propaganda, psychological warfare, and other ideological weapons'.[9] The fear of brainwashing had its origins in American anxieties over communist mind control during the 1940s. The term was brought to public attention by the American journalist Edward Hunter, who published a *Miami News* article on the subject in September 1950, roughly three months after the start of the Korean War.[10] A year later, Hunter, who was a propagandist fascinated by the Far East, published *Brain-Washing in Red China: The Calculated Destruction of Men's Minds*, which warned of a vast Maoist system of ideological indoctrination. The Chinese people had, Hunter claimed, been subjected to a coercive 'thought-reform', a process that used mind-numbing repetition to convert the entire population into conforming puppets. As he said, 'Unrevealed tens of thousands of men, women, and children had their brains washed'.[11] The notions raised by Hunter disturbed a broad audience, but panic became palpable in 1952, when a group of American Air Force PoWs publicly confessed to releasing various biological agents including anthrax, cholera, typhus and plague on North Korea. These confessions were then accompanied by further confessions from another 35 captured pilots, while 5,000 of 7,200 American PoWs signed confessions or petitioned the United States government to end the war. In addition, a further 21 PoWs refused repatriation.[12] The nature of these confessions seemed too fantastical; the communists had to be using some secret method to control the minds of these soldiers. President Eisenhower articulated the response to this threat when he stated, privately, that it was a 'basic truth' that 'the minds of all men are susceptible to outside influence'.[13] The United States, he told a San Francisco crowd in October 1952, was locked in a 'struggle for men's minds', and what was needed in order to combat this was a 'psychological effort put forth on a national scale'.[14]

Yet there is a distinction to be made here. In the early 1950s, when Hunter first published *Brain-Washing in Red China*, he drew a line between two terms that would become entwined later in the decade (something that is still the case today). He wrote that 'Brain-washing is indoctrination, a comparatively simple procedure, but brain-changing is immeasurably more sinister and complicated'.[15] 'Brain-changing', for Hunter, represented the wholesale transformation of an individual's beliefs and memories. In effect, it amounted to the creation of a completely new personality and became the type of Cold War fantasy that haunted America in the 1950s and 1960s, becoming a stock feature of popular culture across Western society. While the extent to which Britain and France shared in America's hysteria over the fear of communist 'brain-changing' is debatable, the two countries were nevertheless influenced by the ideas of mass indoctrination and psychological vulnerabilities associated with brainwashing. Mass indoctrination could be achieved, as Hunter showed, through a mix of processes that took advantage of physical suffering and psychological pressure, a blend of political torture through self-criticism meetings and propagandist theatre.[16] This was a process against which there was thought to be no defence; citizens from all walks of life and all levels of society could fall victim to this form of brainwashing. As such, Western military and security forces would have to pay greater attention to mass indoctrination and devise ways to combat and replicate these methods for their own purposes. However, they were not alone in their increased concern for the mind's perceived vulnerability and the manipulation of the masses' psychological states.

Vulnerable minds

The immediate postwar period experienced a significant increase in the ambitions of psychiatrists and social scientists on an international level for promoting global harmony. The European experience of fascism had left a scar on the minds of many. Never before had the ideals of democracy seemed more vulnerable and so tightly bound to ideas about collective mental health. Nazi Germany, it was believed, had shown that not only individuals but entire nations could become mentally ill. As such, future liberty, peace and international cooperation increasingly required the intervention of medical professionals and human scientists to help protect democracy from what Daniel Pick referred to as 'the renewed bouts of popular authoritarian "sickness"'.[17] As the Statement by the International Preparatory Commission of the International Congress on Mental Health, held in London in August 1948, made clear:

> [t]here can be no world community until individuals and groups have learned to live at peace with themselves and one another, and until they have ceased to struggle for their own sense of group solidarity at the expense of hostility and violence against others.[18]

The assumption underlying the discussions at the Congress, as well as informing many contemporary international and interdisciplinary research efforts, was that the mind and its associated beliefs, attitudes and ideals were not innate or fixed. The mindsets that led to the formation of violent nationalism could and indeed should be made to change. In order to effect this change, one needed to appreciate the ways in which attitudes and ideals were formed, the cultural values that informed them and an appropriate way to (re) educate individuals and groups.[19] Who better to engineer and direct this type of activity than those with expertise in the ways in which minds work? As John Rawlings Rees, the chairman and President of the World Federation for Mental Health, suggested, it was time for psychiatry and the scientists of the mind to apply 'our various skills in the mental health field to "sick groups", to communities and to national tensions, rather than limiting ourselves to the day-to-day developments of psychiatric and mental health work'.[20]

Against this backdrop, the rise of anticolonial nationalist sentiments in the colonies was regarded with suspicion and concern. Britain and France were keen to portray empire as a model of transnational solidarity and even a world government, which made anticolonial movements appear more than a little reminiscent of the violent European nationalism that had traumatised the world.[21] This anxiety was most clearly expressed by the political theorist Martin Wight, who warned of the dangers of letting 'the tyranny of some little African Hitler' take advantage of the Africans' desire for independence.[22] The minds of Africans, as well as other non-white races, were thought to be inherently vulnerable to manipulation. Unlike the European mind, which was rational and intelligent, and had a keen sense of justice, decency and civilisation, the black African was irrational, unintelligent, indecent and primitive.[23] Similarly, the Muslim population of North Africa was seen as being temperamental, apathetic and lazy, fatalistic, superstitious and ultimately possessing criminal impulsivity – an image captured clearly by the knife-wielding Arab in Albert Camus's *The Stranger*.[24]

For much of the first half of the twentieth century, the differences between races were thought to be biological. These assumptions were supported through the views and findings of prominent eugenicists and anthropologists who saw the Africans' 'innate' limitations as crucial factors to be understood when supplying welfare, development, education, and related medico-legal resources to colonial subjects. For example, in the British context, during a speech given at the Annual Dinner of the Kenya Branch of the BMA in 1931, the then President of the organisation and one of Kenya's foremost mental experts and eugenicists, Dr H. L. Gordon, stated that:

> Native backwardness could never be made to disappear under the mere trappings of civilization. No prevention of disease, bonification, education or religion could enable them to gather grapes off thorns or figs off thistles.[25]

A few years later, Gordon's colleague, Dr F. W. Vint, found 'empirical evidence' demonstrating the physical difference between African and European brain sizes. This notorious study was carried out on Kikuyu bodies coming from the King George VI Hospital in

Nairobi. According to his findings, Vint concluded that 'the average weight of the brain of the Kenya native is 10.6 per cent or 152 gm less than the average weight given for the brain of the European'.[26] Meanwhile, French psychiatrists and anthropologists also represented the Algerian as inherently Other, though the Muslim was deemed to be more 'evolved' than the sub-Saharan African, a 'half way between the primitive and the developed Westerner'.[27]

Yet by the 1930s, a mix of psychiatrists, anthropologists and social scientists working in the colonies started to explain the differences between races largely in cultural terms. The affinity between these professions extended into the fabric of the colonial order and shows how medical and social scientists collaborated and shared knowledge and expertise in order to understand the indigenous populations.[28] Together, these scientists of the mind offered an analysis of social evolution and a scientific language for explaining a range of vexing behavioural traits amongst colonised people, from excessive docility to outright criminality and rebellion.[29] The chief concern here was for a scientific understanding of the collective psychology of indigenous populations, not individuals. This is the important point: the indigenous populations were always understood in collective terms, long before the psychiatrists present at the International Conference of Mental Health had met to discuss the psychology of European communities. And like their metropolitan counterparts, these scientists believed their knowledge and expertise should not be limited to the clinic. These professionals sought direct involvement in the administration of the colonies, especially when it came to dealing with rebellious groups.

An issue of considerable concern for colonial administrators, medical psychiatrists and social scientists alike, was the effects Western culture had on indigenous minds. The dominant view was that modernity and 'civilisation' exerted profound pressure on the vulnerable minds of the indigenous populations. An indigenous individual who went mad in a 'native' fashion was relatively harmless; it was just another example of their innate irrationality. An indigenous individual who underwent education and had been influenced by Western civilisation, however, was seen as posing a greater threat to the colonial administrators.[30] 'Madness' in these individuals, some believed, could manifest in violent ways that challenged the colonial order itself. This condition was referred to as 'acculturation' or 'detribalisation' and became the subject of numerous psychiatric, psychological and social scientific studies.[31] The question was, what was 'normal' for indigenous populations? Indigenous minds were thought to be dysfunctional even when healthy; as such, the 'normal' colonised mind was somehow pathological. This was brought about by the administrators' inability to differentiate the pathological behaviour of the genuinely sick from the unusual or 'un-European' nature of indigenous habits. As Megan Vaughan asks, '[w]as it "normal" for Africans to have visions, for Malays to suffer group hysteria, for colonized subjects more generally to be "paranoid"?'[32]

And then there was the subject of faith. For the colonial authorities, there was nothing more confounded than indigenous religion and superstitious expression. As was demonstrated in Chapter 1, Kikuyu religious practices were not only regarded with suspicion but were also pathologised as dangerous and unhealthy. Similarly, colonial perspectives on Algerian culture blamed Islam as being an essentially corrupting and degenerative religion that was both physiologically and psychologically pathological.[33] This prejudice was apparent from the earliest days of occupation. As early as the 1840s, influential individuals like Dr Emile-Louis Bertherand, a doctor in Algeria who became a medical-legal expert at Algiers courts, an editor of Algerian medical journals and founded the Société protectrice de l'enfance algérienne, was arguing that Islam was not only a lesser religion to Christianity but was a source of disease. Whereas his contemporaries regarded the climate as being a danger to health, Bertherand shifted the emphasis to Algerian society and used scientific ideas to justify what was essentially a racial hierarchy in Algeria built on the idea of Islam as debilitating. 'The Algerian question', he wrote, 'is above all one of hygiene and anthropology'. It was only secondarily one of 'inhospitable climes'.[34]

But if Islam and other non-Christian religions were regarded with suspicion under normal circumstances, the colonial authorities became practically frantic when religious exuberance was coupled with political activism. In both Kenya and Algeria, the colonial authorities could not accept nationalist groups who placed their ethnic and religious identities above the benefits of empire's civilising mission.[35] For British and French security forces, nationalists in all their colonies were criminalised as 'thugs', 'gangs', 'bandits' and 'terrorists'.[36] But in Kenya and Algeria, these terms coexisted with psychological explanations about the indigenous population's peculiar mindsets. Such groups were regarded as inherently unstable and suffering from a psychological condition that forced them to take refuge in their primitive cultures and religious heritages. Here the Cold War fear of mass indoctrination and brainwashing, an *esprit du temps*, met with the colonial psychiatrists' beliefs in indigenous mental vulnerabilities and religious enthusiasm. What it generated was a hybrid interpretation of Mau Mau and the FLN as psychologically criminal terrorists who had been manipulated and indoctrinated by sinister agents in similar ways to those inspired or supported by the communists. It also, as Marouf Hasian Jr notes, transformed them into the kind of political outcasts that Giorgio Agamben called *homo sacer*, a pariah who can be dehumanised or killed with impunity.[37]

The myth of Mau Mau

In November 1953, a secret report on Mau Mau activities was sent by the District Commissioner for Nakuru to the District Officer in the Londiani Forest Division in Kenya. The report was written with the aim of presenting a counter-argument to individuals 'of both races African and Europeans who continually criticise the effort of government agents to supress the evils of Mau Mau'. In it, the District Commissioner provided a metaphor for understanding the perceived situation facing Kenya's security forces:

> A doctor will not discharge a patient and send him to the convalescent ward, until he is convinced that he is cured. The Kikuyu Tribe is suffering from a terrible disease – it is undergoing a gradual treatment by expert doctors.[38]

The 'terrible disease' mentioned in the above quote refers to Mau Mau itself and perfectly sums up a view of the nationalist movement that has become known as the 'myth of Mau Mau'. In this fabricated version of events, the image of the rebels as a pathological Other formed the cornerstone for the colonial authority's response to the emergency.

The myth of Mau Mau goes like this: prior to the rise of nationalism in Kenya, the Kikuyu were viewed favourably. Europeans in Africa were fond of racial stereotypes, and those applied to the Kikuyu were almost completely positive. The tribe was noted for 'its devotion to education, its ability to work hard, and its intelligence'.[39] For the most part, the Kikuyu were celebrated for having taken to Christianity, accepted wages for their labour and for being entrepreneurial. In all cases, it seemed like the Kikuyu were racing towards civilisation and embracing its benefits.[40] Their transformation into the savage killers of the Mau Mau movement was thus seen as having something to do with this enthusiasm for progress. This was the quintessential example of 'acculturation' described above. The pressures of civilisation had profoundly influenced the collective psychology of the Kikuyu people and trapped them somewhere between their tribal past and a civilised future. Mau Mau, with its 'pagan' oaths and brutal violence, was the expression of the Kikuyu's flight from modernity. The infamous oath-taking ceremonies used to convert previously 'loyal' Kikuyu into barbarous killers were described as perversions of traditional Kikuyu oath-taking practices, an unholy blend of ancient and modern elements.[41] Once administered, the oath would exploit this mental weakness and effectively brainwash the tribesperson into following the instructions of devious troublemakers, such as Jomo Kenyatta, who had always rejected civilisation. This image of Mau Mau quickly came to dominate the official government analysis of Kenya's troubles. There were no grievances or justifiable claims to be aired; the Kikuyu had been infected with what the prominent white settler, Michael Blundell, summed up as 'a mind-destroying disease'.[42]

This interpretation of African politico-religious groups as mentally unstable had a longer history predating the rise of Mau Mau. As Sloan Mahone has convincingly demonstrated, the colonial administration in Kenya had encountered several prophetic movements during the first half of the twentieth century that were seen as inspiring 'epidemic hysteria' among the African populations and were frequently documented by Kenyan officials and anthropologists. African psychological disturbances were seen as contagious and capable of assuming epidemic proportions. The most notorious Kenyan prophet was Dini ya Msambwa, a popular religious movement of the 1940s, which sought primarily to protect or reclaim lands that were being encroached upon by white settlers. Inspired by 'the mad prophet' Elijah Masinde, they became one of the largest movements of this kind in East Africa, causing much concern for the Kenyan government.[43] Doctors and administrators classed the prophesies and desires of movements like Dini ya Msambwa as being fantastic, an echo of African 'magical' modes of thinking. Such millenarian groups demonstrated, to colonial medical and administrative staff alike, that African populations were subject to periodic spats of mass madness or psychic epidemics just as they were vulnerable to tropical diseases that afflicted the body.[44] When it came to initial reports of Mau Mau's manifestation in Kenya, the colonial government naturally resorted to the time-tested interpretation that it was just another example of African religio-political thinking.[45]

Yet the chief exponent of Mau Mau's cultic roots was the paleoanthropologist and self-appointed Kikuyu expert, Dr Lewis S. B. Leakey. Raised by missionary parents, Leakey had grown up among the Kikuyu and boasted that he was even fluent in their language. Colonial officials were so convinced by his self-proclaimed knowledge of the Kikuyu that they permitted him to attend a private meeting at the Colonial Office in London to discuss the troubles brewing in Kenya on 15 September 1952. In the course of the Emergency, Leakey published two influential books, several magazines and news articles and delivered numerous public speeches in Britain and Kenya. His interpretation dominated the terms of serious intellectual discourse about Mau Mau until the late 1960s and, according to Bruce J. Berman and John M. Lonsdale, is still accepted by some anthropologists.[46] It is through his work that the idea of Mau Mau as an evil cult would receive wide circulation; Leakey's trajectory also demonstrates how selected anthropological knowledge could be useful for the colonial authorities who cherry-picked ideas and theories that supported their existing prejudices.

In his 1952 book, *Mau Mau and the Kikuyu*, speedily written and published a month after the state of emergency had been declared in Kenya, Leakey explains to an all-white readership how Kikuyu's customs '[broke] down under the impact of European civilization'.[47] Although he evoked the idea of acculturation as causing 'mental unrest and instability' among the Kikuyu, which made them vulnerable to manipulation by 'an unscrupulous few',[48] he did not initially subscribe to the belief that Mau Mau was an atavistic return to a savage psychological state.[49] However, if Leakey's earlier work was milder in its appraisal of the Kikuyu, these views would prove short-lived. In November 1954, Leakey published *Defeating Mau Mau*, which described the rebellion as nothing short of an anti-Christian and perverse religion. Admitting that the movement was '*to some extent synonymous with* [earlier Kikuyu] *political organisations*', Leaky now saw the truth: Mau Mau '*was in fact a religion and that it owed its successes to this fact more than to anything else at all*' (emphasis in the original text). The arrival of European culture, and thus Christianity, had persuaded many Kikuyu to turn away from their traditional beliefs. This was only a superficial conversion, though; a spiritual void remained to be exploited by the leaders of Mau Mau. By making the movement a religion, its manipulative creators could gain the support of thousands of adherents: it was Mau Mau as a religion and not a political group that 'turned thousands of peace-loving Kikuyu into murderous fanatics'.[50]

Leakey's work was taken seriously by the colonial authorities, who not only circulated copies of his work to police and security personnel, but also relied on his expertise for devising a policy to deal with the crisis in Kenya. In 1953, the newly appointed Governor, Evelyn Baring, set up a working group to report on the sociological causes underlying the Mau Mau movement. On this committee was Leakey himself, Thomas Askwith, a liberal officer who had been Municipal African Affairs Officer in Nairobi, and Sidney Fazen, secretary of the Kenya Land Commission. This special committee would create the 'Rehabilitation' programme. This programme targeted the Kikuyu population at large, while the military, security and police forces suppressed the guerrillas fighting in the forests. For all intents and purposes, this was the government's social counter-revolution.[51] The aim was to combat Mau Mau indoctrination and return the Kikuyu to being progressive citizens of the modern world.

The basis of discussion for this committee was a report submitted by Askwith on 27 August 1953 upon returning from Malaya, where he investigated the 'methods adopted in connection with the detention and rehabilitation under the Emergency Regulations' in that economically important colony.[52] Since 1948, the British had been engaged in a guerrilla war against the Malayan National Liberation Army (MNLA). Here the British were quicker than the French at adapting to their opponent's Maoist guerrilla tactics.[53] The key to this success was the strategy of isolating the rebels from the civilian population. This, according to Lieutenant-General Sir Harold Briggs, who was responsible for devising this plan, cut the rebels off from their vital support networks among the people by resettling substantial portions of the population in what were referred to as Resettlement Areas, while rebels and suspected rebels were detained without trial in smaller detention centres. Consequently, 500,000 Chinese were resettled into 500 heavily controlled camps called 'new villages'.[54] The method of resettlement, known as the Briggs Plan, was deemed so successful that it became the method of choice in Kenya during the Mau Mau emergency. In fact, the British used forced resettlement in Malaya and Kenya to a far greater extent than did the French in Algeria or the Portuguese in Angola and Mozambique. According to David French, the British moved about half of the Chinese population in Malaya and roughly 70 per cent of the Kikuyu, Embu and Meru in Kenya.[55]

In Malaya, the Briggs Plan was continued and expanded under General Walter Robert Templer, who became the High Commissioner of the colony in February 1952, after his predecessor, Sir Henry Gurney, was assassinated. It was he who provided Askwith with briefings on attempts to secure a lasting peace through re-education and the resettlement of the insurgents and their supporters. Askwith was particularly taken by Templer's insistence that 'the hearts and minds of the people must be won'.[56] The phrase 'winning the hearts and minds' of the people, which has often been falsely attributed to Templer and his use of a well-aimed propaganda campaign in Malaya,[57] has come to mean a campaign that balances military force with larger policies aimed at economic and political development. Its focus is on addressing the causes of unrest.[58] By securing the trust of the people, according to this logic, the 'sea' in which Mao's 'fish' swam would be reduced to little more than a puddle, allowing the military to take care of the remaining armed rebels. Askwith, upon returning to Kenya, was keen to stress that the failure to address wider political, economic or social problems in the colony might lead to the work of rehabilitation being 'undone and a wave of communist sympathy [would recur]'.[59]

As such, Askwith did not regard the Malayan detention camps as locations for punishment. Instead, they were sites where the Chinese and Malays could be 'befriended' by the Government officers and shown the benefits of Western civilisation. The hope was that 'the Communist-infected detainees and other detainees of varying degrees of discontent' would see the errors of their ways and 'take their place [...] in the life of the community'. Rehabilitation was seen to be so important that the Malayan government created a temporary Detention Camps Department under the Ministry of Defence and separate from the Prisons Department. This, Askwith explained, was because detainees were not prisoners and to treat them as such would 'detract from the value of the rehabilitation process itself'.[60] But not all detainees could be rehabilitated. Police Interrogation Units were used to screen and classify detainees as 'black' or 'grey', depending on their level of communist indoctrination. 'Blacks' represented the hard-core communists. Deportation was the only option for these irredeemable individuals. 'Greys' could be 'saved' despite having some communist sympathies, but they would require the correct treatment by advancing through a series of rehabilitation stages aimed at providing greater re-education and voluntary or paid employment.

Templer's approach to the Malayan Emergency is commonly regarded as setting the standard for a less coercive form of counter-insurgency that could be replicated elsewhere, as it was in Kenya. However, this is also a myth with as much substance as that of Mau Mau being a mental infection. The British approach in Malaya and eventually Kenya involved high levels of force and both physical and psychological coercion. In fact, it seems the 'success' in Malaya depended on an effective propaganda campaign that took place in an environment where a range of illegal transgressions and human rights abuses were permissible. In addition to Templer's 'hearts and minds' campaign, the British security forces in Malaya also relied on mass arrests; the death penalty for carrying arms; detention without trial for up to two years (which between 1948 and 1957 led to a total of 34,000 people being held without trial for more than twenty-eight days); deportations; movement restrictions; control of foods and shops; censorship; collective punishment in the form of fines and curfews; arson against the homes of communist sympathisers; treating prisoners as criminals and hanging hundreds of them; and the forced resettlements mentioned above.[61] When Templer took control in 1952, these methods of control and intimidation had already defeated much of the rebel forces.

By the time Askwith made his journey to study Templer's 'hearts and minds' campaign, Kenya had already witnessed mass arrests. Some 1,400 persons had been detained under the Emergency Regulations, along with 9,000 convicts imprisoned for Mau Mau offences and 'the many ex-squatters, and person returned to the reserves as a result of screening, together with the waverers normally domiciled in the reserves'.[62] Settler opinion had been hardened by the brutal killings of several families in the White Highlands and the horror of the Lari Massacre which could only be answered with greater violence. In fact, many conservative observers believed total war with the Kikuyu was the only solution. Under pressure, the governor, mirroring the Malaya example, issued Emergency regulations that transformed Nairobi into a totalitarian space with full control of the Kikuyu's existence.[63] Emergency assizes were established to enforce the new penal code. The tally of executions reached 1,200 by June 1953, with hundreds more awaiting the gallows. Many thousands more were found guilty of lesser Mau Mau offences and consigned to imprisonment for terms that ranged from several months to a lifetime. Yet the sheer number of suspects meant that the Emergency justice system was unable to deal adequately with the crisis. Baring was forced to issue mass detention orders under the Emergency Powers Regulations 1953. Fearing international criticism for detaining so many Africans without trial, the Conservative government in London stressed the word 'rehabilitation' in the hope that it would convey a greater sense of humanitarian concern. Askwith's report and the subsequent work of his colleagues on the special committee was thus the government's liberal veneer providing a reformist face to otherwise extremely coercive measures taking place in Kenya.

Askwith was in a position to learn from many of the precedents set by the Malayan Emergency as well as British experience in 'readapting' communists on the Greek island of Makronnissos.[64] Yet there were two features of the Kenya Emergency that made it distinct from other colonial emergencies: Mau Mau were not in fact communist, and their oath-taking practices were uniquely African in nature. For the rehabilitation process to succeed in Kenya, something had to be done about the oaths.[65] It was at this point that Dr Leakey came to the front line. His recommendations, discussed explicitly in *Defeating Mau Mau*, bring to mind the statement made by the British

Home Secretary Charles Clarke, on 2 October 2005, when he recommended 'treating' Islamic terrorists, whom he likened to members of 'religious cults', with 'anti-brainwashing techniques' to 'deprogramme' their fanaticism.[66] Whereas Clarke wished to have modern terrorists 'deprogrammed', Leakey advocated a programme to 'de-oath' Mau Mau initiates for the same purpose: to correct their thinking. Those who had taken the lower-level oaths – there were thought to be six or seven levels in total – could be 'rehabilitated' by a 'full and free confession followed either by a traditional cleansing ceremony, or by a genuine return to Christianity'. For the hard-core Mau Mau, however, those who had taken the 'more advanced and bestial and foul oaths', he was more doubtful. These individuals may be beyond salvation and would need to be segregated 'for the rest of their lives, so that the evil they have done and the knowledge of it eventually dies with them'.[67] Leakey's recommendations were first put into action in the Bahati and Sabukia Resistance Movement Centres, which were run by local farmers. Here government 'witch doctors' or Kikuyu traditional cleansers would aid in the confession and cleansing ceremonies. Upon touring Bahati, Askwith was to say that the process was 'psychologically sound, and moreover, successful'.[68]

Confession and cleansing would quickly become the precondition for detainees to move through 'the pipeline', a series of detention, transit and work camps created for the purposes of cleansing Mau Mau from the minds of the Kikuyu. In order to be effective, so official policy stated, confession had to be voluntarily given and publicly if necessary where 'the population is more obdurate'.[69] The standard view was that confession was 'a great relief to those concerned, and renders them receptive to an attractive allegiance' to the government. Despite Askwith's liberal aims, detention officers and warders would use the need to obtain confessions from Mau Mau suspects as an excuse to commit extensive violence. What was initially meant to be a therapeutic act quickly became an opportunity for torture and other abuses designed to coerce detainees into subordination. The British authorities in Kenya had used the supposedly scientific insights of an anthropologist to legitimise what was becoming a standard treatment for insurgent forces in various colonial settings: coercive force used to aid in political (re)indoctrination. As such, the conditions in the pipeline quickly came to resemble those experienced by the US PoWs in the detention and re-education camps of Korea or, as will be discussed in the next section, French PoWs in Indochina.

While the Governor's Reconstruction Committee, established in November 1953 to ensure the proper direction and coordination of all matters affecting the reconstruction of Kenyan society, officially endorsed the rehabilitation plan at the end of January 1954, Askwith wanted more.[70] He sought the approval of an acknowledged expert on Kikuyu psychology, Dr John Colin Carothers, an ethnopsychiatrist and former head of the Mathari Mental hospital, Nairobi. Carothers was recognised as the founder of the 'East African school' of psychiatry and the most important authority on the 'African mind'. In 1953, he produced *The African Mind in Health and Disease* for the World Health Organization (WHO), which drew similarities between African patients at the Mathari hospital and leucotomised Europeans.[71] He concluded that African inferiority was the result of their having underdeveloped frontal lobes.[72] The hope was that he could extend his special knowledge of the African mind to help the government win and maintain the support of loyal Kikuyu, Embu and Meru.[73] If Leakey offered the scientific legitimacy for the Kikuyu's need to confess their crimes and Mau Mau allegiances, it was Carothers who established the myth of Mau Mau as justification for the liberal ideal of rehabilitation and the continued need for British stewardship of Kenya.

The Psychology of Mau Mau was the only study of its kind commissioned by a colonial government to be written by a psychiatrist. It therefore represented a landmark in the history of ethnopsychiatry.[74] The twenty-eight-page document sought to explain the psychology of the African, the effects of acculturation that 'shocked' the Africans out of their habitual gradual approach to cultural transition and the rise of Mau Mau. It also offered recommendations for treating the problem over the long term. With this document, psychiatry had certainly escaped the confines of the clinic. Conceding that no biological difference between Africans and Europeans existed, Carothers stressed that important distinctions were still evident. Culture was the determining factor and, despite European presence in Africa, the belief in magic and the supernatural persisted. Christianity, the cultural underpinnings that influenced the development of European thinking, allowed what he described as an individual's ability to

> build a balanced understanding of oneself and the world; an understanding which is not afraid to see the weakness in oneself, for one can also see the strength; an understanding which enables one to view events as governed by forces which are indifferent to oneself and not by 'wills' that love or hate one; an understanding which need not be grossly undermined by living among alien people.[75]

In contrast, the Africans' animism meant that 'misfortunes are seldom seen as one's own fault. They are seen as the work of evil "wills" and since the power of these wills is now largely replaced by the power of the European, the latter is apt to be regarded nowadays as the sole author of all evil'.[76] The Kikuyu's political grievances were therefore not legitimate but part of the African's inability to practise the type of self-reflection produced by a mind raised in a Christian culture.

Carothers compounded this view of the irrational African psyche by likening the Mau Mau oaths to Early Modern European witchcraft. What the Kikuyu and past practitioners of witchcraft had in common was a 'desire to achieve some personal aim which they could not achieve within the "righteous" social framework of their time'. Instead, these people made bargains with the Devil in order to gain their wishes. Carothers was not shy in identifying Jomo Kenyatta as the Mephistophelean figure in this context: 'if one substitutes pagan culture and Christianity for the Catholic faith, and Jomo Kenyatta for the Devil, the two are often virtually identical'.[77] Continuing to tap into contemporary anxieties over mind control as well as subjects of scientific research, Carothers speculated that the Fourth Mau Mau oath contained 'the essential ingredients for hypnosis'. Through monotonous repetition of the ceremonies delivered by a prestigious administrator who commands absolute attention, multiple attendees could fall victim to this altered state of consciousness. This was because 'groups are hypnotized more easily than individuals'. It was therefore 'most likely that hypnosis plays a part in these assembles, and that the suggestions and commands imparted there may govern the subject's thinking and behaviour afterwards in varying degrees, as happens in hypnosis'.[78]

Education, or a lack of it, was a principal concern for Carothers. Western education had largely been delivered through religious institutions provided by missionary societies, but as Carothers continued to state, 'only about half of all Kikuyu boys complete 4 years of schooling and only a tenth complete 8 years even in recent years'. The figure for girls was even smaller.[79] Consequently, the majority of African children were educated at home, where they were taught the magical and animistic principles and supernatural-based morality by their mothers. It was within the home context that the psychological conflicts caused by the clash between Western civilisation and traditional African culture came to a head. A man who had received some education and Christian teaching would find himself in 'a world in which the beliefs he learned in childhood had become inapplicable and ineffective'. Yet 'internal conflict' was 'perpetually aggravated by the presence of the women' who, due to not receiving proper education, tempted him back to the 'old ways', like some latter-day Eve.[80]

The fact that Carothers paid considerable attention to the role of women is significant. Prior to the rebellion's outbreak, African women were thought to be passive, peaceful and uninterested in politics. But Kikuyu women played a fundamental role in administering Mau Mau oaths. They also took an active part in combat, while women in the civilian 'passive wing' served as 'couriers, scouts and spies who provided food, ammunition and information to the guerrilla forest fighters'.[81] By 1953, Askwith had to conclude that women played a pivotal role in 'keeping Mau Mau alive'.[82] The British administration's surprise at these militant women may explain why Carothers emphasised their role in his report. In fact, he believed their lack of education combined with the patriarchal nature of Kikuyu society provided a psychological explanation for their enthusiasm. Accepting Mau Mau would not only bring them closer to 'their men', it would also give them 'unprecedented power', power that would only grow in the promised land free of Europeans.[83]

When it came to recommending possible solutions for these problems, Carothers suggested the establishment of a series of educational programmes aimed at teaching home hygiene as well as moral instruction to install notions of truthfulness and accountability among the young. Above all, the Kikuyu had to learn that the right to political power could only be obtained by being responsible. Carothers also endorsed the development of a Malayan-style resettlement scheme to create new villages where the Kikuyu families could come together. The stability of the family was key. Crime and mental instability in Europe and America, he asserted, were most rife in areas with 'floating populations and where parental influence is weakened and unsettled'. To be civilised, the African would need to have the opportunity to develop a family lifestyle conducive to those aims. Yet most importantly for our purposes, Carothers poured explicit praise on Askwith's rehabilitation programme. After visiting a number of Resistance Movement Centres, Transit and Detention camps, Carothers felt Askwith had shown 'masterly psychological insight' and continued to 'endorse unhesitatingly all the observations and recommendations it contains'.[84]

Together, Leakey and Carothers provided settlers and colonial administrators with the scientific arguments they needed to justify their treatment of the Kikuyu and the purging of the enemy's mind-set. Although it is tempting to see the use of the expertise provided by Leakey and Carothers as evidence of the partnership between state ideals and ambitious scientists, the case is not that simple. British psychiatrists and human scientists such as anthropologists did develop deeper relationships with government officials during this period, but that is not to say that tensions did not exist and that everyone agreed with their interpretations.[85]

In 1954, the *East African Medical Journal* published an article by Dr John Wilkinson of the Church of Scotland Mission Hospital in Tumutumu, Kenya. According to this physician, far from being an insane cult, Mau Mau was 'primarily a political movement', and a 'virtually [...] totalitarian system' with a 'well-organised and disciplined army' that used terror to force conformity from other Kikuyu.[86] In the same year, the anthropologist Max Gluckman argued in the *Manchester Guardian* that Mau Mau was caused by labour exploitation, land alienation and the proscription of African unions and political parties by the British.[87] But one of more cutting critics was Peter Worsley, a contemporary anthropologist, who challenged both Leakey's and Carothers's pathological arguments. Worsley argued that they not only perpetuated a myth of white settlers as misunderstood paternalistic liberal conservatives, but also the image of Mau Mau as a vicious cult.[88] Instead, Worsley stressed that Mau Mau was a political response to the atrocious treatment Africans received in the colony. Worsley even went as far as questioning Leakey's qualifications: 'he can by no stretch of the imagination be called a trained anthropologist'. The fact that Leakey had served as an intelligence officer during the Emergency and had been an interpreter at Kenyatta's trial put his objectivity in question. For Worsley, '[Leakey's] general involvement and sociological ignorance oblige the reader to examine his conclusions very critically'.[89] On the subject of Carothers, Worsley was even more scathing, referring to his work as 'racist nonsense disguised as scientific "psychology"' which 'has already been exposed for what it is by both anthropologists and psychologists'.[90]

When it came to implementing the rehabilitation programme, the psychological recommendations put forward by Leakey and Carothers were applied by police, detention staff and colonial administrators. One reason for this could be that psychiatry, and any other form of psychological medicine as a discipline, was poorly represented in the colonial context of East Africa. It seems an ad hoc professionalism grew out of a small network of asylums in Kenya, Uganda, Tanganyika and Zanzibar which gave rise to an 'East African school' of psychiatry. But although it had a degree of intellectual autonomy and authority within the colonies, it was still a largely underrepresented discipline with few qualified staff.[91] As such, the pipeline detention centres were staffed by non-experts who replaced the scientific ideas in circulation with their own interpretations of the detainees' psychology. This would often be used to justify their use of violence.

The 'Algerian mind' and its violence

The French psychological community in Algeria was more involved in operations against the FLN than their British counterparts were in Kenya. Generally speaking, French colonial psychiatry enjoyed a more active role for its expertise among the colonial administrations and the military, especially in North Africa. This could be explained by the relationship between the psychiatric profession in the metropole and their colonial colleagues. The story of what became known as the Algiers School of French psychiatry, founded by Professor Antoine Porot, stands in stark contrast to the general pattern of colonial psychiatry. While psychiatric institutions in British colonies largely languished due to poor funding, with their staff feeling more like frustrated prison warders, psychiatry in North Africa was at the cutting edge of French medicine.[92] Between 1911 and 1954, psychiatrists in Algeria embarked on a programme of radical institutional reform. They codified ideas about the relationship between ethnicity and psychopathology while pushing the limits of experimental treatment. In many ways, their ambitions shifted the intellectual and institutional gravity of professional psychiatry from France to North Africa.[93] They were the brave new face of French medicine and provided the intellectual and professional milieu in which Frantz Fanon would practise his psychotherapy and develop his damning criticism in *The Wretched of the Earth*. Yet the most important point of distinction between the role of psychology in Kenya and Algeria is that, in the latter context, psychiatry was always closely bound up with the military. From the First World War, its practitioners articulated their mission in the language of battle and struggle against the North African indigenous population. As Richard Keller explains in *Colonial Madness*, 'the historical development of the Algiers School presents a crucial example of colonialism's discordant logic in practice, where a nuanced, detailed, responsive, and even progressive scientific circle with utopian ambitions was simultaneously an uncomprehending, violent entity driven by militant racism'.[94]

By the 1950s, psychiatry and especially ethnopsychiatry were, as the military doctors Gallais and Plangues put it, undergoing a 'revolution'. No longer bound to simple 'armchair ethnographies', such as those of the French anthropologist Lucien Lévy-Bruhl's theory of primitive mentality, the brave new psychiatry could rely on modern techniques: psychological testing, psychoanalysis, narcoanalysis (the use of barbiturates to produce altered states of consciousness in psychotherapy), electroencephalograms and hormonal studies.[95] Ethnopsychiatry, according to Gallais and Plangues, as well as Porot and his student Dr Jean Stutter, should not be limited to the hospital but used for the political administration of the indigenous population.[96] The ultimate manifestation of this commitment to the military operations in Algeria would be in France's psychological warfare programme aimed at the Algerian rebels during the War of Independence.

The French had earlier come to appreciate the (imperative) value of psychology in the aftermath of their bitter defeat in Indochina. Here the Vietnamese Liberation organisation, under the leadership of Hồ Chí Minh and General Võ Nguyên Giáp, succeeded in mobilising mass support from the population and managed to end France's colonial rule in Southeast Asia with its victory at Diên Biên Phu in 1954. This victory, according to the French military theorists, was due to the communists' ability to control the population. For example, Colonel Charles Lacheroy, a French official engaged in the conflict and eventually the pioneer of revolutionary-war theory, believed that the Việt Minh's success lay in the creation of a totalistic environment. Here all aspects of the Việt Minh's social relations were rationally and systematically controlled by what he called 'parallel hierarchies' – overlapping networks of communist groups in various committees and associations.[97] These parallel hierarchies, Lacheroy explained, formed the physical means by which 'the Vietminh system [...] bends the masses to obedience, to work and to the war effort'. But this was only part of the first step in waging a 'total revolutionary war'. By controlling and monitoring the physical activities, the population would be open to 'psychological warfare' which controlled what they thought. As he said, 'when you hold a glass firmly, you put what you want in it'.[98]

Within this context, Lacheroy regarded the indigenous masses as docile and passive. This was a view shared by other French theorists: although the indigenous masses may have some desire for independence, according to such theorists, they also argued that this seemed to be less likely. As the French army official Roger Trinquier stated in his 1964 book on counterinsurgency, *Modern Warfare*, 'Such support may be spontaneous, although that is quite rare and probably a temporary condition'.[99] Instead, the indigenous population were seen to be generally amenable to manipulation, regardless of the ideological content, which made them the ideal targets of subversive propaganda and terrorism.[100] This passivity is similar to the image of the brainwashed Chinese subjected to Mao's thought-reform as described by Hunter; it may have also influenced Jean Lartéguy's portrayal of the Việt Minh in his novel *The Centurions*, where he described them as 'a hive of sexless insects [that] seemed to operate by remote control, as though somewhere in the depths of this enclosed world there was a monstrous queen, a kind of central brain which acted as the collective consciousness of the termites'.[101]

Although a work of fiction, Lartéguy's description, taps into the view that the conversion to communism necessarily destroyed an individual's autonomy and stripped away liberty. It also helped to popularise the idea that was widespread in Western society and felt keenly by the French military: international communism was a threat not only to French values but to Western civilisation itself. Faced with the prospect of this 'insect hive' spreading across the Third World, colonial rule came to be seen, in Maria Lazreg's words, as 'a bulwark against an immoral and shadowy adversary'.[102] A war against this 'subversion' was thus a legitimate and worthy cause, but also a mission to save France and Western Europe from destruction. Once the signs of revolution appeared in North Africa, the French authorities were quick to interpret it as part of the same phenomenon, the tide of communist subversion. As stated by the French military: 'This Algerian revolution, led by the pan-Arab movement, risks setting fire to Europe and America'.[103] Thus, to fend off such an existential threat, the military would need to use any means necessary. In order to fight an enemy who used psychological manipulation to force conformity from the vulnerable minds of the population, the French would need to use their own form of psychological action to overturn the revolutionaries' influence on the Algerian masses.

Yet Lartéguy's novel also captured another feature of the French experience in Indochina that was to have a lasting impression on the military's mindset and the methods they would ultimately use in Algeria – the experience of French PoWs in Indochina. As Marie-Catherine Villatoux notes, 'Any serious study of the psychological treatment of rebel prisoners in Algeria can hardly ignore the influence exerted by the Indochinese experience on a large section of the French officer corps of the 1950s and 1960s'.[104] Lartéguy's account of his fictional soldier's imprisonment in the Việt Minh's re-education camps illustrated the idea that enemy combatants or particularly recalcitrant groups, such as military officers, would need to undergo specific indoctrination methods that blended physical discomfort with psychological coercion. In Lartéguy's version of the Việt Minh's notorious Camp No. 1, 'the Voice', the communist functionary responsible for overseeing the conversion of the French soldiers to Communism, is described as 'behaving like a scientific chemist'. He 'regulated [the soldiers'] hunger, their fatigue and their despair so as to reduce them to the exact point to which, broken and deranged he could at last work on them and drill them against their past by concentrating on what still remained: the elementary reflexes of fear, fatigue and hunger'.[105] Lartéguy's description of these officers' experiences fits eerily well with the accounts of French officers incarcerated in Việt Minh prisons.

For example, in 1956 Captain Prestat of the Service historique de la Défense compiled some of these accounts and narratives into a report titled *L'Endoctrinement des prisonniers de guerre*. In this document, Prestat described the indoctrination methods used on French officers as attaining 'a sort of perfection in "moral techniques"'. These techniques could be broken down into five phases which, according to an unnamed officer,[106] consisted of 'brainwashing, obsession, compromise, creation of collective consciousness, and denouncement and hope'.[107] Under the section for 'brainwashing', the report described how prisoners had to be put into a receptive condition in order to 'listen sympathetically to the doctrines and the teachings of the [Communist] party'. This involved, for instance, maintaining a high mortality rate in the camps to frighten the remaining prisoners; separating them from news sources and reading material in order to give them a 'thirst for reading, to stir up [their] appetite' to read even communist propaganda; stripping all officers of their ranks and isolating them to stop them 'from having the slightest bit of influence'; and the 'writing and signing of a manifesto' by the prisoners (which many refused to sign). Although the report notes that '[t]here was no brutal punishment' in the camp, it continues to explain how the prisoners' conditions deteriorated 'almost scientifically' – a line that is extremely reminiscent of Lartéguy's above quote. And similar to that quote, the prisoners found their food rations increasingly restricted while their guards became more aggressive and abusive: 'They beat us with cudgels, they slapped us'. Any particularly recalcitrant prisoners were then subjected to isolation for a number of days, depending on the perceived infraction or the will of 'the higher authorities of the camp'. These techniques amounted to what Lacheroy called the 'flattening', a process that broke down an individual's resistance: 'when the prisoner has nothing to hang on to, he is ready' for indoctrination.[108]

This unique experience, generating deep trauma, led many officers returning from the camps to question the meaning of their commitment and the very nature of the conflict they had been confronted with.[109] But for some officers, the lesson learnt in Indochina would be valuable for combating the FLN in Algeria. The French military had to concede that the 'disintegration of personality by psychological aggression is today as dangerous a threat as the disintegration of matter by thermonuclear aggression'.[110] The indoctrination of prisoners in the colonial wars in Indochina and Algeria were thus part of the Cold War writ large. For example, on 7 February 1956, General Lorillot, Commander of the Tenth Military Region, sent a document to the Resident Minister in Algeria that explained how lessons taken from China, Indochina and Korea had shown that psychological warfare was particularly useful for dealing with prisoners of war. These techniques had been honed by the Office of Psychological Action of the Tenth Military Region and were used to formulate a plan for the 'detoxification of prisoners' who could be turned to aid the French in their propaganda efforts.[111]

Detention played a fundamental role in the military's counterinsurgency strategy. The avowed aim, as in Kenya, was to isolate the rebellious elements from the passive members of the population. Although the creation of detention camps was prohibited under the Emergency Law issued in Paris for Algeria on 3 April 1955, the first camps in Algeria were opened in May 1955 as part of the law's provisions for placing suspects under house arrest.[112] The military soon established a network of detention and internment centres that would become the sites of extreme violence and torture that seemed, in part at least, to be coterminous with efforts to brainwash or 'detoxify' the prisoners. Several camps were created: CTTs, concentration camps named *centres d'hébergement* (accommodation centres), military internment camps and the shadowy re-education centres.[113] It was especially within confines of the latter centres that the military focused attention on turning specific enemy combatants to the French cause. Nevertheless, the indoctrination of detainees was not limited to the re-education camps. In the end, the entire Muslim population were the target of France's psychological warfare programme. Faced with the seemingly insidious threat of the communist indoctrination tactics, the French responded by institutionalising their own psychological warfare programmes for offensive and defensive purposes.[114]

Responding to the communist psychological tactics in Indochina, the French established the Bureau de la guerre psychologique in

1953, but its actions remained relatively modest; it focused on the distribution of propaganda in the form of leaflets, newspaper broadcasts and loudspeaker messages.[115] It was in 1957 that the Cinquième Bureau (Fifth Bureau) came into being with the specific mission of combating the FLN's propaganda. For the Bureau, the struggle against the enemy was understood in psychological terms. As a previously classified report notes: 'Why do we say psychological warfare? Because war consists in imposing one's will on the adversary. Formerly it was imposed by material violence. Today it is possible by psychological violence'.[116]

This approach to warfare demanded 'scientific and technical intelligence' to inform the Bureau of 'the evolution of psycho-sociological knowledge' of their opponents.[117] As such, its tactics were separated into two forms. On the one hand, there was *action psychologique* (psychological action) aimed to 'train, develop, support morale and immunise personnel against psychological attacks'.[118] On the other hand, *guerre psychologique* (psychological warfare) targeted enemy combatants and the indigenous population, seeking to disrupt, modify and control their attitudes and behaviours.[119] Although propaganda was used in *guerre psychologique*, it was deployed to convert detainees and other Muslims to France's cause. They utilised censorship, loudspeaker announcements, graffiti, images and radio to convince the Algerians of the benefits of French civilisation and to take advantage of their mass psychology. Ultimately, the aim was, as the Bureau put it, 'to remotely control the spirits, from the outside'.[120]

In order to deliver a viable psychological warfare programme, the Bureau explored various academic traditions and compiled a bibliography of influential research into the human mind.[121] Yet the dominant theme running through this research was the psychology of groups or masses. The military's experience in Indochina and their encounter with the logic of brainwashing formed the context in which they sought to understand group and mass behaviours. In a general sense, military thinkers turned to the work of Gustave Le Bon and Serge Chakotin to guide their thinking. Le Bon was among a group of French thinkers who believed democracy ushered in the rule of the mob. His work influenced Freud's conception of group psychology but was also being taught in the Ecole supérieure de guerre before the Second World War.[122]

For counter-revolutionary thinkers, Le Bon's concepts reduced revolutions to a dynamic where psychologically vulnerable people in crisis situations were exploited by manipulative leaders.[123] The crowd alone, Le Bon claimed, is a-rational. In order to create action within the crowd, revolutionary leaders tap into perceived inequities and political grievances. This is what he referred to as the rational logic for a revolution, but it accounts for only one part of the process. The leaders have to overrule the mass's reason by awakening 'different forms of logic', which included 'affective logic, collective logic and mystic logic'.[124] Although all these logics played a role in creating and moving the masses, Le Bon saw mystic logic as being particularly troubling. The 'mystic temperament' attributed mysterious power to superior beings or forces and was thought to be 'at the bottom of all religious and most political beliefs'. 'Buddhism, Islamism, the Reformation, Jacobinism, Socialism [...] seem very different forms of thought', he argued, 'yet they have identical affective and mystic bases, and obey a logic that has no affinity with rational logic'. Properly manipulated, mystic logic constituted the might of the great popular movement. It was the means by which a non-violent person could be brought to arms or even motivated to die for the cause.[125]

Reading Le Bon's work makes it clear why members of the Cinquième Bureau became convinced that Islam sat at the heart of the Algerian problem. In their minds, communists had taken advantage of the efforts of some Islamic religious men who were exploiting the religious consciousness of the population in order to 'fight against the integration of Algeria with France'.[126] The masses were being mobilised through, if Le Bon was correct, their mystic logic. As such, an effective counter-revolutionary campaign would need to account for the psychology of the Muslim group. It was on this point that the Bureau turned to the Algiers School for their expertise.

Fortunately for the French military, the Algiers School had been producing published research on the subject of the Muslim masse for decades. While the Cinquième Bureau wanted to create 'mass man' for *guerre psychologique*, Porot had already produced a psychological account of the Muslims as, like Kenya's Africans, extremely suggestable multitudes.[127] In 1918, while describing conscripts, Porot avowed that the indigenous population, due to their religiously inspired docility, formed 'ignorant masses'.[128] As such, the military set about trying to gather as much data as possible on the psychology, sociology, ethnography, politics, customs and culture of the Muslim population; essentially it sought to codify their souls in order to pinpoint the best means for understanding, controlling and modifying their temperaments. The extent to which the military relied on this information is evidenced in a conference paper circulated by the Centre d'instruction à la pacification et à la contre-guérilla during the war, which provided a detailed overview of these features.[129] It shows how much the military relied on the work of Porot and his colleagues. The document is saturated in the psychological stereotypes of Muslims that had been common to the Algiers School since the early part of the twentieth century. Although it tries to distance itself from ideas that portray the indigenous population – referred to as French-Muslims – as inferior to Europeans, the document nevertheless describes them as instinctive, impulsive, lacking a developed faculty for reasoning, imagination and a critical mind, and as ultimately being credulous and superstitious.[130]

The French military were particularly keen to identify a psychological explanation for the FLN's use of violence, which they described as corresponding 'to a specific character of the Arab temperament'.[131] This was an old stereotype that saw North Africans as inherently violent and homicidal. In 1932, Antoine Porot and his student Don Côme Arrii attempted to explain what they believed to be a behaviour peculiar to the 'North African race', what they called the frequency of criminal impulsivity'.[132] The article, which was a revised version of Arrii's thesis, examined forty criminal cases heard in French-Algerian courts and concluded that the '*indigene*' – a category that made no distinction between Kabyles, Arabs and Moors – possessed a flawed mindset that predisposed them to violent impulses. Porot and Arrii believed the aetiology for this 'impulsivity' lay in two categories. The first, 'morbid pathology', included 'alcoholism and other intoxicants', 'delirious or demented states', '*crisis excito-motrices* [crisis of motor excitation]' and 'epilepsy', which accounted for half of the sample population. Yet the most significant group, in the authors' view, were the members of the second group. These individuals suffered from 'constitutional impulsivity' derived from 'the elements of personality related to race, morals, beliefs [and] instincts'.[133] Violent criminality in this group was generated through mental debility caused by the tropical environment, coupled with natural credulity and suggestibility, the tendencies to stubbornness and mental perseverance leading to poor judgement or logic. These Muslims experienced a 'weakness of social feeling in its altruistic forms', had a 'contempt for human life' and were jealously possessive.[134] This view of the criminally impulsive Muslim became so influential that Fanon even recalled speaking with his psychiatrist colleagues who stated: 'It's a hard pill to swallow, but it's been scientifically established'.[135]

Despite its popularity among French psychiatrists, the study presented a rational flaw that was consistent in Porot's reasoning: his research focused on individuals facing criminal charges, mainly for murder, and his task as a forensic psychiatrist was to determine degrees of criminal responsibility. Porot and his colleagues often extrapolated more general statements about the Muslim population from their limited data. There was also no attempt to use a control group for his studies.[136] Yet this research also demonstrates the ambitious aims of the Algiers School. For Porot and Arrii, psychiatry offered a means for shaping policy towards Algerians generally, but also those immigrating to mainland France. While conceding that the pathological cases in their study were not legally culpable for their actions, the cases under 'constitutional impulsivity' should be treated harshly. In the interest of the 'educational value of punishment', the authors argued, 'justice in such cases must take its course'. It was only 'through examples and sanctions that those unkind and instinctive beings will be taught that human life must be respected'. In their view, French North Africa required intense policing.[137]

The FLN's terrorism, like Mau Mau's, was regarded as indicative of a mental pathology brought about by a reversion to past savagery. In 1956, Dr F. Lagrot and Dr J. Greco published an article in *La Presse medicale* containing thirty photos of people who had been mutilated by FLN members. These individuals had had their noses, ears and lips cut off.[138] For many, this article showed the 'true face' of the terrorists and was eventually distributed worldwide to health organisations and medical associations.[139] Yet for the psychiatrists, these mutilations demonstrated something more general. According to doctors A. Fourrier, P. Michaux and J. Thiodet of the laboratory of Forensic Medicine at the University of Algiers, the mutilations committed by the terrorists were 'the serial and stereotyped reproduction of [...] criminal acts that have always been practised in this country'. These atrocious disfigurements were 'suggestive of the tenacity of a collective atavism', or '*paléophrénie réactionnelle*',[140] 'that could be thought to have vanished'.[141] Islam, they argued, was the source of this atavism. As they explained, to stand before Allah, Muslims had 'to appear intact in the Celestial Court', and therefore victims of mutilation would be forbidden to take part in posthumous experience.[142] The FLN's mutilations were thus seen as evidence of a reversion to this ancestral violence, an explanation that was not dissimilar to those used to account for Mau Mau's return to primal aggression. Yet when it came to the subject of mass insanity in the Algerian population, members of the Algiers School had a different explanation to their Kenyan counterparts.

As late as 1960, Porot and Dr Charles Bardenat believed that the Algerian nationalism stemmed from a pathological form of North African 'xenophobia'. This was because the FLN's violence was directed against 'subjects belonging to an occupying race and generally of a different religion'.[143] There were no political motivations for these attacks; they were just the acts of 'solitary [lunatics], deeply committed to the mystique of their religion which dictates to them a hostile behaviour towards the foreigner'.[144] But Porot and Bardenat were careful to state in a footnote that 'xenophobia' in this case 'is only a strictly individual behaviour or reaction to subjects of another race or religion and not a collective movement or uprising against occupants'. This seems difficult to reconcile with the situation taking place in Algeria in 1960, when the number of FLN supporters was reaching new heights. If terrorism was only the pathological xenophobia of the few, how did these scientists understand the sheer number of supporters who had taken part in the uprising?

Although Porot and Bardenat only briefly discuss the 'Algerian terrorists', they nevertheless provide a subtle explanation of the psychological mechanisms at play in leading the masses to support the FLN; an explanation that not only accounts for why so many Algerians joined together but may also provide a theoretical justification for the military's use of detention and segregation. The section on xenophobia is followed by a discussion of 'family and collective psychosis'. According to the authors, families or collections of people can suffer from 'deliriums' whereby the delusions of 'an isolated individual', usually delusions of persecution, are shared by one or more individuals.[145] Building on earlier ideas about contagious delusions, such as Professor J. Delay's use of the term 'personality in several persons', a condition where each participant contributes to a common delirium 'according to the extent of his means', these delirious groups acted like a cohesive cell. But Porot and Bardenat are careful to state that 'this applies mainly to family psychoses where the number of deliriants is quite limited'. In these cases, the 'cure' for the family's delusions is to break up the group and to separate the 'passive subjects' from the solitary lunatics responsible. Although they do not mention the political situation unfolding in Algeria at the time, the discussion acknowledges that 'collective psychoses' concerning the reaction of crowds or social masses 'are not without analogies with certain family psychoses'. The influence of individual xenophobic zealots among crowds, if this logic is extended, could thus operate in a similar way to those with persecution delusions within a family unit. Although the authors do not continue with this line of thought, if the relationship between family members is the microcosm of the masses, then it is conceivable that the 'cure' for mass psychosis would also rest in separating the agitators from the passive population. This would represent a very close affinity between the ideas of the Algiers School and the counter-revolutionary theorists.

Although it is not possible to assess the extent to which the military used this particular part of Porot's works for their own aims, there are nevertheless clear indications that they read his work. Moreover, there is evidence to suggest that Porot supported, at least to some extent, the military's use of mass detention in Algeria. A top-secret memorandum titled *Sur le problème de la mentalité des Musulmans* produced on 1 June 1959, shows that the Cinquième Bureau sought the expertise of 'Drs Porot and Sutter'[146] with the explicit aim of developing a psychological programme to speed up the 'recuperation of *fullagha* detainees'.[147] Their expertise, along with those of other experts on Islamic culture,[148] was sought for an 'objective study of the mentality of Muslims' to 'produce evidence for stereotypes' about 'the most profound element of Muslim culture'. Experiments were devised to gather information on Muslim self-perception, the effects of education and personal experience on cognitive development, the role of religion in shaping Muslim psychology, the archetypal content of their culture (in keeping with the military's interest in Jung's psychoanalysis) and whether it influenced their perception of the government's work in Algeria. The experiments even envisaged using 'projective tests' of the type designed by Dr Ombredane for the Congolese population.

It is currently unclear whether this research project delivered usable data for the military, but it at least shows that a range of civilian experts, especially psychiatrists, were actively involved in devising potential 'treatments' for 'rehabilitating' Algerian prisoners of war. However, it should be stated plainly that these research programmes do not implicate these scientists in any of the violent activities known to have taken place in the Algerian detention camps at this point. Their connection to the French military's activities does not mean these were the individual psychiatrists whom Fanon described as being in the 'habit' of 'flying to the aid of the police' and subsequently aiding in the torture and interrogation of FLN suspects.[149] Nevertheless, the evidence reveals close affinities between the military's aims and the beliefs and ambitions of the psychiatric communities in Algeria. As with the situation in Kenya, eminent ethnopsychiatrists like Porot and his colleagues provided scientific explanations for the rebels' behaviour that reinforced older stereotypes about the natives' criminal propensities and their roots in religious thinking, in this case Islam. Unlike their Kenyan counterparts, however, the Algerian psychiatrists did not advertise their associations with the government to the same extent as Leakey and Carothers. Nevertheless, the link between their views of North African psychology reveals something of the extent to which the Algiers School participated in the military's psychological warfare campaigns. Although the military had learnt the value of mass detention through their experience in Indochina, their use of it on the Algerian population took on a specific local flavour through their collaboration with these psychiatrists.

Conclusion

This chapter has argued that the postwar confidence in the power of psychiatrists, psychologists, sociologists and anthropologists to explain and 'treat' a plethora of social issues, combined with the paranoia induced by the Cold War, placed greater emphasis on the vulnerability of minds to subversive 'brainwashing' and ideological manipulation. These complicated forces came together in an untidy way during the wars for liberation in Kenya and Algeria, where the counterinsurgency strategies of the respective colonial security forces were given a scientific veneer by ethnopsychiatrists and anthropologists to help legitimise them. As such, the British and French governments were able to explain away the political grievances of the Kikuyu and the Algerians by identifying them as religiously insane and mentally unstable. While Mau Mau initiates were understood to be suffering from collective epidemic hysteria brought on by the stresses of the modern world, the Algerians who joined the ranks of the FLN were expressing an innate criminal impulsiveness rooted in Islam. Typically regarded as inherently violent and criminal, these older stereotypes about Muslim behaviour were updated to represent the terrorists as religiously radical murderers, something that is reminiscent of the stock image of the terrorist in the modern War on Terror.

While both the British and French colonial forces relied upon the expertise of psychiatrists to inform their responses to their respective insurgencies, the extent to which these practitioners collaborated with the government varied. In Kenya, Leakey and Carothers were far more open in their support and cooperation than their French colleagues were, as they both published accounts of their explanations and advice for public consumption. Although the Algiers School of ethnopsychiatry did not publicise their role in the counterinsurgency efforts against the FLN, the long-existing links between the School and the French military meant that their research and views found a close affinity with the latter's aims. Evidence even demonstrates how Porot and his colleagues worked with the military in the detention camps in an effort to research techniques for rehabilitating FLN supporters.

As such, these scientists not only promised to diagnose the rebellious condition, but they also offered new weapons against the enemy mindset. In Kenya, this would take the form of the government's 'Rehabilitation' programme designed specifically to remove the 'disease' of Mau Mau from the misled and corrupted Kikuyu population, while in Algeria, the French military would wage their *guerre psychologique* against the terrorists and the population in order to break down and recreate new French-Muslim citizens. In both cases, extensive systems of detention centres and resettlement villages were used to separate the indigenous population from the guerrillas, who were then subjected to 're-education', a blend of psychological and physical coercion techniques used to 'shock' them into subservience. Every aspect of life within these totalistic environments, from the availability of food, the supply of medical care, access to reading material, news or correspondences with family loved ones, was carefully monitored and administered to help break down the detainees' psychological resistance and political allegiance. As such, this chapter provides a foundation for understanding the coercive activities, including the systematic use of torture, to be discussed in subsequent chapters. The ultimate aim of these counterinsurgency programmes was to create new model subjects who respected colonial rule; but in conflicts regarded as wars for the survival of empire as well as Western ideals, those responsible for creating these new citizens would use any methods they could.

Notes

1 Diek Walter, *Colonial Violence: European Empires and the Use of Force* (London: Hurst, 2017).
2 This perception was influenced by Khrushchev's new assertiveness towards the 'Third World', whereby Russia would provide financial support to newly independent states as they made the transition to Communism. See Karl Moore and David Charles Lewis, 'Globalization and the Cold War: the Communist dimension', *Management & Organizational History* 5 (2013), pp. 10–11.
3 Corfield, *Historical Survey of the Origins and Growth of Mau Mau*, p. 219.
4 SHD 1 H 2411/d.1. 'Les missions de l'armée française dans la guerre révolutionnaire d'Algérie', presented as part of the Conférence donnée à S.H.A.P.E. par le général de corps d'armée Allard commandant le corps d'armée d'Alger avec l'assistance des colonels Godard et Goussault, 15 November 1957.
5 Roger Trinquier, *Modern Warfare: A French View of Counterinsurgency*, trans. Daniel Lee (Westport and London: Praeger Security International, 2006), p. 5.

6 Mao Tse-tung, *On Guerrilla Warfare* (Chicago: University of Illinois Press, 1961), p. 8.
7 Michael Fitzsimmons, 'Hard hearts and open minds? Governance, identity and the intellectual foundations of counterinsurgency strategy', *Journal of Strategic Studies* 31 (2008), p. 339.
8 Within the last few years, a range of studies have turned their attention to 'brainwashing' and ideas around the science of persuasion in the Cold War context. In particular, Daniel Picks's Hidden Persuaders project has mapped out how psychologists and other scientists of the mind helped ideas about brainwashing become so pervasive in Cold War culture.
9 Fitzsimmons, 'Hard hearts and open minds?', p. 21.
10 There is currently a debate over whether Hunter was in fact employed by the CIA to popularise the idea of brainwashing as an imminent threat, as the term has been found in government documents that appear to predate Hunter's own publications. However, this could just mean that both Hunter and the CIA picked up the idea from Chinese sources, independently. See Timothy Melley, 'Brain warfare: the covert sphere, terrorism, and the legacy of the Cold War', *Grey Room 45* (2011), pp. 18–40; Charles S. Young, *Name, Rank, and Serial Number: Exploiting Korean War PoWs at Home and Abroad* (Oxford: Oxford University Press, 2012). See also Marcia Holmes, 'Edward Hunter and the origins of "brainwashing" ', produced as part of the Hidden Persuaders project: www.bbk.ac.uk/hiddenpersuaders/blog/hunter-origins-of-brainwashing/
11 Edward Hunter, *Brain-Washing in Red China: The Calculated Destruction of Men's Minds* (New York: The Vanguard Press, 1953), p. 4.
12 Melley, 'Brain warfare', p. 24.
13 From Kenneth Osgood, *Total Cold War: Eisenhower's Secret Propaganda Battle at Home and Abroad* (Lawrence: University of Kansas Press, 2006), pp. 53–54, quoted in Melley, 'Brain warfare', p. 24.
14 Melley, 'Brain warfare', p. 24.
15 Hunter, *Brain-Washing in Red China*, p. 10.
16 David Seed, 'Brainwashing and Cold War demonology', *Prospects* 22 (1997), p. 538.
17 Daniel Pick, *The Pursuit of the Nazi Mind: Hitler, Hess and the Analysts* (Oxford: Oxford University Press, 2012), pp. 182–183.
18 Anonymous, 'Statement by the International Preparatory Commission of the International Congress on Mental Health' (1948), p. 80.
19 Anonymous, 'Statement by the International Preparatory Commission', pp. 79–84.

20 J. R. Rees, 'The International Congress on Mental Health', *British Medical Bulletin* 6 (1949), p. 5.
21 Linstrum, *Ruling Minds*, p. 157.
22 W. Arthur Lewis, Michael Scott, Martin Wight and Colin Legum, *Attitude to Africa: A Survey of the Main Problems of British Africa, Suggesting the Lines of Policy That Any British Government Should Follow in the Years Ahead* (Middlesex: Penguin Books, 1951), p. 36.
23 Vaughan, *Curing Their Ills*, p. 101.
24 Albert Camus, *The Outsider* (London: Penguin Books, 2013), pp. 53–54.
25 Quoted in Chloe Campbell, *Race and Empire: Eugenics in Colonial Kenya* (Manchester: Manchester University Press, 2007), p. 39.
26 F. W. Vint, 'The brain of the Kenya native', *Journal of Anatomy* 68 (1934), pp. 216–223.
27 The explanations blended ideas about the North African's psychical being, Arab and Muslim social culture more generally, and their ethnic identity, all of which was presented rather confusingly. See Jean-Michel Bégué, 'French psychiatry in Algeria (1830–1962): from colonial to transcultural', *History of Psychiatry* 7 (1996), pp. 544–545.
28 Shane Doyle, 'Social disease and social science: the intellectual influence of non-medical research on policy and practice in the Colonial Medical Services in Tanganyika and Uganda', in Greenwood (ed.), *Beyond the State*, pp. 126–127.
29 Megan Vaughan, 'Introduction', in Megan Vaughan and Sloan Mahone (eds), *Psychiatry and Empire* (Basingstoke: Palgrave Macmillan, 2007), p. 1.
30 Vaughan, *Curing Their Ills*, p. 108; Sloan Mahone, 'The psychology of rebellion: colonial medical responses to dissent in British East Africa', *The Journal of African History* 47 (2006), pp. 242–244.
31 For example, see Leonard H. Ainsworth and Mary D. Ainsworth, 'Acculturation in East Africa. I. Political awareness and attitudes toward authority', *The Journal of Social Psychology* 57 (1962), pp. 391–399; and Mary D. Ainsworth and Leonard H. Ainsworth, 'Acculturation in East Africa. IV. Summary and discussion', *The Journal of Social Psychology* 57 (1962), pp. 417–432. Alternatively, see Homer G. Barnett, 'Acculturation: an exploratory formulation. The Social Science Research Council Summer Seminar on Acculturation, 1953: comment', *American Anthropologist* 56 (1954), pp. 1000–1002.
32 Vaughan, 'Introduction', p. 1.
33 Ellen J. Amster, *Medicine and the Saints: Science, Islam, and the Colonial Encounter in Morocco, 1877–1956* (Austin: University of Texas Press), pp. 55–61.

34 Quoted in Amster, *Medicine and the Saints*, p. 59.
35 David French, *The British Way in Counter-Insurgency, 1945–67* (Oxford: Oxford University Press, 2011), pp. 59–60.
36 In Algeria, they were also called the *fellagha*, an Arabic word for 'head-splitters' or just 'bandits' which was borrowed from the Tunisian nationalist struggle. See Marnia Lazreg, *Torture and the Twilight of Empire: From Algiers to Baghdad* (Princeton and Oxford: Princeton University Press, 2008), p. 112.
37 Marouf Hasian Jr, 'The development of ethnographic science and psychological warfare during the suppression of the Mau Mau Rebellion', *Journal of Medical Humanities* 34 (2013), p. 338.
38 TNA FCO 141/6750/64. Author redacted, 'Resistance Movement Centre, Bahati, Nakuru, Report on Mau Mau Activities: Maji Mazuri – Eldama Ravine Area', C. November 1953.
39 Ian Henderson, *The Hunt for Kimathi* (London: Hamish Hamilton, 1958), p. 16.
40 Anderson, *Histories of the Hanged*, p. 279.
41 Anderson, *Histories of the Hanged*, p. 279.
42 Blundell, *So Rough a Wind*, p. 171.
43 Mahone, 'The psychology of rebellion', p. 251.
44 Mahone, 'The psychology of rebellion', p. 243.
45 In fact, evidence that the British suspected a connection between Mau Mau and Dini ya Msambwa in the early days of the uprising emerged in 2011, when previously hidden documents on the Kenya Emergency were released as part of the Hanslope Park disclosure. In June 1953 the Director of Intelligence and Security reported to the Kenyan Commissioner of Police and the Chief Secretary that Mau Mau members had met with Dini ya Msambwa adherents who advised them to conduct oath-taking ceremonies in the Trans Nzoia area of Kenya. According to this report, Dini ya Msambwa had also allegedly 'advocated stronger oaths' for adherents in order to 'expel the European from Kenya'. Although this document does not contain any references to pathology or mental disturbances, it nevertheless demonstrates that earlier prophetic movements had indeed impacted on interpretation of Mau Mau and that the oath-taking ceremonies needed to be monitored in order to limit the spread of their doctrine. See TNA FCO 141/5877. 'Dini ya Msambwa/Mau Mau Link-up', 1952.
46 Bruce J. Berman and John M. Lonsdale, 'Lewis Leakey's Mau Mau: a study in the politics of knowledge', *History and Anthropology* 5 (1991), p. 144.
47 Lewis S. B. Leakey, *Mau Mau and the Kikuyu* (London: Methuen, 1952), p. vii.

48 Leakey, *Mau Mau and the Kikuyu*, pp. 17, 85.

49 Instead he recognised the Kikuyu's genuine grievances over their loss of land to the white settlers, the insecurity of jobs on white farms, overcrowding in the remaining Kikuyu lands, the terrible wages of urban workers and the social insult of the colonial colour bar. The government's inability to take these issues seriously made the Kikuyu vulnerable to political agitators, such as the KCA and the Kikuyu African Union (KCU) from whom Mau Mau was understood to have developed. The oath-taking ceremonies, which Leakey regarded as corrupted and illegitimate versions of traditional Kikuyu practices, were designed to subvert Kikuyu values and were the means by which the rebels 'forced Mau Mau on the masses'. See Leakey, *Mau Mau and the Kikuyu*, pp. 105–115, 85–93 and x.

50 Lewis S. B. Leakey, *Defeating Mau Mau* (London: Methuen, 1954), pp. 41, 43.

51 Caroline Elkins, 'The struggle for Mau Mau rehabilitation in late colonial Kenya', *The International Journal of African Historical Studies* 33 (2000), p. 25.

52 FCO 141/5666/303/p. 1. Thomas Askwith, 'Detention and Rehabilitation', 27 August 1953.

53 Klose, *Human Rights in the Shadow of Colonial Violence*, p. 110.

54 Klose, *Human Rights in the Shadow of Colonial Violence*, p. 110. See also Simon Smith, 'General Templer and counter-insurgency in Malaya: hearts and minds, intelligence, and propaganda', *Intelligence and National Security* 16 (2001), p. 62.

55 David French, 'Nasty not nice: British counter-insurgency doctrine and practice, 1945–1967', *Small Wars & Insurgencies* 23 (2012), p. 752.

56 FCO 141/5666/303/. Thomas Askwith, 'Detention and Rehabilitation', 27 August 1953, p. 3.

57 The phrase was first used by Lieutenant-Colonel C. E. Bruce of the Indian Political Department in 1938 in his book about the North-West Frontier of India.

58 Paul Dixon, '"Hearts and minds"? British counter-insurgency from Malaya to Iraq', *Journal of Strategic Studies* 32 (2009), p. 368.

59 FCO 141/5666/303/. Askwith, 'Detention and Rehabilitation', p. 3.

60 FCO 141/5666/303/. Askwith, 'Detention and Rehabilitation', pp. 2–4.

61 Dixon, 'Hearts and minds'?, p. 368.

62 TNA CO 822/489/83. Telegram from Baring to Lyttleton, 13 July 1953.

63 Elkins, 'The struggle for Mau Mau rehabilitation', p. 36.

64 Elkins, 'The struggle for Mau Mau rehabilitation', p. 36.
65 TNA FCO 141/5666/303. Thomas Askwith, 'Detention and Rehabilitation', 27 August 1953, p. 10.
66 Anonymous, 'Clarke wants terrorists treated like victims of cult brainwashing', *Daily Telegraph*, 2 October 2005.
67 Leakey, *Defeating Mau Mau*, pp. 85–86.
68 TNA CO 822/794/1. 'Rehabilitation', 6 January 1954.
69 TNA CO 822/794/52. Savingram from Governor Baring to the Secretary of State for the Colonies, 3 January 1956.
70 Elkins, 'The Struggle for Mau Mau Rehabilitation in late colonial Kenya', p. 40.
71 Fanon was particularly critical of Carothers's leucotomy argument in *The Wretched of the Earth*, where he denounced it as being an example of the same form of overt racism espoused by members of the Algerian psychiatry community. See Fanon, *The Wretched of the Earth*, p. 244.
72 John Colin Carothers, *The African Mind in Health and Disease: A Study in Ethnopsychiatry* (Geneva: World Health Organization, 1953), p. 157. See also John Colin Carothers, 'Frontal lobe function and the African', *Journal of Mental Science* 97 (1951), p. 12.
73 Jock McCollock, *Colonial Psychiatry and 'the African Mind'* (Cambridge: Cambridge University Press, 1995), p. 67.
74 McCollock, *Colonial Psychiatry and 'the African Mind'*, p. 67.
75 John Colin Carothers, *The Psychology of the Mau Mau* (London: Government Printer, 1954), p. 4.
76 Carothers, *The Psychology of the Mau Mau*, p. 12.
77 Carothers, *The Psychology of the Mau Mau*, p. 16.
78 Carothers, *The Psychology of the Mau Mau*, p. 18.
79 Carothers, *The Psychology of the Mau Mau*, p. 7.
80 Carothers, *The Psychology of the Mau Mau*, p. 10.
81 Katherine Bruce-Lockhart, '"Unsound" minds and broken bodies: the detention of "hardcore" Mau Mau women at Kamiti and Gitamayu Detention Camps in Kenya, 1954–1960', *Journal of Eastern African Studies* 8 (2014), p. 593.
82 Thomas Askwith, *From Mau Mau to Harambee* (Cambridge: University of Cambridge, African Studies Centre), p. 106.
83 Carothers, *The Psychology of the Mau Mau*, p. 17.
84 Carothers, *The Psychology of the Mau Mau*, p. 23.
85 Linstrum, *Ruling Minds*, p. 157.
86 John Wilkinson, 'The Mau Mau movement: some general and medical aspects', *The East African Medical Journal* 31 (1954), p. 299.
87 Linsturm, *Ruling Minds*, p. 183.

88 Peter Worsley, 'The anatomy of Mau Mau', *The New Reasoner* 1 (1957), p. 15.
89 Worsley, 'The anatomy of Mau Mau', p. 15.
90 Worsley, 'The anatomy of Mau Mau', p. 22.
91 Sloan Mahone, 'East African psychiatry and the practical problems of empire', in Vaughan and Mahone (eds), *Psychiatry and Empire*, p. 41.
92 Vaughan, 'Introduction', p. 6.
93 Richard C. Keller, 'Taking science to the colonies: psychiatric innovation in France and North Africa', in Mahone and Vaughan (eds), *Psychiatry and Empire*, p. 18.
94 Keller, *Colonial Madness*, p. 123.
95 P. Gallais and L. Planques, 'Etude sur les déficiences mentales dans les territoires d'Outre-Mer. Perspectives ethnopsychiatriques dans l'Union Française', *Médecine tropicale* 11 (1951), pp. 9–25. See also Alice Bullard, 'The critical impact of Frantz Fanon and Henri Collomb: race, gender, and personality testing of North and West Africans', *Journal of the History of the Behavioural Sciences* 41 (2005), p. 231.
96 Gallais and Planques, 'Etude sur les déficiences mentales dans les territoires d'Outre-Mer', p. 6. See also Antoine Porot and Jean Stutter, *Le "Primitivisme" des indigènes nord-africains, ses incidences en pathologie mentale, par le professeur* (Marseille: Impr. marseillaise, 1939).
97 SHD 1 H 2411/d.1/. Colonel Lacheroy, 'La guerre révolutionnaire: Conférence no.1 Leçons de l'Action Viet-Minh et Communiste en Indochine', p. 7.
98 SHD 1 H 2411/d.1/. Lacheroy, 'La guerre révolutionnaire', p. 10.
99 Trinquier, *Modern Warfare*, p. 6.
100 Lazreg, *Torture and the Twilight of Empire*, p. 24.
101 Jean Lartéguy, *The Centurions* (London: Penguin Books, 2015), p. 20.
102 Lazreg, *Torture and the Twilight of Empire*, p. 21.
103 SHAT 1 H 2411/d.1. 'Les missions de l'armée française dans la guerre révolutionnaire d'Algérie', presented as part of the Conférence donnée à S.H.A.P.E. par le général de corps d'armée Allard commandant le corps d'armée d'Alger avec l'assistance des colonels Godard et Goussault, 15 November 1957.
104 Maria-Catherine Villatoux, 'Traitement psychologique, endoctrinement, contre-endoctrinement en guerre d'Algérie. Le cas des camps de détention, *Guerres mondiales et conflits contemporains* 208 (2002), p. 48.
105 Lartéguy, *The Centurions*, p. 96.

106 This officer may be Captain Alain de Braquilanges, who was imprisoned in the actual Camp No. 1 until 1954. The extract contained in the report seems to have come from his *Méthode psychologique utilisé pour forcer l'adhésion des esprits*, see Villatoux, 'Traitement psychologique', p. 49.
107 SHD 1 H 2411/d.1/. *L'Endoctrinement des prisonniers de guerre*, conference of Captain Prestat, 10 March 1956, Centre d'instruction de guerre psychologique, p. 1.
108 SHD 1 H 2411/d.1. *L'Endoctrinement des prisonniers de guerre*, 1956, pp. 5–6.
109 Villatoux, 'Traitement psychologique', p. 49.
110 SHD 1 H 2411/d.1. *L'Endoctrinement des prisonniers de guerre*, p. 1.
111 SHD 1 H 2573/d.1. 'Centre-endoctrinement des fellagha: Project général', *c.* July 1956.
112 Thénault, 'L'Internement en France pendant la guerre d'indépendance algérienne'.
113 Lazreg, *Torture in the Twilight of Empire*, pp. 46–47.
114 Paul Villatoux, 'L'Institutionnalisation de l'arme psychologique pendant la guerre d'Algérie au miroir de la guerre froide', *Guerres mondiales et conflits contemporains* 208 (2002), pp. 36, 39. See also Lazreg, *Torture and the Twilight of Empire*, p. 61.
115 Villatoux, 'L'Institutionnalisation de l'arme psychologique pendant la guerre d'Algérie au miroir de la guerre froide', p. 36.
116 SHD 1 H 2524/d.1. 'La guerre psychologique. Conférence no. 1', *c.* July 1956, p. 5.
117 SHD 1 H 2411/d.1. 'Conférence. Le Renseignement psychologique', *c.* June 1957, p. 3.
118 SHD 1 H 2524/d.1. 'L'Action psychologique dans les forces armées', date unknown, p. 5.
119 Lazreg, *Torture in the Twilight of Empire*, p. 61.
120 SHD 1 H 2524/d.1. 'La Guerre psychologique. Conférence no.1', *c.* July 1956, p. 6.
121 Their exploration of this psychological literature can be separated into two categories: what they referred to as 'the Soviet school', defined by the work of Ivan Pavlov, and 'the American school', based on Carl Jung's collective psychoanalysis (which they conflated with behaviourism). According to the Bureau, the Soviets had used Pavlov's classical conditioning techniques to wage a war of words in their propaganda campaigns, but while they considered it instructive, the French military ultimately deemed it to be passé. The American school, however, caught the Cinquième Bureau's attention. They were particularly interested in Jung's ideas of collective psychoanalysis,

determining the extent to which Muslim culture contained the type of archetypes in his theories, and whether they pertained to his concepts of the 'the sacred'. See SHD 1 H 2524/d.1. 'La Guerre psychologique. Conférence no. 2', *c.* 1957, pp. 1–8.

122 Lazreg, *Torture and the Twilight of Empire*, p. 62.

123 SHD 1 H 2411/d.1. 'Note sur le rapport du Capitaine Prestat', 1955, p. 1.

124 Gustave Le Bon, *The Psychology of Revolution*, Project Gutenberg www.gutenberg.org/cache/epub/448/pg448-images.html

125 Le Bon, *The Psychology of Revolution.*

126 SHD 1 H 2411/d.1. Capitaine Jacques Mercier, 'La Guerre révolutionnaire en Algérie', May 1958, p. 15.

127 Keller, *Colonial Madness*, p. 155.

128 Antoine Porot, 'Notes de psychiatrie musulmane', *Annales médico-psychologiques* 74 (1918), p. 380.

129 SHD 1 H 2524/d.1. 'Sociologie musulmane. Causerie no. 9', *c.* 1957–1958.

130 SHD 1 H 2524/d.1. 'Sociologie musulmane', pp. 1–2.

131 SHD 1 H 2409/d.1. 'Action psychologique du conflit', *c.* 1957, p. 14.

132 Antoine Porot and Don Côme Arrii, 'L'Impulsivité criminelle chez l'indigène algérien. Ses facteurs', *Annales médico-psychologique* 14 (1932), p. 589.

133 Porot and Arrii, 'L'Impulsivité criminelle chez l'indigène algérien', pp. 588–611.

134 Porot and Arrii, 'L'Impulsivité criminelle chez l'indigène algérien', pp. 610–611.

135 Fanon, *The Wretched of the Earth*, p. 241.

136 David Macey, 'The Algerian with a knife', *Parallex* 4 (1998), p. 165.

137 Porot and Arrii, 'L'Impulsivité criminelle chez l'indigène algérien', p. 611. See also Keller, *Colonial Madness*, p. 140.

138 F. Lagrot and J. Greco, 'Les Mutilations facials au cours du terrorisme en Algérie et leur réparation', *La Presse médicale* 51 (1956), pp. 1193–1198.

139 Klose, *Human Rights in the Shadow of Colonial Violence*, p. 218.

140 The term *paléophrénie réactionnelle* was coined by C. A. Pierson in 1955 to serve as a new label for the long-held assumptions about North African primitivism and their 'ancestral' tendencies towards impulsive criminality and violence. As he stated, *paléophrénie réactionnelle* referred 'to a less evolved ontology and a sensitivity that has changed little since the [North Africans'] distant ancestor'. See C. A. Pierson, 'Paléophrénie réactionnelle. Physiopathologie de l'impulsion morbide en milieu nord-africain', *Maroc medical* 360 (1955), pp. 642–647.

141 A. Fourrier, P. Michaux and J. Thiodet, 'Aspects particuliers de la criminalité algérienne', *Algérie médicale* 61 (1957) quoted in Antoine Porot and Charles Bardenat, *Psychiatrie médico-légale* (Paris: Maloine, 1959), p. 305.
142 A. Fourrier, P. Michaux and J. Thiodet, 'Aspects particuliers de la criminalité algérienne'.
143 Antoine Porot and Charles Bardenat, *Anormaux et malades mentaux devant la justice pénale* (Paris: Librairie Maloine, 1960), p. 155. See also Keller, *Colonial Madness*, p. 152.
144 Porot and Bardenat, *Anormaux et malades mentaux devant la justice pénale*, p. 155.
145 Porot and Bardenat, *Anormaux et malades mentaux devant la justice pénale*, p. 159.
146 Presumably a misspelling of Dr Stutter.
147 SHD 1 H 2460/d.1. 'Sur le problème de la mentalité des Musulman', 1 June 1959.
148 These experts included Professor Philippe Marçais, the French Arabist and politician, and Professor Louis Massignon, an influential Catholic scholar of Islam and pioneer of Catholic–Muslim mutual understanding.
149 Fanon, *A Dying Colonialism*, p. 138.

3

Behind the barbed wire

Disease in Britain's carceral archipelago

On 21 October 1952, security forces in Kenya arrested 183 leading African politicians as part of Operation Jock Scott. These individuals, including Jomo Kenyatta, were thought to be the masterminds behind Mau Mau, and the colonial authorities hoped their arrest would stop the movement entirely. However, the operation merely radicalised the younger and more militant members of the African resistance.[1] This led the colonial authorities to treat all Kikuyu as potential Mau Mau adherents, and resulted in the widescale arrest of suspects who were forced into newly erected transit camps from December 1952 onwards. From here, the detainees were to be deported en masse to the reserves, a process that began in earnest in early 1953. The authorities created a series of screening centres throughout the Rift Valley and Central Provinces, through which thousands of Kikuyu were channelled by local settlers and colonial officials, who subjected the repatriates to intense interrogation that could last for days at a time.[2]

Then, in April 1954, the situation became more complicated with the launch of Operation Anvil. The purpose of Anvil, as described by Henry Hopkins, the then Minister of State, was 'to remove the active and passive supporters of Mau Mau from Nairobi to holding camps where a thorough screening will take place on an individual basis'.[3] The result was that a further 24,000 Kikuyu living in Nairobi were arrested and deported to detention camps. In many accounts of the Kenya Emergency, this was the pivotal moment when detention and forced villagisation became a central feature of the story of the Mau Mau uprising.[4] Operation Anvil rapidly expanded the camp system and led to the creation of new prison camps at Langata, Mackinnon Road and Manyani.[5] The pipeline was now in operation. Each detainee was meant to pass through Langata, where they would be interrogated and classified depending on the intensity of their presumed Mau Mau affiliation. Those thought to be actively involved in the movement were transported to either Mackinnon Road or Manyani for further assessment, while the less 'indoctrinated' inmates were taken to other camps or resettlement villages in the reserves.[6]

By the time Operation Anvil came to an end, Kenya was home to the largest network of detention and prison camps ever established in a British colony.[7] By December 1954, 71,346 people had been arrested as part of the Emergency, a number that would eventually reach 77,000 people, according to official British statistics.[8] It is likely that these figures have been greatly underestimated, as at least one in every four male Kikuyu was imprisoned or detained for some time during the Emergency.[9] With the influx of detainees brought in by Operation Anvil, the nascent detention camp system was put under sudden and unprecedented strain. The new centres at Langata, Mackinnon Road and Manyani were not prepared to accommodate so many new inmates. Resources were already stretched beyond their limits and soon the cramped and unhygienic conditions became unbearable.[10] At the Manyani Camp, for example, 16,000 people were kept in a site intended for 6,000 prisoners – a situation that earnt it the dubious honour of being the largest detention camp outside the Iron Curtain.[11] The combination of these factors – poor sanitation, overcrowding, insufficient diets and a low quality of medical care – inevitably led to the outbreak of infectious diseases like typhus, dysentery and tuberculosis, as well as deficiency diseases such as scurvy and pellagra.[12]

What is interesting about the outbreak of these diseases, when compared to claims about beatings and torture throughout the Emergency, is that medical officers and professionals took them far more seriously. For instance, on 9 May 1954, Dr H. G. Waters, the deputy director of the Kenyan Medical Services, wrote a report warning that Manyani Camp's condition was so poor that, if action was not taken immediately, there would soon be cases of epidemic disease among the detainees.[13] Waters explained how the kitchens that prepared food for the inmates were filthy and fly-infested, bins were not emptied sufficiently, unclean latrine buckets were left to pile up around the camp and night-soil was not disposed of correctly. He soon discovered that an entire area close to the camp had been 'heavily and extensively fouled and contaminated with excreta and every form of indiscriminate dumping' which meant there was 'a very dangerous threat from typhoid, dysentery and diarrhoea to the camp inmates'.[14] Despite making multiple recommendations, Waters's report was largely ignored.

A few days after his visit, the Kenya press heard a rumour that typhoid was already present in Manyani and the Mackinnon Road camps. Responding to this, the Government completely denied the claims. The tactic here was to issue an outright denial of the situation in the camps. For this to work, the colonial administration rallied the Medical Department to add weight to their counter-claims. According to a Press Office handout issued on 10 May 1954 by the Medical Department in Nairobi, 'there [was] no type of epidemic at either of the camps'.[15] According to Dr J. R. Walker, Assistant Director of Medical Services, he and Dr Farnworth Anderson, the Director of Medical Services, had visited the site the week before and were 'completely satisfied with the arrangements'.[16] Rather than admit the camps were understaffed and poorly prepared, the Medical Department insisted that both camps – Manyani and Mackinnon Road – had fully equipped medical facilities and trained staff. In fact, so the handout claimed, Mackinnon Road had a '60-bed hospital with a doctor, two European nursing sisters, African hospital assistants and dressers'.[17] In addition, European health inspectors shared responsibility of the two camps and there were African staff and a European hygiene officer in each camp.[18]

Despite this being a standard response when faced with questions about ill health in the camps, it was a lie. In reality, these facilities were not in operation at the time the handout claimed; the hospital wards at Manyani were not even opened for use until mid-July 1954.[19] It is also doubtful that the facilities were as well staffed as the doctors suggested, given that the Medical Department was so understaffed that, in August 1954, the War Office gave instructions to prioritise the screening of 'persons such as medical dressers, dispensaries, hospital assistants', who could be put to work in the camps.[20] This statement by the Medical Department not only dismisses the factual basis of the epidemic, it also presents the camps as humane facilities with modern equipment and a fully qualified staff available to treat the detainees. Rather than challenge the conditions within the camps at this early stage in the Emergency, the doctors within the Kenya Medical Department used their positions of authority to support the administration's wider denials. This was the first of many tactics the department adopted to undermine claims of ill health in the camps.

When it came to other health issues among the inmates, the Medical Department were quick to blame the detainees themselves. For instance, the same handout admitted that there had been two cases of typhoid, but far from catching the illness while in detention, these two victims had 'contracted the disease before entering the camps'.[21] Other diseases were also listed by a Dr Walker, but the decision to include them in the press release was perhaps an attempt to further undermine the image of the Kikuyu as 'victims'. For example, at Mackinnon Road in April 1954, Walker explained, there had been 100 cases of illness. Of these, 35 had been dysentery, which had been treated effectively by a 'fully prepared staff', and 25 had been venereal disease. Of the two deaths that occurred in Mackinnon Road camp, one was due to a man who entered the facility with 'cerebral malaria', again not a condition contracted in the camp, while the other died as a result of a fight with another inmate.[22] If this press release was to be believed, Manyani was largely free of illness, though there were some isolated cases of infection. An alternative approach might have been to deny the existence of any form of illness in the facility, but this would have stretched the credulity of even the most determined supporters of the pipeline regime. Instead, the burden of responsibility was placed on the inmates whose lifestyles had led to their conditions. The inclusion of the venereal disease cases is particularly illustrative of this, as the social stigmas surrounding these conditions would have contributed to the image of Africans as unclean.

Despite the Medical Department's efforts to conceal the conditions in the camps, it was clear by September 1954 that Manyani was experiencing a full-blown typhoid outbreak. By October, the infection had claimed at least eighty-six lives, while hundreds of others were to be infected before it ended towards December that year.[23] The epidemic soon spread to Langata camp as well as Mackinnon Road. Interestingly, the epidemic caught very little attention within the British press. If it was discussed in news reports, the significance and extent of the epidemic was played down. For instance, on 21 September, the *Manchester Guardian* published a short article which touched on the situation in Manyani. According to a small paragraph in the text, Dr Anderson 'announced to-day that 35 Mau Mau suspects had died in the typhoid epidemic in the Colony's biggest detention camp'.[24] This account came with no commentary or explanation for the situation. It was merely a statement of facts regarding the number of victims among the surviving detainees. Instead of expanding on the conditions that led to the epidemic, the article moves swiftly onto the number of Kikuyu who were sentenced to death on the same day for their Mau Mau crimes. All these statements, however, were preceded by the main story of the article which focused on a Dr William Mackintosh, a sixty-two-year-old retired director of veterinary services in Uganda, who had 'fought off four [Mau Mau] terrorists who attacked him' on his farm and stole his automatic pistol.[25] In comparison to the story of a heroic doctor and the executed Kikuyu, the details of the typhoid epidemic were of tertiary concern. If anything, the juxtaposition of the piece concerning the daring behaviour of the retired veterinarian attacked by a gang of 'terrorists', like the reference to venereal disease above, further highlighted the image of detainees as violent thugs, which may have further detracted from any sense of concern or outrage for the conditions in the camp.

Back in Kenya, however, the authorities were responding with urgency. Since June 1954, the Army Hygiene Unit had been assisting with sanitary control at the camps. In July, with fifty known cases, the hospital wards at Manyani were finally opened and by August, four additional hospital wards were in use.[26] Yet the full extent of the epidemic was not understood until the first weeks of September 1954, four months after Dr Walters first submitted his report. As David Anderson has shown, the whistle-blower in this instance was Dr Hugh Stott, a medical adviser to the Labour Department.[27] His initial suspicions were raised after receiving the weekly medical returns for Manyani and noticing a sharp increase in the death rate for cases of 'malaria'. This seemed unlikely to him given that the blood culture tests from the camp returned as negative. Soon after, Stott visited Yatta Works Camps, where he saw two cases of typhoid in the camp hospital and, on his way back to Nairobi, witnessed a further three cases in the Thika Hospital. All these cases were recorded in patients who had recently left

Manyani.[28] Stott noted that the conditions at Manyani were overcrowded, which was contributing greatly to the unhygienic situation; buckets intended for drinking water were placed next to those used for defecation in the huts. As later investigations confirmed, contaminated water was indeed responsible for spreading typhoid in the camps. Manyani was subsequently quarantined for over two months but was soon opened again for the transport of prisoners towards the end of 1954.[29]

Despite this outbreak's severity, typhoid and other infections such as tuberculosis and leprosy continued to occur in the camps throughout the Emergency.[30] Standards of hygiene and well-being were consistently low, even after Dr Stott produced his reports on the Manyani incident. For its part, the Colonial Medical Department was generally understaffed, which meant the colonial authorities struggled to supply camps with sufficient personnel and effective care in all instances. However, after his tour of multiple camps, Stott came to the decision that the rules were simply ignored by camp commanders and staff.[31] Yet Stott's protests at the conditions within the camps remained, to a large extent, an internal matter. At no point did a member of the Colonial Medical Department attempt to raise wider awareness of these conditions outside government circles. As such, those professionals employed by the Colonial Office to safeguard the health of the detainees in the detention camps often failed to deliver on their mission. In fact, prominent figures within the Medical Department explicitly aided the administration by denying the presence of infection within the camps.

This became the preferred method for dealing with sensitive events that could cause embarrassment for the colonial authorities and the British government more generally: they were treated as internal issues. Yet while those employed within the Colonial Medical Department helped to maintain the culture of secrecy surrounding the camps, there were others outside the government's employ who tried to raise concerns about the typhoid epidemic.

On 28 September 1954, the Socialist Medical Association in London wrote to the Secretary of State for the Colonies, Alan Lennox-Boyd, to raise grave concerns over the rumours that typhoid had broken out in the Manyani Camp and that fifty detainees had already died. Comparing the situation in Kenya with 'Camps of this nature in Germany during the war', the Association wanted to 'protest most vigorously and [insist] that emergency action be taken to end this system of detention, before the outbreak spreads and becomes completely out of our control'.[32] It is currently unknown whether the Secretary of State for the Colonies replied to this letter. However, he demonstrated the extent of the wider cover-up later during a debate on Manyani Camp in the House of Commons on 2 October 1954. While being asked for an update on the 'steps he has taken to curb the outbreak of typhoid in Manyani Camp' by James Johnson, a Labour MP, he responded:

> I am satisfied that conditions in the camp are good, and that the outbreak at Manyani camp, which I visited last Saturday, was not due to the camp water supply or sanitation, or to any [failure] to take proper health measures. The probable cause was the spreading by personal contact of infection from a number of detainees who had the disease in a mild form and did not report sick. All necessary steps to control the outbreak and to prevent a recurrence have been taken, including reinoculation, isolation of sufferers and provision of more medical staff.[33]

While Dr Stott had specifically connected the epidemic to the poor conditions in the camp, especially the contaminated water sources, Lennox-Boyd had continued the method of blaming the detainees and to portray them as unhygienic and negligent for not reporting their illness, meaning that neither the government nor the Medical Department could be held accountable for the outbreak.

The government's efforts to cover up the squalid conditions in the camps received another blow in 1956 when the Quaker social worker turned whistle-blower Eileen Fletcher published *The Truth About Kenya*. This document explained the state of the camps she witnessed during her service as a Rehabilitation Officer at Athi River and Kisumu camps, among others, from December 1954. Fletcher described an atmosphere of horror where unhygienic and overcrowded facilities, some exceedingly crude in design, were filled with men, women and children who were detained without trial, some for years at a time. Prisoners were abused indiscriminately, and torture was rife. Moreover, prisoners were often forced to carry out heavy labour while ill and severely malnourished.[34] When it came to disease, Fletcher noted how a contractor at Kisumu had suggested that allowing detainees to die from malaria and Blackwater Fever was the next best thing to having them all shot.[35] The connection between disease and punishment was not just limited to the camps. In another report produced in July 1956, Fletcher noted that, due to draconic curfew conditions placed on a new village in the Embu reserves, seventy people had died from typhoid in mid-1955 as a result of not being allowed to fetch clean water.[36] These villages were meant to function as part of the rehabilitation programme's mission to modernise the underdeveloped reservations and raise the standard of living among the Kikuyu deported back to the reserves. However, according to Fletcher, they functioned as another form of prison in which the Kikuyu, especially women, were taken hostage and subjected to coercion, torture and rape at the hands of the African Home Guard.[37]

Although Fletcher's report paints a grizzly image, it would likely be too much to suggest that disease was deliberately fostered as an explicit means of punishment in the Kenya camps. It is more probable that such conditions were exploited by unscrupulous security officers who took advantage of a badly organised and severely underfunded punitive system. Disease in the Kenya camps may have been a useful adjunct to the torturer's toolkit rather than a consciously created weapon, but that does not mean it was any less pernicious. It might also be tempting to think about the medical situation within the camps as being static throughout the Emergency, but there is actually evidence that some aspects of the Colonial Medical Department did try to improve conditions in the camps, albeit to a limited extent.

Malingering and resistance

Between May and October 1954, while the typhoid epidemic was underway, Dr Stott was touring the detention camps during a secondment from his role with the Labour Department. His terms of references were comprehensive and included, among other things, 'an endeavour to standardise the hygiene arrangements' in the camps, to 'determine any potential diseases likely to arise within them and to take measure to prevent them', and 'to introduce a standardised system of notification of disease'.[38] In particular, Stott was addressing the fact, so he claims, that the Medical Department had received very little information on the state of health and hygiene in most of the camps up until that point, which was the main reason for his appointment.[39]

Stott's report reveals much about the ways that medicine and medical practitioners interacted with the camp system, but, crucially, it shows just how chaotic the early phase of the Emergency was when it came to matters of health and hygiene. For one thing, the report admits that the camps were initially run by 'at least three different departments – The Administration, the Prisons and the Police' and that 'the African Land Development Board', Stott noted 'had considerable influence on the policy, finance and general running of the camps'.[40] He also struggled to identify just how many camps were actually in operation and that, 'even after obtaining what was considered to be a full list', he 'came upon other camps, previously unknown to me'.[41]

This 'multi-headed method of organisation' made it difficult to get any medical recommendations put into action or to introduce standards of practices. The situation only improved 'to a certain extent', Stott claimed, in July 1954, when the whole camp system came under the control of the Commissioner of Prisons. Even then, the camps in Fort Hall and Embu districts wanted independent control. Regardless, Stott's report explains that the main camps of Langata, Manyani and Mackinnon Road had a European Medical Officer in charge of their operations, while camps at Embakasi, Athi River, Kajiando and Lukenia were under general charge of the Senior Medical Officer of Nairobi. These camps were, he claimed, visited 'almost daily' by an Asian Medical Officer.[42] However, all the other camps were left to the supervision of Medical Officers in charge of the districts where they were situated and were visited far less frequently, because they and their staff were 'overworked with extra burdens of the Emergency'.[43]

In fact, the paucity of medical care was significant enough for comment from the delegation of the International Committee of the Red Cross (ICRC). During their first visit to the Crown Colony between March and April 1957, Drs Louis A. Gailland and Henri-Philippe Junod visited fifty-two detention camps and eighteen 'new villages' where they had freedom to speak to detainees away from the guards and to inspect the overall conditions of each site. Junod's role within these conflicts will be discussed in more detail in Chapter 4, but for now it is worth noting that his and Gailland's findings were consigned to a confidential report that was given to the British government. In general, the delegates were satisfied with the camp system and made no comment on any forms of abuse that may have been present in the camps.[44] However, Gailland and Junod expressed astonishment at 'the rarity of medical visits' and the fact that in multiple camps, the medical officer made only 'one visit per month or six weeks'.[45] Rather than press the matter further, the delegates were persuaded by the fact that the medical officers were also in charge of the districts surrounding the camps, which contained hundreds of thousands of inhabitants, and that consequently, detainees were 'better placed than the general population for receiving medical care'.[46] In particular, the ICRC delegates were impressed by the camp authority's treatment of detainees suffering from tuberculosis, which was apparently endemic in the Reserves. Even though most detention medical centres were not equipped with radiological facilities to enable the systematic examination of potential tuberculous patients, the delegates believed the detainees received better medical care than the Kikuyu outside detention. In fact, Gaillard expressed disappointment that more could not be done. He felt the mass internment of the Mau Mau supporters in the camps and the resettlement villages offered a 'unique' opportunity to screen and treat the 'entire population', to eliminate tuberculosis more generally.[47]

The first visit from the ICRC has been criticised for its ineffective approach to the situation playing out in the detention camps, in particular their reticence on the widespread use of violence against prisoners.[48] The subject of abuse and violence will be considered later, but is worth noting that their concerns over the infrequent medical visits may highlight a factor that contributed to the violence in the camps. With fewer visits from doctors, detainees were left at the mercy of their guards, who had little interest in improving the conditions they experienced in detention, though this should not suggest that the presence of a medical expert in the larger camps necessarily guaranteed protection or fair treatment. Aside from medical complicity in overt forms of violence such as torture, the clinical gaze could also overlook evidence of ill health or medical need if they thought a detainee was malingering.

For instance, on 24 January 1954, detainees at Athi River wrote a petition to the British Parliament listing various grievances, including the accusation that they were forbidden access to proper medical care and that their doctor would give them doses of saline for their complaints.[49] Moreover, they claimed that a detainee called Stephen Kiunjuri had died due to medical neglect. According to the petitioners, Kiunjuri had reported ill with a 'temperature' but the Medical Officer 'alleged he was malingering and hence ordered the wardens to put him in cells'. He apparently died in isolation soon after.[50] In response to the petitioner's claims, the Commissioner of Prisons simply stated that Kiunjuri had died of natural causes in hospital.[51]

While it is not currently known whether Kiunjuri died in detention or in hospital, there are other features of the detainee's complaints that are worth attention, in particular the subject of malingering, which was a consistent concern for camp authorities.[52] Malingering has received very little historical attention, especially within the context of the detention camps, but it represents a specific instance where detainee resistance and medical authority met. For a detainee, as Anne Applebaum notes when discussing doctors working in the Soviet gulag, sympathetic doctors could be 'guardian angels'. 'Everyone else – the guards, the camp commander, the brigadiers – constantly told the [inmates] to work harder', she notes, but the doctor alone was not obliged to do so.[53] The evidence of such 'angels' being present in Kenya is sparse, but this does not mean doctors had nothing to say on the subject.

In 1958, a paper titled 'Psychological reaction of detainees to internment and its causes' was circulated by the Director of Medical Services in the hope of instructing detention staff on how to understand the mind of the detainee. The paper, which was written by Dr A. G. Ubaya, an assistant surgeon who had been working at Mara River camps, sought to provide a guide on how to understand the behaviours and reactions of African detainees who were 'subject to [the] mental stresses inevitably associated with detention or imprisonment'.[54] Rather than relying on any form of psychological data or objective evidence, Ubaya's explanations mixed older racial ideas about the African mind with first-hand anecdotal evidence that medicalised specific acts that others may have interpreted as detainees exercising conscious resistance.

For example, uncooperative or evasive inmates were not reacting to a potentially hostile environment, they were merely expressing a form of psychological repression produced by the same innate 'primitive reflexes' that led them to join Mau Mau in the first place.

The only cure for this mental repression, Ubaya believed, was through a process of 'expression', where detainees confessed their involvement with Mau Mau to rehabilitation officers.[55] Another behaviour to fall under Ubaya's clinical gaze was the act of writing 'anonymous letters' to government officials or the press that complained about systemic abuses and poor conditions within the camps. Rather than interpreting this as a genuine point of concern or asking questions about the veracity of these claims, the assistant surgeon dismissed them: the detainees were not drawing attention to any actual incidents of abuse, but rather trying to 'remove [...] mental stress through writing'.[56] In fact, the authors were acting out of anger and guilt for having made a confession to the rehabilitation officers. What they needed, Ubaya believed, was time to reflect on their actions, to rationalise the situation and see their suffering as an outcome of their own poor behaviour.

But while Ubaya's paper dealt with several forms of detainee resistance, he spent the most time writing about malingering. According to Ubaya, detainees were like a 'spoilt child' hiding from responsibility by 'avoid[ing] the parent'. Their mental stress, brought on by the guilt of their Mau Mau crimes, eventually developed into either 'an anxiety neurosis' or 'disgruntled malingering'. The anxious neurotic, essentially a hypochondriac, turns up at the doctor's clinic insisting their everyday complaints are serious infectious diseases or other dangerous conditions. For these patients, the assistant surgeon noted, 'only a full expression or confession is the absolute cure'.[57] Then there were the disgruntled malingerers. Whereas the anxious neurotic malingered due to imagined illnesses, which Ubaya did not see as their fault, these more hostile inmates were a different matter. These individuals made up the vast majority of the camp population, Ubaya believed, and 'had no social standing, educational background nor Christian influence' prior to internment. Their level of aggression towards the colonial order led them to resist every apparent effort to help them:

> When such a person carries a psychological burden which he is unable to shed, every condition of his environment, irrespective of its nature or environment, appears distasteful. Thus every duty, whether heavy or light, every beneficial approach made to him by the Rehabilitation department, any necessary diet prescribed by the medical authorities, all are equally hateful to him.[58]

If such a disgruntled detainee cannot find a legitimate excuse to avoid work then they 'creat[e] one by easy recourse to malingering'. Ultimately, Ubaya believed, the detainee's 'unreasonable and flimsy excuses' did more harm to them than anything else as it prevented rehabilitation and a chance to resolve their unconscious stresses through confession.

While Ubaya's paper shines a rare light on the views and approaches of a doctor operating within the detention camps as well as the stern, sceptical approach to potential malingerers, it also provides some support to the claims made by the detainees at Athi River. As, according to Ubaya himself, a useful way to deal with a potential malingerer was to administer a fake dose of 'alkaline mixture as a reward for his wasted trouble and send him away as "fit"'.[59] This admission corresponds with Ubaya's wider approach, as he frequently advises on the best ways to manipulate and manoeuvre detainees who he sees as credulous and deceitful. It seems that Ubaya saw no harm in providing detainees with placebo medication, supporting the claims made by the detainees at Athi River concerning the injection of saline. While they seem to regard this as evidence of misconduct and a refusal to treat their ailments, it is possible the doctor responsible was addressing what they believed to be a case of malingering.

But why would detainees seek to avoid work? During the Emergency, all types of detainees were expected to undertake some form of labour during their incarceration, but it was in the 'hard-core' camps where the heaviest workloads were expected. Although work was seen as a fundamental step in the rehabilitation process, in many instances the situation translated into arduous forced labour. This was a preferred punitive measure for warders seeking to tame the prisoners. As the settler Sir Richard Woodley saw it, forced labour was 'slavery from dawn to dusk, on a ration sufficient to keep [the detainee] alive and working but no more'.[60] This was not new; the reliance on forced labour reflected an older colonial tradition of exploiting convicts as a source of cheap labour.[61] As a result, it was not uncommon for detainees to organise work strikes in protest to their conditions, something that the British saw as the greatest example of defiance to their authority.[62] Food restrictions and rationing, in addition to routine beatings, were often employed to break detainee resolve.[63] This was ultimately in keeping with the types of coercive methods favoured by British security and intelligence agencies in the Cold War, as will be discussed in more detail in Chapter 4. For now, it is sufficient to stress that 'underfeeding' was regarded as an easy way to enforce compliance. Although poor diets and underfeeding was a common practice within Kenyan prisons throughout the colonial period, its use against the Mau Mau brought it into alignment with postwar ideas about coercive manipulation.

It is not difficult to find instances where poor diets and restrictive rationing were used as a punishment during the Emergency. According to Fletcher's report, an unnamed Rehabilitation Officer had detainees transferred to Manyani from an unspecified camp during the early part of its existence. These individuals were 'in very poor shape physically. Very thin and appeared under-nourished'.[64] The detainees later told the Rehabilitation Officer that they were always hungry as they were only receiving half of the rations to which they were entitled. When the Rehabilitation Officer explained to the Prison Commandant at Manyani that the men could not work, the latter apparently replied 'Send them to me: I'll make them work all right'.[65] In another incident, recorded by Mohamed Mathu and Don Barnett in *The Urban Guerrilla*, a camp commander at Showground Camp, in the Nyeri District, was so fond of this type of punishment that the prisoners called him 'Famine'.[66] But it was in the complaints made by detainees themselves where we see the impact this had on their lives.

On 10 April 1956, in an effort to draw attention to their plight, detainees at Manyani sent a letter to the Secretary of State for the Colonies and a copy to the Editor of the *Daily Mirror*. The letter, handwritten on official government paper, decried the 'high tendency of discrimination in the schemes by which the detainees are fed'.[67] The detainees identified stark variations in the standard of diets offered at different camps and cited the systematic reliance on supplements, such as ascorbic acid (vitamin C) and boveast (a vitamin preparation originally designed to feed cattle in Africa), as solid evidence that detainee's diets were insufficient.[68] 'The issue of Ascorbic and Boveyeast [*sic*]', they claimed, 'is an unrefutable [*sic*] proof of the prevailing malnutrition, and the foodstuffs given contain no pinch of the required mineral constituents requisite to health'.[69] Later, on 8 June 1958, the *Observer* published a letter it had received from detainees at the camp which stated, among other grievances, that 'It now appears to us that it is the intention of the Kenya Government to starve us to death and to this we say we are prepared to fight for our human rights up to the end and we shall never give up our national struggle'.[70]

The issues caused by poor diets were raised throughout the Emergency, especially when malnutrition led to various deficiency diseases. This subject took up a significant portion of Dr Stott's report into the medical and sanitary conditions in the camps in 1954. Even at this relatively early phase of the Emergency, he raised concerns about unstandardised diets present in the different camps. According to Stott, the diet scales had been drawn up by 'the Government Biochemist' and reflected the minimal standard necessary for detainees to live well, depending on their situation. For instance, there was one diet prescribed for male and female detainees undertaking 'moderate work', one for 'hard work', which was only for men, one for 'pregnant women' and one for 'lactating women'.[71] However, Stott noted that the Prison Department had published an 'abbreviated form of this diet' in the *Kenya Gazette*, which was not wide enough in scope to apply to all areas of the colony. Although it was recommended that this be changed, 'owing to a misunderstanding in the Office of the Minister for Defence the formula became distorted'.[72] He hoped this would soon be corrected but added that some camps, especially in the Central Province, still refused to comply. By 1957, the ICRC confirmed that 'no arrangements for diet meals had been made in any of the camps'.[73]

Scurvy was a common issue throughout the Emergency, which resulted in many detainees being given 25 mg of ascorbic acid each day to supplement their poor diets. Similarly, pellagra appears to have been endemic in the camps, though admittedly at consistently low levels. The deficiency diseases was particularly present throughout the Prison and Work camps in 1954, as well as at Lokitaung in 1958.[74] In 1955, the instructions were issued to all prison and camps about the provision of boveast to counteract pellagra.[75] During their first visit, the ICRC expressed surprise at the low quantities of fats, vitamins and proteins in the government's prescribed diet and decided to follow up with Dr Demole, a lecturer in dietetics at the Faculty of Geneva, to see if the caloric value was sufficient.[76] Although it is unclear what the results of this enquiry were, concerns over the state of detainee diets remained high throughout the Emergency and were a persistent question raised by the Opposition in Parliament.[77]

'You came here to die'

The use of detention in Algeria was also a key tool in the war against the nationalists and, just as with their East African counterparts, the camps became sites of torture and suffering. In a similar move to the British authorities in Kenya, the French security forces started by arresting and confining known agitators or people they considered suspicious. They arrested the former members of the militant Organisation spéciale (OS), a paramilitary group established in 1947 to prepare for armed struggle against the French, the supporters of the nationalist politician, Messali Hadj, and members of the Algerian middle classes who supported Ferhat Abbas's more moderate nationalism. As Klose notes, the 'arrest of this [latter] political group robbed Algerian nationalism of its countervailing influences', a move that pushed the chances of a peaceful resolution into 'the distant future'.[78] The detention centres started out as the euphemistic *centres d'hébergement*, which became the central hubs from which the rest of the camp system expanded across the colony.

Initially, internment was practised with restraint while the camps were overseen by the civil authorities. Between 17 April 1956 and 7 January 1957, there were only 1,500 known cases of detention. However, this quickly changed when the military took control. Massu and the 10th Paratrooper Division arrested 950 suspects the day after they took control of Algiers and soon institutionalised a widespread carceral system to detain thousands of FLN supporters and operatives.[79] This was achieved by empowering the local prefects and the military with the extraordinary powers created by the emergency regulations, which allowed them to create the CTTs across the colony. As with their East African counterparts, these camps were ostensibly designed to sift suspected FLN members and sympathisers from the otherwise 'loyal' population. Here members of the police, army and gendarmerie took advantage of the interrogation centres to question suspects. If an individual was thought to be innocent, they were released. If not, they were transferred to the *centres d'hébergement* for long-term detention.[80] This approach was so enthusiastically embraced that, by September 1957, the military had interned around 24,000 people in Algiers alone.[81]

Officially, the camp system was to be a place of rehabilitation and re-education, just as it was in Kenya, and so the colonial and security authorities advised against the use of violence. As early as 1956, Robert Lacoste, the then Governor General of Algeria, recognised how the use of physical force on detainees would be counterproductive: eventually, he argued, the detained population would be released, and they could easily revert to nationalism again if the French authorities failed to counter the revolutionaries' propaganda.[82]

This is why re-education was crucial and best served through persuasion rather than abuse. How else could they demonstrate the virtues of French society and culture? Each camp was meant to have a member of the *action psychologique* team on hand to meet and interact with detainees as they arrived. Speed was of the utmost importance here but so was a light touch, as General Raoul Salan, the then Commander-in-Chief of the French forces in Algeria, made clear: 'the contact, by erasing fear of death or ill-treatment, can provoke a "reaction" during which the interested person indulges without reluctance'.[83] This, he believed, was the only way to convince rebels of the 'the vanity of their cause'. Later, in 1958, the General even advocated treating some rebels caught in action as worthy of a status similar to official prisoners of war, but this was not to be extended to those deemed to be actively engaging in terrorism.[84] For Salan, these captured militants could still be re-educated and turned to French military service as potential Harkis (Algerian Muslims who sided with the French) or at least they could be made to conform as model colonial citizens: 'We must, therefore, use the time of detention to teach the cause of France to the internees and to transform them into convinced partisans of New French Algeria', he stated in a directive in March 1958.

In reality, the detention centres were sites of explicit cruelty and violence. In the CTTs, detainees were essentially held for indeterminate amounts of time and circulated between different camps. Each time they arrived in a new camp, they were interrogated again, which meant an individual could be tortured numerous times while imprisoned. In addition to the officially 'known' centres, there were also secret and semi-secret centres, some of which were privately owned, along with mobile centres that consisted of tents to be used during operations.[85] As with Kenya, there was a distinct difference between what was *officially* permitted and expected, and what actually happened on the ground. The same is true for the state of medical treatment within this system of incarceration.

'Unsuitable for housing human beings'

The relationship between medicine and military was more complicated than it was in Kenya, as civilian and military boundaries were blurred to a greater extent. Medical oversight of the *centres d'hébergement* was meant to lie with civil authorities, while the other centres were run by the military. In addition, both sets of institutions were expected to transfer any serious or chronic patents, as well as any suspected cases of epidemic disease, to the nearest civilian hospital.[86] The result was a division of medical oversight within the Algerian context, with the civilian and military authorities working in tandem to deal with their respected detainees while relying on the hospitals for support. This connection will be explored in more detail in subsequent chapters, but it is important to note here that, although there had always been a tacit relationship between military and civilian healthcare providers in the French colony, the power dynamic between the two shifted significantly in favour of the former during the Emergency. The military also took advantage of its connections with the hospitals, especially those operated by the army even during peacetime, which allowed them to use their facilities as improvised interrogation centres.[87] In the process, they co-opted resources, equipment and, willingly or otherwise, hospital staff for their purposes.

There are a few closely related reasons why this relationship is so distinct to the situation in East Africa. Firstly, hospitals were less common in Kenya and the remote nature of the camps may have made it impractical for detainees to be transported across large regions of open country to the nearest facility. This often meant that, as we have seen in the larger camps like Manyani and Mackinnon Road, there were rudimentary hospital wards and isolation options for both chronically ill detainees and those with infectious diseases, such as tuberculosis and typhoid. Although it is certainly true that Mau Mau detainees would sometimes be transferred to hospitals if their condition was urgent, it is not clear how often this happened nor how this arrangement was managed.[88] The relationship between detention and hospitals in Kenya was therefore more ad hoc. In Algeria, however, hospitals played an established and prominent role in detainee treatment.

Secondly, given that the Algerian War was also in part an urban war, there was increased military activity around towns and cities, which could have made it easier, and probably cheaper, for them to interact with hospitals. The extent to which the military relied on hospitals is most evident towards the end of the conflict in January 1962, when the Prefect Director of the National Security in Algeria wrote to Commander Guyard to complain about the inadequate methods being used in the camps to track detainees transferred to hospital. This, the Director felt, made it difficult to properly track the costs incurred for their treatment and who had responsibility for paying.[89]

This tripartite relationship between the civilian-run camps, the military and the hospitals may also explain why the Algerian detention system did not suffer any serious outbreaks of epidemic disease throughout the Emergency. According to the existing evidence gathered by both the military and the ICRC reports, there does not seem to be any sign of an equivalent epidemic to the typhoid crisis that plagued Kenya throughout 1954. However, this should not suggest that the camps in Algeria, especially the CTTs, were healthy locations. Indeed, infectious disease was a constant concern for the detainees, and many conditions, as with Kenya, were endemic throughout the camp system, as will be shown below. Nor should we assume, just because the camp authorities had the ability to transfer patients to hospitals for urgent care or isolation, that they always did so.

The camps in Algeria, as with their Kenyan counterparts, were often overcrowded and primitive locations. It is true that some were built in places that could accommodate larger numbers of detainees, such as in old forts, abandoned barracks or, in the case of the *centre d'hébergement* at Lodi, a summer camp, but others were rapidly and poorly developed with wooden structures or tents planted in the desert and cordoned off by barbed wire.[90] The conditions within the camps therefore varied in location and across time. Even the governmental agency responsible for overseeing the civilian camps, the Service central des centres d'hébergement, admitted on 17 August 1956 that the conditions at the camps were often far from perfect.[91]

One of the recurrent issues for the civilian camps was the staffing. It was often difficult for the commanders of the *centres d'hébergement* to find doctors willing to work at the sites on a permanent basis. This meant there were regularly large gaps between medical visits as the authorities relied on visiting civilian practitioners to travel great distances to treat inmates. This situation was a point of concern for the Service central des centres d'hébergement, as many of these visiting physicians had to use isolated roads that made them vulnerable during the 'insecurities' of the Emergency. Still, these doctors were meant to visit no 'less than three [times] per week'.[92] In contrast, the military camps were overseen by the Commandants, who were responsible for maintaining hygiene and sanitation. This involved providing detainees with adequate bedding and sufficient food. They were also meant to ensure camp discipline and to protect detainees from abuse.[93] When it came to medicine, the military camps were administered by the local military doctor. These individuals had complete control of all medical and health-related decisions in the camps. They not only decided how detainees were treated but, more importantly, whether they could be transferred to a hospital.[94] These individuals could therefore act as gatekeepers between the harsh realities of camp life and the 'relative' safety of a hospital.

A significant issue, which seems to have had more of an impact on the Algerian detainees than Mau Mau ones, was discomfort generated by the local climate, especially in the desert regions. An example of how intolerable such conditions could be is summed up in tragic detail by Nadji Abbas Tarqui, a detainee who was arrested in his home in March 1957. Tarqui, like many others, made his way through various detention camps during his internment where he and his fellow inmates were subjected to beatings and torture, but while detained at Paul-Cazelles, a military camp, Tarqui also experienced the harshness of the desert climate:

> This desolate region, very hot during the day, is freezing at night. Our old, worn tents, perforated with countless holes, also bear tears that the camp administration never bothered to have repaired. Thus, a few days after my arrival, showers fell at night on the camp. In the morning, we found ourselves covered with a layer of solidified hail.[95]

If this was not miserable enough, Tarqui's account adds that the detainees also had to contend with infestations of various pests and dangerous animals, such as 'rats which swarm at night, scorpions and vipers which show themselves more during the day, and finally fleas and lice'.[96]

There were other contemporary reports that drew specific attention to the intolerable conditions in the camps. In 1956, the magazine *Saturne*, published by the International Commission Against Concentration Camps (CICRC), reported many details that were similar to those Tarqui experienced. For example, in the camp at Aïn el Amara, located in a desert about 400 miles south of Algiers, the CICRC noted how the temperatures regularly reached 45 to 50 °C 'in the shade', and then plummeted during the nights. The report added that, at the time, the number of inmates in the camp was manageable, but if they increased then it would put a severe strain on the amount of water available for everyone.[97] Similarly, at the camp at Guelt Es Stel, around a hundred kilometres from Boghar, south-west of Algiers, the inmates were plagued by scorpions and had to content with the desert winds that buffeted their tents, sending sand and dust into every corner.[98]

The inhospitable climate was not the only concern raised in this report. At the camp in Aflou, the CICRC explained, sick detainees were neglected and left 'shivering with fever in their beds', their only treatment being 'aspirin tablets'. At the same time 'poor old people crippled with rheumatism' were left to suffer with no aid.[99] The report added that at the camp at M'sila, which they regarded as 'by far the worst' camp, the detainees frequently reported being beaten, extorted for labour and insufficiently fed. In fact, it seems the prescribed rations were drastically cut from '200 grams of pasta to 25 or 30 grams'. The report added that 'many internees were ill, and if no provision was made for them, it was certain death for several of them'.[100] Tarqui made similar observations while held at Paul-Cazelles, where a 'number of tuberculosis patients were subjected to the common diet'. Not only were these individuals not in isolation, they were visibly 'wasting away'. Tarqui added that 'some dared to complain to the chief guard, who answered them in these terms: "you came here to die" '.[101]

Far from being an isolated situation, negligence towards sick detainees was quite common. According to a telegram written by the detainees, some of whom were themselves doctors, at a camp in Berrouaghia, south of Algiers, the 'concentration camp' was overcrowded, with 700 inmates who ranged from 'sixteen to eighty', including several invalids 'from all social strata' living in 'deplorable hygienic conditions'. In particular, detainees with tuberculosis, diabetes and cardiac issues were left to suffer with minimal care and were not transferred to the hospitals. Moreover, the visiting doctor only saw patients for four hours every two weeks, while the site itself had an 'insufficient stock of medicines'. If patients wanted specific treatment, the internees claimed, they had to pay for it themselves.[102] Finally, in January 1956, the former director of the camp at Djorf published a letter in *Témoignage chrétien* and then in *Le Monde* which decried the situation he saw in that camp. According to this letter, in addition to miserable living conditions, disease was rife, with 'dysentery reigning in this camp' and internees 'afflicted with chronic tuberculosis and various other contagious diseases without any provision being made for their isolation'.[103]

In many ways, the situation at Djorf symbolises the conditions within the camps more generally. Throughout the War, this camp was consistently described as unhygienic and as a breeding ground for infection.[104] But in late 1961, the situation became so drastic that the French authorities had to take notice. What is particularly telling about this case, however, is that the whistle-blowers were not only a group of doctors who had been interned at the camp, they were also European, a fact that confused and surprised the ICRC.[105] The details of their account were damning but familiar.

On 14 September 1961, seven doctors from both France and Algeria described the situation they faced in Djorf. They explained how, having been detained 'against [their] will', they were interned with 200 others 'without any specific reason having been given to us'.[106] Djorf was located, as they said, 'in a near-desert area in the extreme south of the department of Sétif on a dusty plateau' which was 'open to all winds, exposed to intense sunshine, practically without vegetation' and 'where the risks of heatstroke, sunstroke and dehydration are very serious'.[107]

According to the doctors, the facilities at the camp were 'in a deplorable state and unsuitable for housing human beings worthy of the name'. They were cramped, covered in dust and dirt, and, so the doctors claimed, could not be cleaned due to 'the absence of water'. The overcrowded conditions and the poor quality of space created 'a suffocating and exhausting atmosphere preventing rest and sleep'. There was no fixed lighting in most of the blocks, the bins were ripped open and 'garbage scattered around' and the latrines were 'insufficient', with excrement left out to 'attract flies and parasites'.[108]

It is no surprise that the doctors claimed to witness evidence of serious infection in the camp. Firstly, there was no running water, so the entire supply for all the camp inhabitants came from storage tanks that were described as 'insufficient'. Despite only being given small quantities to drink, the imprisoned professionals reported their first case of diarrhoea within 24 hours of being interned. More concerning, however, was the presence of other diseases. The doctors 'detected, among other things, three forms of tuberculosis which, in addition to the risks they run personally, can contaminate those around them'.[109] As with other camps, the elderly and infirm were left to suffer without any support and, despite their qualifications, the doctors were unable to treat their fellow inmates because they had no access to an 'infirmary, nor medicine, nor medical equipment of any kind'.

The seven doctors concluded that all 'these elements create morally and physically dangerous living conditions for the internees'. Soon, they argued, the lamentable conditions would cause serious epidemics, not just of tuberculosis, but also typhus due to the prevalence of 'parasites' in the camp, typhoid and dysentery due to the unclean water supply, and 'contagious dermatosis' due to the proximity of so many people crowded together.[110] Ultimately, they reasoned:

> Such living conditions sadly reminded us of the concentration camps against which many of us once fought in the hope of seeing them abolished. They are incompatible with the most elementary human dignity. They are all the more inadmissible for people who have committed neither crimes nor misdemeanours and whose only fault is perhaps to love their country too much.

Throughout the emergency, various detainees and concerned parties outside the military tried to raise awareness as to the plight of those residing in the camps, but they rarely succeeded in affecting meaningful change. We will discuss some of the more high-profile cases in subsequent chapters, but it is telling that the final nail in the coffin for the story of Djorf should be made by European doctors who encountered the realities of Algerian detention, even though they themselves were not subjected to torture like many of their Muslim counterparts. At no other point in the war did a set of complaints lead to such quick reactions.

The letter caused an outcry, especially from fellow doctors, who took up the pen in defence of the seven convicts. At the end of September that year, the President of the Departmental Council of Medicine of Bône wrote to the President of the ICRC to plead for an investigation into the conditions at Djorf and for the ICRC to intercede with the French Government to 'put an end to this scandalous situation'.[111] Then, on 2 October 1961, representatives of the Federation of Medical Unions of Algeria, as well as representatives of the Ordinal and Trade Union Professional Organisations of Dental Surgeons and Pharmacists of the Igamie of Algiers, gathered in an 'extraordinary assembly' to condemn the situation. They stated that they were '[p]ainfully affected by the alarming news of those of their own who share the life and the risks of the human beings detained in the Djorf camp' and were 'appalled by the realities of their precarious living conditions'. The representatives called on the 'Public Authorities' to make every effort to 'ensure that the treatment of these French people' was 'quickly humanised'.[112]

Eventually, in October 1961, a French government commission visited Djorf and witnessed the conditions for themselves, which led them to recommend closing the camp.[113] Although word of the hardships experienced by the Algerian detainees held within the wider camp system had regularly appeared within press reports, it was the plight experienced by European doctors, these 'French people', that aroused their concern. It is notable that at no point in their letters to the ICRC do they raise objection to reports of torture that had been rife for many years prior to this, nor do they express additional concerns for the Muslim population of these institutes more generally. These doctors, in the end, were mostly concerned with protecting their own.

Conclusion

This chapter has explored the nature of medicine within the networks of detention camps in Kenya and Algeria. As has been well known for some time, these locations were a far cry from being the humanitarian facilities they were 'officially' intended to be. In reality, the detention camps in both East and North Africa were often primitive, overcrowded locations that were diseased and punitive in nature. Yet, the role medicine played in supporting such conditions, and how medical professionals operated on a day-to-today basis, has rarely been considered despite their consistent presence in many aspects of everyday camp life. Contrary to much of the existing historiography on the subject, the detention camps in both Kenya and Algeria were often fitted with medical facilities, to a greater or lesser extent, and doctors featured in multiple aspects of the camps' administration, frequently in ways that were fundamental to their operation.

In the Kenyan pipeline, conditions became difficult after Operation Anvil, which put unprecedented pressure on the already disorganised and poorly funded rehabilitation system. The impacts were fast-hitting with the emergence of the typhoid epidemic that spread through the main camps that year, even though the colonial authorities had been warned that the sanitation measures in many camps were not suitable and were liable to lead to disaster. But while a doctor had tried to draw some internal attention to the pending crisis, once it broke out, the Colonial Medical Department added to the Government's culture of denial by covering up the true extent of the crisis. This outbreak, its severity and the fact it was known to the public, is a unique element of the Kenya Emergency when compared to Algeria. Although there was certainly a significant and consistent level of disease in the North African camps, there was no comparable epidemic in that context.

The typhoid outbreak revealed many of the fault lines within the nascent camp system, many of which would persist throughout the Emergency, but it was one of the rare instances where medical practitioners actively tried to improve conditions in the camps, though these efforts remained limited and mostly confined to internal discussions among the colonial authorities. In most instances, the doctors who attended the camps were either unaware of the true levels of privation surrounding them or they did not care. In many ways this indicates a culture of mistrust that was persistent within the detention camps and cut both ways. In particular, Dr Ubaya's instructions on how to deal with and manipulate recalcitrant and malingering detainees – or at least those perceived to be malingering – goes some way to illustrate how detainee complaints could be dismissed by unsympathetic doctors and potentially, in the case of Stephen Kiunjuri, to fatal consequences.

Malingering was a concern for the colonial authorities as it represented a form of resistance whereby detainees attempted to avoid the hard exploitative labour they were required to conduct as part of their incarceration. In this instance, doctors played a vital role as agents of this exploitation, as they were the only ones who could distinguish between legitimate illness and fraudulence. These same individuals were responsible for monitoring detainees' fitness to work, which extended to their diets. But heavy rationing and starvation were common forms of punishment in Kenya prisons generally, and it was a tactic used with impunity within the detention camps. As such, many detainees were extremely malnourished and suffering from deficiency diseases such as scurvy and pellagra.

In Algeria, the overall situation was not dissimilar. The network of camps in North Africa were equally deprived and unsophisticated. In fact, in some cases where they consisted of simple tents and barbed wire fences, they appear to be more so than in Kenya. This issue could be explained by disparities in how detention camps were run in this context. Whereas the Kenyan pipeline was overseen by the civilian authorities with no interference from the military, responsibility for the camps in Algeria was split between civilian control and the military, with both relying on the hospitals (civilian and military) as needed. This division of control was frequently blurred throughout the war, but it also meant the standards of provision within the camps were dangerously inconsistent. Moreover, the necessities of the ongoing war often meant that the military could make demands of the civilian institutes for its own purposes.

Another feature of camp life in Algeria, one that seems to have been more frequently cited as a source of complaint by the detainees and concerned organisations like the CICRC and the ICRC, was the ambient conditions surrounding the different camps. In particular, camps located within desert regions were often too hot for habitation and had poor water supplies. At night, the temperatures in these areas would plummet, causing additional complaints among the detainees. Then there were the plagues of insects and venomous animals, such as snakes and scorpions. The military-run CTTs were particularly horrendous locations and were not only inhospitable and unhygienic, they were also home to detainees suffering from debilitating, chronic and often contagious diseases. Multiple reports addressing the conditions within these camps pointed out how sick people were left without appropriate support and were not taken to hospital, despite there being provisions in place to enable these transfers. As with Kenya, it seems that there was just a culture of negligence within these camps whereby the authorities in charge turned a blind eye to the suffering they perpetuated.

The camp at Djorf was an illustrated representation of the issues that occurred throughout the war, but it also serves as a reminder of the racial factors that underpinned much of the conflict. The camp was consistently criticised for its poor standards of care for its detainees but the situation only received cogent attention when the conditions threatened the health of white European doctors who were interned there towards the end. Their letter highlighting the plight of the detainees finally led to the camp being closed in 1962, but it only occurred because European doctors were now the ones being subjected to its abuses.

Notes

1 Elkins, *Britain's Gulag*, pp. 35–36.
2 Elkins, *Britain's Gulag*, p. 63.
3 Hansard, House of Commons Debate. 'Kenya (anti-Mau Mau operations)', Henry Hopkinson, 28 April 1954, paragraphs 1620–1621.
4 Caroline Elkins, 'Alchemy of evidence: Mau Mau, the British Empire, and the High Court of Justice', *Journal of Imperial and Commonwealth History* 39 (2011), p. 734.
5 Anderson, *Histories of the Hanged*, pp. 200–203; Klose, *Human Rights in the Shadow of Colonial Violence*, p. 156.
6 Anderson, *Histories of the Hanged*, p. 203.
7 Anderson, *Histories of the Hanged*, p. 313.
8 Anderson, *Histories of the Hanged*, p. 313.

9 Anderson, *Histories of the Hanged*, p. 313.
10 Anderson, *Histories of the Hanged*, p. 313.
11 William Baldwin, *Mau Mau Man-hunt: The Adventures of the Only American Who Has Fought the Terrorist in Kenya* (New York: Dutton, 1957), p. 183.
12 This latter illness was brought about by a deficiency in vitamin B3 and resulted in dermatitis, diarrhoea, and mental disturbances.
13 TNA CO 822/801/244. Dr H. G. Waters, 'Public Health Report – Manyani Camp', 9 May 1954.
14 TNA CO 822/801/244. Waters, 'Public Health Report – Manyani Camp', p. 4.
15 TNA CO 822/801/2. Press Office Handout No. 568: 'Medical Arrangements at Detention Camps', 10 May 1954.
16 TNA CO 822/801/2. Press Office Handout No. 568.
17 TNA CO 822/801/2. Press Office Handout No. 568.
18 TNA CO 822/801/2. Press Office Handout No. 568.
19 TNA CO 822/801. Anonymous, 'Typhoid – Manyani Camp', 13 October 1954.
20 TNA FCO 141/6166/115a. Secret Registry File, 7 August 1954.
21 TNA CO 822/801/2. Press Office Handout No. 568.
22 TNA CO 822/801/2. Press Office Handout No. 568.
23 TNA CO 822/801. 'Manyani Camp Typhoid Epidemic: Report by Director of Medical Services', 13 October 1954.
24 Anonymous, 'Knife attack repulsed: Man's Escape from Mau Mau', *Manchester Guardian*, 21 September 1954.
25 Anonymous, 'Knife attack repulsed: Man's Escape from Mau Mau', *Manchester Guardian*, 21 September 1954.
26 TNA CO 822/801. Anonymous, 'Typhoid – Manyani Camp', 13 October 1954.
27 Anderson, *Histories of the Hanged*, p. 318.
28 TNA CO 822/801. Dr Stott, 'Typhoid Outbreak at Manyani', 14 September 1954.
29 TNA CO 822/801. Anonymous, 'Typhoid – Manyani Camp', 13 October 1954.
30 Anderson, *Histories of the Hanged*, p. 319; Fabian Klose, *Human Rights in the Shadow of Colonial Violence*, p. 158.
31 Anderson, *Histories of the Hanged*, p. 319.
32 TNA CO 822/801/18. Letter from the Assistant Secretary of the Socialist Medical Association to Alan Lennox-Boyd, 28 September 1954.
33 Hansard, House of Commons Debate. 'Manyani Camp', Mr Lennox-Boyd MP, 20 October 1954, paragraphs 1192–1193.

34 Eileen Fletcher, *The Truth About Kenya: An Eye Witness Account* (London: Movement for Colonial Freedom, 1956).
35 Fletcher, *The Truth About Kenya.*
36 SOAS CBMS, Eileen Fletcher, 'Report on my period of employment in the community development department of the Kenya Government', 24 July 1956, p. 12.
37 Klose, *Human Rights in the Shadow of Colonial Violence*, p. 161.
38 London School of Tropical Medicine Archive (LSTM), GB 0809 Nutrition/17/01/04/02. Hugh Stott, 'Report on Health and hygiene in Emergency Camps', 1954, p. 1.
39 LSTM, GB 0809 Nutrition/17/01/04/02. Hugh Stott, 'Report on Health and hygiene in Emergency Camps', 1954, p. 4.
40 LSTM, GB 0809 Nutrition/17/01/04/02. Stott, 'Report on Health and hygiene in Emergency Camps', p. 2.
41 LSTM, GB 0809 Nutrition/17/01/04/02. Stott, 'Report on Health and hygiene in Emergency Camps', p. 2.
42 LSTM, GB 0809 Nutrition/17/01/04/02. Stott, 'Report on Health and hygiene in Emergency Camps', p. 3.
43 LSTM, GB 0809 Nutrition/17/01/04/02. Stott, 'Report on Health and hygiene in Emergency Camps', p. 3.
44 Klose, *Human Rights in the Shadow of Colonial Violence*, pp. 131–132.
45 ACICR B AG 251 108–007. 'General Report on the Mission of the International Committee of the Red Cross to Kenya, February 20 – April 18 1957', pp. 15–16.
46 ACICR B AG 251 108–007. 'General Report on the Mission of the International Committee of the Red Cross to Kenya', p. 16.
47 ACICR B AG 251 108–007. Dr Louis Gailland, 'Rapport General', 11 April 1957, p. 13.
48 Klose, *Human Rights in the Shadow of Colonial Violence*, p. 128.
49 TNA FCO 141/5667/57. Letter from detainees, 20 January 1954.
50 TNA FCO 141/5667/57. Letter from detainees, pp. 5–6.
51 TNA FCO 141/5667/57. Commissioner of Prisons, 'Detainee's Petition, 23 January 1954, p. 2.
52 TNA CO 822/1267. Record of the Proceedings of an Enquiry under Colonial Regulation 60 into Charges against Superintendent M.G. Sullivan, M.B.E., and Assistant Superintendent A.C. Coutts, both of the Kenya Prison Service, 7 July 1959, p. 11.
53 Anne Applebaum, *Gulag: A History of Soviet Camps* (London and New York: Penguin Books, 2003), p. 337.
54 TNA. FCO 141/6519/200. A. G. Ubaya, 'Psychological Reaction of Detainees to Internment and Its Causes: As a Doctor Sees it', p. 2.

55 TNA FCO 141/6519/200. Ubaya, 'Psychological Reaction of Detainees to Internment and Its Causes', p. 3.
56 TNA FCO 141/6519/200. Ubaya, 'Psychological Reaction of Detainees to Internment and Its Causes', p. 7.
57 TNA FCO 141/6519/200. Ubaya, 'Psychological Reaction of Detainees to Internment and Its Causes', p. 7.
58 TNA FCO 141/6519/200. Ubaya, 'Psychological Reaction of Detainees to Internment and Its Causes', p. 7.
59 TNA FCO 141/6519/200. Ubaya, 'Psychological Reaction of Detainees to Internment and Its Causes', p. 10.
60 Woodley quoted in Robert B. Edgerton, *Mau Mau: An African Crucible* (New York: Free Press, 1989), p. 80.
61 Florence Bernault, 'The shadow of rule: colonial power and modern punishment in Africa', in Frank Dikötter and Ian Brown (eds), *Cultures of Confinement: A History of the Prison in Africa, Asia, and Latin America* (New York: Cornell University Press, 2007), pp. 71–72.
62 Anderson, *Histories of the Hanged*, p. 317.
63 Klose, *Human Rights in the Shadow of Colonial Violence*, p. 158.
64 Fletcher, *The Truth About Kenya*.
65 Fletcher, *The Truth About Kenya*.
66 Mohamed Mathu, recorded by Don Barnett, *Urban Guerrilla: The Story of Mohamed Mathu* (Richmond, BC: LSM Press, 1974), p. 79.
67 TNA FCO 141/5667. The Secretary of Defence, 'Irregular Correspondence: Manyani Camp', 4 May 1956.
68 TNA FCO 141/5667. 'Petition on Detainees [*sic*] Grievances', 10 April 1956, pp. 1–2.
69 TNA FCO 141/5667. 'Petition on Detainees [*sic*] Grievances', p. 2.
70 Hansard, House of Commons Debate. 'Kenya (Prisoners, Lokitaung)', Mr Patrick Wall MP, 16 June 1958, paragraphs 854–855.
71 Stott, 'Report on Health and Hygiene in Emergency Camps', Appendix 3.
72 Stott, 'Report on Health and Hygiene in Emergency Camps', p. 13.
73 ACICR B AG 251 108–007. 'General Report on the Mission of the International Committee of the Red Cross to Kenya', p. 13.
74 TNA FCO 141/6777. 'Decode of Telegram to Secretary of State: Your Telegram No. 460, Lokitaung', 7 July 1958.
75 TNA FCO 141/6777. 'Parliamentary Question At (d/93)', 7 July 1958.
76 ACICR B AG 251 108–007. Gaillard, 'Rapport General', p. 9.
77 Hansard, House of Commons Debate. 'Prisons and Detention Camps, Kenya', Barabara Castle MP, 24 February 1958, paragraphs 1040–1041.

78 Klose, *Human Rights in the Shadow of Colonial Violence*, p. 163.
79 Jacques Vergès, Michel Zavrian, and Maurice Courrégé, *Les Disparus. Le Cahier vert* (Lausanne: La Cité, 1959), pp. 95–105.
80 SHD 1H 1492/2. Raoul Salan, 'Note de Service', 3 June 1957, p. 1.
81 This figure was stated by Paul Teitgen, the Police Prefect of Algiers, who recorded it in his resignation letter in 1956, when he objected to the frequent use of torture by the military. He also noted that, as well as the people in detention, an additional 3,024 individuals were 'missing'. Klose, *Human Rights in the Shadow of Colonial Violence*, p. 164; Aussaresses, *The Battle of the Casbah*, p. 163.
82 ACICR B AG 225 008–003. Robert Lacoste, 'Circulaire', 23 August 1956.
83 SHD 1H 1492/2. Raoul Salan, 'Note de Service', 3 June 1957, p. 5.
84 SHD 1H258 D1. 'Rebelles fait prisonniers les armes à la main. Camps d'internes militaires', 10 March 1958.
85 Lazreg, *Torture and the Twilight of Empire*, p. 48.
86 SHD 1 H 1492/2. Colonel Boyer Vidal, 'Note d'Information sur le règlement des problèmes des personnels assignes à résidence surveillée dans les centres militaires', 27 April 1959, pp. 4–5.
87 Colonel Vidal, the Inspector General of the detention centres in Algeria, explicitly noted that rebels injured when captured could be taken to the nearest military hospital for initial treatment, before being transferred to a CCT. SHD 1 H 1492/2. Vidal, 'Note d'Information sur le règlement des problèmes des personnels assignes à résidence surveillée dans les centres militaires', 27 April 1959, pp. 4–5.
88 As was allegedly the case with Stephen Kiunjuri, who was apparently taken to hospital, where he died, contrary to what his fellow detainees recorded in their petition to the British Government. TNA FCO 141 5667. 'Detainees' Petition', 23 January 1954, p. 2.
89 SHD 1H 1492-1. Prefect Director of the National Security in Algeria, 'Assignés des CH et CTT Hospitalisés', 18 January 1962.
90 Sylvie Thénault, 'Personnel et internés dans les camps français de la guerre d'Algérie. Entre stéréotypes coloniaux et combat pour l'indépendance', *Politix* 69 (2005), p. 66.
91 ACICR, B AG 225 008-002. Director of the Service central des centres d'hébergement, 'Situation des Assignés à Résidence', 17 August 1956.
92 ACICR B AG 225 008-002. The Director of Services Central des Centres d'Hébergement, 'Situation des Assignés à Résidence', 17 August 1956, pp. 3–4.
93 SHD 1H 1492/2. Raoul Salan, 'Note de Service', 3 June 1957, p. 4.
94 SHD 1H 1492/2. Raoul Salan, 'Note de Service', 3 June 1957, p. 5.

95 Testimony of Nadji Abbas Tarqui, in Hafid Keramane, *La Pacification. Livre noir de six années de guerre en Algérie* (Paris: Les Petits Matins, 2013), p. 126.
96 Testimony of Nadji Abbas Tarqui, *La Pacification*, p. 126.
97 CICRC report on the situation at Aïn el Amara, in Robert Barrat and Denise Barrat, Algérie, 1956, *Livre blanc sur la répression* (La Tour-d'Aigues: Editions de l'aube, 2001), pp. 28–29.
98 CICRC report on the situation at Guelt Es Stel, in Barrat and Barrat, *Livre blanc*, p. 29.
99 CICRC report on the situation at the camp at Aflou, in Barrat and Barrat, *Livre blanc*, p. 26.
100 CICRC report on the situation at the camp at M'sila, in Barrat and Barrat, *Livre blanc*, p. 31.
101 Testimony of Nadji Abbas Tarqui, *La Pacification*, p. 125.
102 A telegram from the interns at Berrouaghia, 1956, in Barrat and Barrat, *Livre blanc*, p. 41.
103 'Le Directeur d'un camp s'indigne des conditions faites aux détenus', 6 January 1956, in Barrat and Barrat, *Livre blanc*, pp. 43–44.
104 In addition to the complaints raised by individuals like Tarqui, the ICRC also believed that Djorf needed 'improvements' to its 'hygiene measures' and overall water supply when they visited in 1956. ACICR, B AG 255 008-004.02. 'Mission du Comité International De La Croix-Rouge en Algérie. May to June 1956', pp. 4–5.
105 ACICR, B AG 255-008-032. Paul Gaillard, 'Plainte relative au camp de Djorf', 2 October 1961.
106 ACICR, B AG 255-008-032. Letter from seven doctors held at Djorf camp, 14 September 1961.
107 ACICR, B AG 255-008-032. Letter from seven doctors held at Djorf camp, pp. 1–3.
108 ACICR, B AG 255-008-032. Letter from seven doctors held at Djorf camp.
109 ACICR, B AG 255-008-032. Letter from seven doctors held at Djorf camp, p. 3.
110 ACICR, B AG 255-008-032. Letter from seven doctors held at Djorf camp, p. 3.
111 ACICR, B AG 255-008-032. Letter from the President of the Departmental Council of Physicians of Böne to the President of the ICRC, 27 September 1961.
112 ACICR, B AG 255-008-032. Letter from representatives of the Federation of Medical Unions of Algeria sent to the President of the ICRC, 5 October 1961.
113 Klose, *Human Rights in the Shadow of Colonial Violence*, p. 165.

4

First, do no harm?

Torture and postwar medical ethics

In 1847, Victor Hugo, the French poet and novelist, asserted that torture had 'ceased to exist'.[1] From the eighteenth to the early nineteenth century, statutory abolition of torture in criminal law had swept through virtually all of Europe. In this time, the evaluation of evidence on its own merits replaced the need for forced confessions. Yet by the 1920s, torture had reappeared. Under Hitler's Third Reich and Stalin's Soviet Union, along with fascist Italy and Spain, brutal force returned to interrogation rooms across Europe. Old techniques were updated by new methods to expand the intensity and diversity of pain. As a consequence of the extensive use of this form of violence and other grave violations against human rights during the Second World War, the international community sought to establish an absolute ban on torture in a series of new international human rights conventions, treaties and international laws. Yet while documents like the United Nations' Universal Declaration of Human Rights, passed on 10 December 1948, and the codification of the European Convention on Human Rights (ECHR) in 1950 sought to enact a general ban on torture, it was not until the creation of the Declaration of Tokyo in 1975, as mentioned in the Introduction to this book, that the medical community received one specifically addressing interrogation and torture. Nevertheless, it is worth examining the evolution of international medical codes of conduct in the immediate postwar period as they provide a foundation for understanding how medical involvement in violent interrogation and torture detracted from international norms.

In September 1947, the newly formed WMA held its first official meeting in Paris. At this meeting, the WMA devoted 'some time to the consideration [of the] betrayal of the traditions of Medicine' by the Nazi doctors who served in the concentration and death camps during the Second World War. Representatives of the medical profession from across the world attended the meeting to condemn German doctors who had conducted widescale human experiments that took place without the prisoner-subjects' consent and often resulted in their deaths as a planned outcome.[2] At the meeting, particular attention was paid to the findings of what is commonly referred to as the Nuremberg Doctors' Trial, which started on 9 December 1946. The Doctors' Trial exposed and judged the attitudes and atrocities apparently committed in the name of medical science by Nazi doctors. At its conclusion on 20 August 1947, sixteen physician-scientists were found guilty of gross human rights violations, of whom seven were executed. Responding to the results of the Doctors' Trial, the WMA sought a number of ways to prevent such atrocities and professional shame from occurring again. One of these was to reconsider the Hippocratic Oath, which, it was felt, was being taken for granted 'in many medical schools'. The WMA therefore argued that 'the restoration of the taking of the *Hippocratic Oath* or of a suitable modern substitute as a serious part of the graduation or licensing ceremony would help to impress on newly qualified doctors the fundamental ethics of medicine and to raise the general standard of professional conduct'.[3]

The problem with the Hippocratic Oath was that its loose and vague language could be used to justify inhumane activities, such as when Karl Brandt, the Nazi physician, defended the Nazi euthanasia programme as an extension of Hippocratic ethics.[4] As such, the WMA devised the Declaration of Geneva to modernise it and to be taken by new doctors 'at the time of being admitted as a member of the medical profession', so that they could pledge their '[lives] to the service of humanity'.[5] With the Declaration, the doctor vows that 'the health of my patient will be my first consideration', to 'respect the secrets which are confided in me', not to 'permit considerations of religion, nationality, race, party, politics or social standing to intervene between my duties and my patient' and to 'maintain the utmost respect for human life from the time of conception; even under threat, I will not use my medical knowledge contrary to the laws of humanity'.[6] The rest of the Declaration pledges doctors to respect their teachers, to practice their profession with dignity, to maintain the profession's honour and traditions and to ensure fraternity among its members.

A year later, in October 1949, at the Third General Assembly in London, the WMA adopted the International Code of Medical Ethics into which the Declaration of Geneva was to be incorporated. The International Code is subdivided into three parts. Under the first section, labelled 'Duties of Doctors in General', the International Code sought to protect the standard of professional conduct. In particular, it addressed the anxieties expressed by the Medical Chamber of Western Germany at the first General Assembly by codifying as unethical any collaboration 'in any form of medical service in which the doctor does not have professional independence'.[7] Physicians were to be free from institutional control, such as the state. When it came to patient care, the International Code stated that 'Any act, or advice which could weaken physical or mental resistance of a human being may be used only in his interests'. The relationship between doctors and their patients was further outlined in the second section, 'Duties of the Doctor to the Sick'. The doctor 'must always bear in mind the obligation of preserving human life'; 'A doctor owes to his patient complete loyalty and all the resources of his science [...]'; 'A doctor shall preserve absolute secrecy on all he knows about his patient because of the confidence entrusted in him'; and 'A doctor must give emergency care as a humanitarian duty unless he is assured that others are willing and able to give such care'.[8]

Together, the Declaration of Geneva and the International Code of Medical Ethics represented an updated version of the Hippocratic ideal of *primum non nocere* [first, do no harm]. They reaffirmed the responsibility to protect life and to refrain from causing harm as fundamental principles of medical conduct, as had been the case with the Hippocratic Oath. Not only were doctors forbidden from undertaking any act that might weaken the physical and mental resistance of a human being, not necessarily just their patients, they were also to preserve life when it was in their power to do so and to guard the secrets entrusted to them by their patients. However, there were a number of limitations to these codes. Firstly, they held little standing within the legal community. Secondly, as George J. Annas and Michael A. Grodin point out, these two updated codes were consistent with the wider 'physician-protection' goals of the WMA.[9] In these codes, the physician's rights held greater weight than patients' rights. An older sense of medical paternalism, expressed as 'the doctor knows best', was allowed to persist. For example, while a doctor may have been expected to forgo any act or advice that might weaken their patient's physical and mental resistance, this was only when it was contrary to the patient's *interest*. Yet it was ultimately the doctor who decided what these interests were, or were not, in this context. Thus, patients and their bodily autonomy were not necessarily protected by this stipulation.

But one of the more significant limitations of the Declaration of Geneva and the International Code of Medical Ethics was that they were too general in purpose. Although produced in the wake of the Second World War, the text of these two codes sought to guide medical professionals' attitudes and practices in everyday environments. Generally speaking, few doctors are likely to encounter situations where their assistance could be considered cruel or tantamount to torture. The language enshrined within these international medical codes did not necessarily factor in the ambiguities and novelties presented by a conflict environment where the meaning of certain clauses could be harder to interpret. For instance, the International Code obliged physicians to provide emergency care as a humanitarian imperative, but could this be used to justify treating a patient-prisoner who had been tortured in the knowledge that they would only undergo further mistreatment?[10] How should a physician respond when they know their treatment will lead to their patients undergoing further abuse? Such dilemmas regularly played out when doctors were faced with torture victims. The guiding principles of the WMA's codes were therefore not necessarily helpful in the rare, but morally demanding, circumstances created by the emergencies in Kenya and Algeria.

Yet while other postwar humanitarian documents, such as the Universal Declaration of Human Rights and the ECHR, which banned torture outright, were still coming into existence, international efforts were directed towards strengthening existing conventions that protected the rights of individuals involved in wars. In February 1945, Max Huber, the president of the ICRC, addressed a letter to the governments of 'the Big Five' (the United States, Great Britain, the Soviet Union, France and China) as well as to the national Red Cross committees, to raise support for addressing, reaffirming or even expanding 'Hague Law'.[11] The next four years saw various experts drafting revisions to existing international humanitarian law. These were accepted at the Seventeenth International Red Cross Conference in Stockholm in 1948 and finally ratified as the Geneva Conventions by fifty-nine states on 12 August 1949.[12] In addition to updating the terms of the two existing conventions agreed in 1928, two new conventions were added, along with the first codified definition of 'war crimes'.[13] The outcome was a set of conventions that protected the individual rights of soldiers, shipwrecked members of the armed forces, prisoners of war and civilians in war zones.

Although the Geneva Conventions were not specifically directed at the medical community, it was understood that physicians had a particular responsibility for ensuring their application in the field of battle. This was because, according to Jean-Pierre Schoenholzer of ICRC, physicians and the Geneva Conventions shared a common principle: 'the suffering man is sacred'.[14] This meant that the rights of patients, be they soldiers, prisoners or unarmed civilians, were to be protected by the physician before consideration of politics or other external pressures. This was because, so Schoenholzer contended, the medical profession, especially doctors, and the ICRC were both bound by the same ideals: 'to alleviate human suffering [*alléger la souffrance humaine*]'. Without doctors, he argued, the ICRC would be powerless, while the doctors owed the ICRC for having 'imposed on the world' the principles they had long been defending, 'namely the equality of men in the face of suffering'.[15] As such, doctors were meant to be particularly bound by the rules established by the Geneva Convention generally, and were to specifically safeguard the health and well-being of soldiers, prisoners and civilians, who were to be free from harm such as torture, as codified in all four conventions.[16]

Article 3, which is common to all four conventions and is often referred to as the 'convention in miniature', guaranteed the extension of basic humanitarian standards to non-international conflicts, such as civil wars or revolutions, and could be ignored neither by governments nor resistance movements without stepping outside the bounds of civilisation.[17] As such, in internal conflicts, such as the Kenya Emergency and the Algerian War, civilians and combatants no longer actively fighting due to illness, wounds, detention or any other cause were protected under the Geneva Convention.[18] Article 3 ensured that 'violence of life and person, in particular murder of all kinds, mutilations, cruel treatment and torture, taking hostage, outrage upon personal dignity, in particular humiliating and degrading treatment, the passing of sentences and carrying out of executions without previous judgement pronounced by a regularly constituted court, affording all the judicial guarantees which are recognized as indispensable by civilized people' was prohibited under any circumstances.[19] In addition to this general ban on torture, a separate article in each of the four conventions also prohibited torture under any circumstance.

Although the establishment of such fundamental basic standards as those enshrined in the Universal Declaration of Human Rights and the Geneva Conventions marked a breakthrough for international humanitarian law in the postwar period, especially in regard to conduct in internal conflicts, the idea, as Fabian Klose has shown, was not popular among the colonial powers.[20] Britain in particular was keen to oppose adoption of the provision to extend international humanitarian law to internal armed conflicts of any kind, because it feared international intervention in colonial uprisings. Passages in the draft Geneva Convention that banned, for instance, the use of collective punishment caused significant irritation to the Colonial Office, as this was a standard punitive measure used to quash rebellious activities overseas. The deadlock caused by this disagreement over the terms of the Conventions was only broken when the French delegation at the 1949 conference sought to limit the extension of all aspects of Article 3 to a bare minimum in cases of 'internal conflicts'.[21] Klose argues that the French proposal was not an expression of 'heartfelt commitment to the humanitarian protection of the colonial population during internal unrest'.[22] This is because the French had opposed the passage related to 'colonial conflicts' in the conventions. Instead, they were motivated by their experience with German occupation and denial of combatant status to resistance fighters. They ultimately wanted to protect their own population in potential future conflicts.[23]

The human rights established by the various postwar conventions were not to be extended to the colonial conflicts breaking out in East and North Africa. Colonial authorities did not want their own security forces to be impeded by humanitarian norms, nor for the rebels to enjoy protections in their struggles against the colonial order. So, while colonial officials were expressing the need to ensure their colonial subjects were treated in accordance with the Geneva Convention, the unofficial standard was one of brutality and repression. For example, in June 1955, Léon Boutbien, a French MP, asked the President of the Council: 'if, indeed, the Government cannot admit that it is conventionally bound by the [Geneva Convention] with regard to the events of Algeria, which cannot be assimilated to an armed conflict within the meaning of the Convention, France must however apply to the outlaws […] the humanitarian provisions mentioned in Article 3'.[24] Yet even as late as 1958, the French military in Algeria were being told to do the opposite. While discussing treatment of detainees in military camps in Algeria in March 1958, General Salan explicitly stated that 'It is understood that interns should not be considered as prisoners of war'.[25] For Salan, the ability to gain information from suspects was a crucial part of French counterinsurgency tactics; nothing could be allowed to prevent security forces from obtaining it: '[Therefore the] Geneva Conventions are not applicable to [detainees] […] and the search for intelligence by their interrogation is always allowed'.[26] Torture was thus permitted to play a crucial role in the colonial response to insurgents in both Kenya and Algeria.

By refusing to regard the uprisings as legitimate wars and by dehumanising the rebels, colonial authorities allowed their security forces to step outside the agreed standards for civilised combat. To what extent the members of the medical communities in Kenya and Algeria were conscious of this or how they understood their ethical responsibilities is difficult to know, given the extreme paucity of sources reflecting on the subject.[27] However, captured in the recalibrated postwar medical ethics codes were several overlapping standards of conduct that were applicable at the time. Chief among these was the rule that medical practice, knowledge and intervention should not be directed towards any act that detracted from the therapeutic interests of the patient. This even extended to any act or advice capable of weakening the physical or psychological resistance of the patient if it was not in their interests. Moreover, doctors were to remain independent agents free from institutional pressures, such as those imposed by the state, and were to provide care and attention free of prejudice while protecting the covenant of professional secrecy at all costs. It is clear that the failure to extend the minimal protections afforded by the Geneva Conventions and the nascent human rights regime meant that detainees were left with few protections. Moreover, colonial and military doctors were further ill-equipped to understand the highly ambiguous circumstances generated by revolutionary wars, an ambiguity that allowed many to act with impunity.

However, this is not to suggest that the situation would be any different if a sufficient code of ethics had existed at the time. As the WMA acknowledged while discussing the creation of the Geneva Declaration in 1948:

> As a stream cannot rise above its source, so a code cannot change a low-grade man into a high-grade doctor, but it can help a good man to be a better man and a more enlightened doctor. It can quicken and inform a conscience, but not create one.[28]

'A shock which is more psychological than physical'

On 15 January 1955, early into the Algerian War, *L'Express*, a weekly review, published an article by the journalist and writer François Mauriac entitled 'La Question', a French term for torture. Mauriac's article reported the testimony of a friend, referred to as R., a priest with Mission de France living in the north-east Algerian province of Constantine. R.'s account explained the extent to which he had, for unexplained reasons, witnessed the local police using extreme violence in their interrogations.[29] When the Algerian war started, operations were separated between the army, on the one hand, and the police and gendarmerie, on the other. The former had recently returned from their defeat in Indochina, where, as discussed earlier, they had learnt to appreciate the power of torture in a revolutionary war, while the latter were essentially responsible for supressing the uprising in the towns and countryside. The police and gendarmerie, as will be shown below, also had a long history of using excessive violence as part of their practice. As mentioned in Chapter 3, the police's initial response was to systematically arrest known political agitators, such as members of the nationalist organisation known as the Mouvement pour le triomphe des libertés démocratiques (MTLD). Although the MTLD had nothing to do with the FLN's rebellion, members were arrested and subjected to torture at the hands of the police.[30]

The methods used, R. claimed, were a mix of beatings and stealth techniques designed to leave few or no marks on the victim's body. These included techniques that would become common throughout the war: the use of electrocution, simulated drowning, prolonged and exhausting interrogation sessions, and isolation and hunger. In the end, suspects would sign confessions and implicate others as terrorists just to make the interrogation stop. One of the cases mentioned by R. was that of Moulaï Merbah, the Secretary General of a faction of the MTLD, who had been arrested and severely beaten over a five-day period, despite Article 114 of the Penal Code effectively forbidding arbitrary detention. By the time his lawyer was allowed to see him, Merbah's back showed the signs of his treatment: it 'was covered with open or barely covered wounds'. Mauriac continued to explain that, according to R., a 'forensic doctor' had been invited to examine Merbah and, instead of enquiring into the source of these injuries, had certified that he was '*le mieux du monde*' ['the best in the world' or 'in perfectly good health']. The doctor's certificate, R. suggested, subsequently convinced the French Minister of the Interior, François Mitterrand, that Merbah had not been mistreated at all. After their abusive interrogation, suspects were dragged to a magistrate at unusual hours so as to limit the number of witnesses to their trial. In a few cases where suspects' wounds were seen, such as when R.'s wife saw the 'injured chest' of a man named Abd el-Haziz, the judge called for a medical examination but insisted that it not take place in 'the presence of a professor from the Faculty of Algiers'.[31] Presumably, this was to ensure the doctor selected could be trusted to reach the right verdict that would not contradict the police's views.

Mauriac's article brought the realities of France's campaign of suppression to the French public in Paris. It not only highlighted the extent to which torture was already a tool being deployed against suspected rebels, but for our purposes, it also revealed the close connection between torture and the institutions of medicine and law. As noted by Elaine Scarry, although other institutions such as the sports stadium in Chile, the police station in Paraguay, the traffic control office in Greece and even the sweets factory in Algeria might be implicated in torture campaigns, this is usually due to a coincidence of proximity: the torture rooms just happened to be close to a headquarters facility. Yet when it comes to systematic torture, the 'two ubiquitously present' institutions are medicine and law, for, as Scarry notes, 'they are the institutional elaborations of body and state'.[32] As such, when torture is widespread, the doctor and the lawyer are rarely far from sight. In this case, to give institutionalised torture in Algeria legal protection, Mauriac tried to use medical opinion to justify and strengthen his recommendations.

Following the public outcry generated by Mauriac's article, the Mendès-France government responded in two ways. Firstly, they transferred a number of suspected Algerian police officers to Paris and 'integrated' French police officers with their Algerian counterparts. The hope was that the former group would serve as a positive influence on the latter.[33] Secondly, in direct response to Mauriac's article, Mendès-France commissioned an official investigation to ascertain the truth about police and military tactics in the colony. The civil Inspector-General, Roger Wuillaume, was seconded to the Governor General in Algeria, Jacques Soustelle, in order to investigate the nature of Mauriac's accusations. Despite the Mendès-France government collapsing soon after the commission was established, Wuillaume carried out his inquiry and submitted his report to Soustelle on 2 March 1955. Although his investigation was limited to Kabylie and the department of Constantine, he nevertheless felt he had 'sufficient information to form a judgment'.[34] In the process of his investigation he interviewed sixty-one prisoners at Lambèse, Batna, Guelma and Constantine who, he believed, had been carefully selected 'from among those most unlikely to have been urged by their lawyers to make complaints'.[35] Wuillaume concluded that prolonged imprisonment without trial and the use of torture – beatings, electrocution, various water techniques and others – were not just common, but were also 'old-established practices' within the police culture of Algeria, dating back to decades before the Algerian War.[36] Yet despite the evidence indicating the extent to which violence was a routine part of police practice in Algeria, Wuillaume did not recommend punishing suspected police officers. To do so, he feared, would result in a loss of morale among the police at a time when, by his own admission, these regrettable techniques had led to unspecified 'first-class results'.

Instead, Wuillaume recommended that torture be allowed to continue: 'Ought we nevertheless to continue to accept the procedures described above?'[37] Some forms of physical violence, such as the 'well-known beat-up procedure', were to be banned, along with 'mental violence' that publicly humiliated Muslims who were forced to appear naked in front of their families and to 'engage in unnatural acts' (forced sodomy). However, other forms of violence, which Wuillaume referred to as 'essential if the police [were] to do [their] job satisfactorily', were to be permitted. These techniques included prolonged interrogation sessions that caused physical exhaustion and enforcing hunger. They also included 'water and electricity methods', which, according to 'experts', produced a 'shock which is more psychological than physical and therefore do not constitute cruelty'.[38]

Although he did not specify who these experts were, Wuillaume continued to state how 'certain medical opinion' had convinced him that techniques like the water-pipe methods – where a pipe was forced down the throat of a suspect and water was then poured in to simulate drowning – were harmless if applied correctly. He did acknowledge, however, that electricity was a danger to 'anyone whose heart is in any way affected'. Ultimately, Wuillaume regarded these techniques as effective alternatives for the police until 'the introduction into our legal system of the lie detector and the use of pentothal'.[39] By appealing to expert medical opinion in this instance, Wuillaume was trying to add a level of legitimacy and control to these violent acts, perhaps to demonstrate they were not merely the tactics of a brutish police but a seemingly more sophisticated method for obtaining *truthful* statements and intelligence. Interestingly, the claim that these methods were harmless if applied carefully suggested there was a correct way to administer pain which fell under the purview of medical expertise to regulate. There was also a tacit idea that these techniques were acceptable, if crude, substitutes for such 'scientific' alternatives as the lie detector and drug interrogation. What the above remarks suggest, however, is the existence of a seeming correlation between medical supervision and the potential respectability of a given torture technique, especially for its assumed ability to produce truthful statements.

Although Soustelle did not agree with Wuillaume's recommendations regarding institutionalising electric and water tortures, these techniques would nevertheless become established practice among the police and the military during the war. With the military's belief that they were confronted by an entirely new form of subversive warfare in Algeria, the French security forces felt that traditional tactics would not prevail against the Algerian rebels. Unconventional tactics were needed and, from 1956 onwards, torture was not only common practice, but was also professionalised and systematised under the leadership of generals like Jacques Massu, Maurice Challe, and Raoul Salan.[40] Torture was a standard method during the screening of arrested individuals for identity checks or during operations. It served the purpose of coercing confessions from suspects as well as extracting operational intelligence. However, torture soon took on its own logic and became an instrument of terror and suppression used indiscriminately by the French security forces.[41]

The idea that medical knowledge adds a dimension of legitimacy to otherwise inhumane acts inverts the conventional role of the doctor, and transforms them from agents of healing into 'agents of pain'.[42] In fact, the use of their expert knowledge to advise on an activity that was not in a patient's therapeutic interest itself contravened the principles informing the Declaration of Geneva and the International Code of Medical Ethics, as discussed above. Similar measures to medicalise aspects of violence were adopted by the authorities in Kenya, as will be shown below, but in this instance medical personnel were required to check the health of suspects before and after they were tortured. This was not a requirement on which Wuillaume insisted. Instead, medical expertise in Algeria was simply called upon to advise on the nature of the techniques, while their implementation was left to trusted police officers in the presence of their superiors.[43] Ultimately, the controlled use of torture in special circumstances was deemed to be a lesser evil than forbidding its use outright. To do so, Wuillaume insisted, would 'plunge the police into a state of disorder and paralysis'.[44]

The dilution technique

There is currently no evidence of institutionalised or systematic violence in the early phases of the Kenya Emergency. However, this changed with the introduction of a particular form of 'compelling force' into the Mwea camps from 1957 onwards. This method, known as the 'dilution technique', was originally masterminded by the prison staff officer John Cowan at the Gathigiriri Camp (one of the detention centres in Mwea), but was later adapted and extended to the other camps by Terrence Gavaghan, the colonial district officer for the Mwea camps.[45] In practice, the technique used a mix of warders, African home guards and 'turned' rebels to cajole resistant detainees to confess their Mau Mau associations. Its application was brutally simple. Firstly, camp officials would separate the 'hard-core' and other detainees into smaller, more manageable groups. Unrestrained force was then unleashed on the captives, who were subjected to beatings with fists, whips, truncheons, clubs and any other weapons close to hand. The abuse would continue until detainees fell into line, responded to orders and ultimately confessed.[46] A clear description of the technique in action was given by Eric Griffith-Jones, Kenya's attorney general, when he witnessed its use in the Mwea camps in June 1957. In a secret memorandum, Griffith-Jones explained that 'In some cases, [...] defiance was more obstinate, and some officers immediately converged on the man and "rough-housed" him, stripping his clothes off him, hitting him, on occasion kicking him, and, if necessary, putting him on the ground. Blows struck were solid, hard ones, mostly with closed fists and about the head, stomach, sides and back'.[47] Despite the brutality, Griffith-Jones continued to stress that some restraint was observed: 'There was no attempt to strike at the testicles or any other manifestations of sadistic brutality'.[48]

Although originally developed for the detention centres in Mwea, the dilution technique was institutionalised by the colonial government and later exported to other camps in early July 1957.[49] After this, the dilution technique was sometimes referred to as the 'intake procedure', as it was generally used to quickly crush any spark of defiance in new prisoners entering the camps. Such intentions were reminiscent of what Primo Levi noted when describing the concentration camps under the Nazis:

> Remember that the concentration camp system even from its origins [...] had as its primary purpose shattering the adversaries' capacity to resist: for the camp management the new arrival was by definition an adversary, whatever the label attached to him might be, and he must immediately be demolished to make sure that he did not become an example or a germ of organized resistance.[50]

In comparison to other forms of abuse and torture taking place in many of the Kenyan detention camps, the dilution technique was organised and systematised. Its ability to coerce conformity and confession from even the most recalcitrant Mau Mau adherents promised to be the solution the British government needed at a time when they were under increased pressure to empty the pipeline. Governor Baring's enthusiasm for the technique was expressed in a secret and private correspondence to Alan Lennox-Boyd, in June 1957, when he wrote:

> In this covering letter to the enclosed papers, I wish to put before you two ideas. The first is that the so-called 'dilution' technique in the camps for detainees is giving very hopeful results indeed and is in fact the only way of dealing with the more dyed-in-the-wool Mau Mau men who will be our problem in the future. The second is its successful implementation depends on our ability to deal with a small number of very difficult men; and if we are able to do this successfully, risks are unavoidable.[51]

The 'risks' in this context was the dilution technique's potential for killing detainees or causing severe injury. For instance, between 6 and 15 September 1958, three detainees died in three separate incidents at Aguthi Works Camp and at Gathigiriri Camp.[52] Yet despite its potentially fatal outcomes, Baring believed the technique's ability to effect a 'psychological shock', which often led to confessions and cooperation from detainees upon intake, was too valuable to be suspended: 'We have felt that either we must forbid Gavaghan and his staff to proceed in this way, in which case the dilution technique will be ineffective and we will find that we cannot deal with many of the worst detainees, or, alternatively, we must give him and his staff cover provided they do as they say they are doing'.[53] Keen to muster any support for the technique, Baring explained how he had corresponded privately with Dr Junod, delegate to the ICRC. Junod, who had been a missionary and knew Baring from their days together in South Africa, had, Baring explained, 'spent his whole life working with Africans and most of it with African prisoners'.[54] According to Baring, Junod had 'no doubt in his own mind that if the violent shock was the price to be paid for pushing detainees out to the detention camps near their districts, away from the big camps, and then onwards to release, we should pay it'.[55]

He agreed with Junod and went as far as to say he was prepared to ask him 'at the invitation of the Kenya Government, to visit us again and examine the methods used'.

Junod's role in legitimising the dilution technique has been well known for some time.[56] Yet, it is unclear just how much Junod was aware of or supported this technique. In 1957, after trying for several years to gain entry to Kenya, the ICRC was finally allowed to visit the detention camps. During this first visit, Junod and Gailland visited prison and rehabilitation camps over a two-month period. According to Josiah Mwangi Kariuki, famous for *'Mau Mau' Detainee*, an account of his experience in the Kenya detention camps, Dr Junod was 'a very intelligent and quiet man, and listened to all our troubles with close attention'. This earned Junod the nickname *Muthuri wa Itathi*, a title of respect among the Kikuyu for someone who judges actions calmly and dispassionately. Kariuki concluded that Junod was thus 'a truly good man'.[57] According to Gavaghan, however, Junod had given his support to the dilution technique when he saw it in action during his visit to the Mwea camps. Apparently, Junod told him: 'Do not distress yourself [*Ne vous inquiétez pas*]', he said; 'compared to the French in Algeria, you are angels of mercy'.[58] Historians have also noted that Junod failed to mention the use of torture in Kenya in his final report to the ICRC, which they regard as tacit support for its use.[59]

Various scholars have questioned the motives for this omission.[60] Some have concluded that the British tricked Junod and the ICRC in their inspection mission by not showing the delegates all the prisons and the extent of the violence taking place behind the barbed wire. Others suspect that the ICRC omitted a complaint against torture because of prejudice held by the Committee and Junod himself.[61] Fabian Klose has gone so far as to explain the omission as sheer negligence on the part of the ICRC and Junod more generally.[62] However, Eric Morier-Genoud has recently shown that Junod did in fact denounce the torture taking place in the camps in his report to the ICRC, but that a decision was made at the ICRC headquarters to remove it from the final report. He also cautions against accepting Gavaghan's statement concerning Junod's support, given that the latter raised it in passing in a 'self-serving auto-biography which he published just as veteran Mau Mau fighters prepared a court case against the British in London in 1999, forty-two years after the event'.[63] This is plausible, as Gavaghan may well have been trying to deflect responsibility from himself and his role in systematically applying the dilution technique, but Junod's advice to Governor Baring is harder to dismiss. In fact, Morier-Genoud fails to provide a suitable explanation for this. Thus, the fact remains that Junod may well have accepted that torture was a necessary evil if it brought about a faster resolution to the Emergency. While Junod was not a medical doctor, and so he was not bound by the same ethical principles associated with that profession, his relationship to the ICRC was nevertheless significant as, if Dr Schoenholzer's views are correct, the ICRC and the medical community shared a common ideal about suffering victims. As such, Junod's personal views on this torture technique indicate another example where an individual's professional ideals were at odds with their personal ones. Regardless, despite his role within the ICRC, his personal advice to Baring seemed to be one of reassurance and not necessarily expert guidance for the method itself. However, this is not to say physicians had no role to play in the implementation of the technique.

The dilution technique was not to be carried out indiscriminately and without safeguards. According to Griffith-Jones, the method was only to be conducted by conscientious European officers who would assess whether such force was even necessary and appropriate. After this, they would only proceed in a measured manner that was not excessive or would not lead to serious injury. Before these steps were taken, however, detainees were to undergo a medical examination: 'every detainee included in a "dilution" intake should be medically examined before leaving his previous camp and any to whom force is applied should be medically examined again immediately after completion of the intake'.[64] For Griffith-Jones and Baring, the presence of a medical expert was an important safeguard that made the dilution technique's implementation more palatable. The motivation for this is unclear, but perhaps the hope was that the presence of medical oversight would add a humane veneer to torture. Indeed, this is one of the reasons why many efforts to legitimise torturous interrogation, such as with the Wuillaume report and examples in more recent contexts, have stressed the need for doctors to be present during the interrogation procedures.[65]

This is an interesting point which an exclusive focus on the bloody outcomes of torture tends to obfuscate: it is easy to miss the mundane ways in which it was normalised. Medicine played a key part in this process in Kenya. While Wuillaume had merely consulted expert opinion for his recommendations in Algeria, Griffith-Jones had bound physicians to the locations where torture took place. In addition, this prescription for a medical examination prior to and after its implementation made the dilution technique almost indistinguishable from already sanctioned forms of corporal punishment which were still standard practice in the Kenyan penal system of the 1950s. Here the procedure for administering corporal punishment also required detainees to undergo medical examination prior to being flogged. For example, in January 1959, the District Officer in Nyeri, Mr Brookes, requested permission to flog eight detainees at the Aguthi Works Camp for refusing to follow orders. Permission was granted and, on the following day, the detainees were 'examined and certified fit by the Government Doctor, Dr Twigg' before undergoing punishment.[66] It is arguable that by referring to the dilution technique as 'corporal punishment' and institutionalising it with the same requirements for medical examination, the procedure could be hidden behind a more acceptable mantle of established punitive violence.

A good example of the power of this ambiguous phrasing can be seen in a set of new instructions for the 'Intake of Z Detainees'[67] that were circulated by the Commissioner for Prisons to the staff at the Embu camps (Thiba, Kandongu, Gathigiriri and Mewa camps) on 27 July 1957. The instructions were distributed a few weeks after the dilution technique had received official sanction through the approval of Regulation 17 of the Emergency (Detained Persons) Regulation.[68] The instruction for the 'intake procedure' stipulated that, firstly, 'the only force which may be used is "overpowering" force; "beating" force may not be employed'. It is not clear what 'overpowering force' is in the context, but once the new prisoners arrived, had their heads shaved, clothes changed for camp clothes and received a 'pep-talk' from a rehabilitation assistant, they were to be asked, one by one, whether they intended to cooperate. If any said no or remained 'mute of malice', then the 'Officer in Charge of the camp should arrange to make a charge against him under Regulation 17 of, and Item 9 of the Third Schedule to, the Emergency (Detained Persons) Regulation, 1954'.[69] After this, if found guilty of the offence and 'corporal punishment' is needed, 'the detainee should be medically examined to ascertain whether he is fit to undergo corporal punishment', which should 'only be administered in the presence of a medical officer or the Officer in Charge'. The instructions continue to specify the number of strokes permitted under the regulations,[70] which could have related to the type of 'overpowering' force mentioned above (although it is unclear) which regularly relied on the use of batons.[71]

According to Gavaghan, however, this process was too slow, as meting out punishment for each individual could take up to an hour at a time. As such, Griffith-Jones approved Gavaghan's 'streamlined' process, which punished recalcitrant detainees collectively, 'rather than one after the other'.[72] Also, given that the Officer in Charge would be present from the start of each intake, there was no need to gain his approval for subsequent punishment. Nevertheless, the need for a medical officer to be present continued to be stressed.

To what extent, however, did prisoners actually receive a medical examination as part of this intake procedure? The evidence is patchy, but there is enough to show that this safeguard was taken seriously, at least in certain camps. For instance, on 3 October 1957, the then Permanent Secretary of Defence, A. C. Small, wrote to the Commissioner of Prisons to explain that, owing 'to the quietness of the recent intakes at the Mwea Camps the doctor there is no longer fully employed and the Director of Medical Services has asked and it has been agreed that he can be transferred elsewhere'.[73] He continued to stress, however, that should intake increase at any time, then 'a doctor will be made available to accompany and to attend with the Deputy or Assistant Commissioner of Prisons at the intakes and that it will be the responsibility of the Commissioner of Prisons to ensure that his Deputy or Assistant Commissioner going to the Mwea to attend an intake is accompanied by a doctor'.[74] Later, in another confidential correspondence, W. M. Campbell, Small's replacement as Permanent Secretary for Defence, explained to the Director of Medical Services in Kenya that the 'intake procedure', the dilution technique as modified by Gavaghan, was not to be applied to the Athi River detention centre. Because of this, there was no need for a Medical Officer to be present during prisoner intake at this facility.[75]

Yet it also seems the role of the Medical Officer was not always clear. Around the time when the new instructions for implementing the dilution technique were being circulated, Dr Twigg expressed confusion over his duties under the new Regulations. According to R. G. Turnbull, the then Acting Governor, Dr Twigg, was 'under the impression that it was his duty to stand by to ensure that an excessive degree of force was not employed'. This, Turnbull noted, was not the case, as the only force permitted was the force necessary to overcome resistance. Instead, Twigg's role was to 'carry out a medical examination of the detainees after they had been through the intake procedure; and [...] to carry out the responsibilities laid down under section 88 of the Prisons Ordinance in connexion with the administration of corporal punishment'.[76] However, it was crucial that the doctor played no part in the handling of detainees during the 'intake procedure'. In fact, 'He should not be present at that time but should come on the scene after the detainees had been shaved and reclothed'.[77] This seems to be contradictory. According to the instructions discussed above, doctors were expected to examine the prisoners before 'corporal punishment' and to witness it in action, but Turnbull seems to be suggesting that the rough-handling of detainees should take place prior to the head shaving. Despite this uncertainty, it is apparent that medical officers were not called upon to actively engage with the actual process of beating detainees. Perhaps this was an attempt to protect the medical profession's ethical standing, since a direct involvement in the carrying out of violence would have certainly undermined the image of the physician as healer; yet the reasons for this distancing are not made clear in the existing documents.

Although physicians were not required to take part in acts of violence themselves, it is clear that in both Algeria and Kenya, medical expertise was sought to help legitimise efforts to systematise and institutionalise torture in the respective counterinsurgency campaigns. In this regard, these doctors were still on the periphery of the violence, even in Kenya, where their presence was required to monitor detainees' conditions before or after they were abused. There is thus a distinction between monitoring or advising on a set of violent techniques and practically carrying them out. By requiring doctors in Kenya to merely examine detainees after they had been beaten, doctors were not necessarily contravening the ethical principles enshrined in the international codes of medical conduct. Ultimately, they could argue that they were merely doing their jobs by treating these victims. However, there were other instances where physicians took a more direct role in the interrogation process, especially in Algeria.

'The injection that makes you talk'

The use of what was referred to as *sérums de vérité* [truth serums], or sometimes 'truth drugs', to extort confessions or gather information from detained subjects is arguably one of the most significant and disturbing points of distinction between the Algerian and Kenyan emergencies. In the former context, the administration of these drugs by European medical experts assisting the military's interrogation process either made them explicitly complicit in the violence or turned them into de facto interrogators themselves. The situation was straightforward, if not in terms of legal or ethical implications then at least in terms of their application: a reticent suspect thought to have vital information is injected with a substance designed to overcome their conscious resistance. Or, as Fanon described it, the 'principle of [the truth drug] is well known: a chemical substance having hypnotic properties is injected into a vein, which, when the operation is carried out slowly, produces a certain loss of control, blunting of consciousness'.[78]

Since the nineteenth century, psychiatrists had been interested in the potential of various substances (hashish, opium, cocaine and mescaline) to overcome unconscious resistance and bring to light repressed psychological states.[79] Throughout the first half of the twentieth century, doctors and psychiatrists experimented with other types of drugs, such as scopolamine, a sedative derived from the same family as nightshade and mandrake, and barbiturates like sodium pentothal (sometimes sodium thiopental) and sodium amatol.[80] Originally developed for anaesthesia, barbiturates were found to make patients more suggestible in the pre-comatose stage or during recovery from unconsciousness. Once relaxed, the subject would be open to 'narcoanalysis', that is, psychotherapy conducted on a patient in a dream-like state. For the therapist, narcoanalysis could help diagnose psychosis and treat amnesia and neurosis.[81] However, it was also believed that, in this suggestible state, patients would feel more inclined to offer truthful statements about their past experiences.[82] The apparent ability of these drugs to render an individual incapable of lying was therefore of obvious appeal to criminal investigators or intelligence officers.

The use of truth drugs by medical professionals involved in interrogation marks the transition from passive contribution to torture to torture itself. It also highlights an area of historical research that has gained remarkably little attention, especially in the case of the Algerian War of Independence. In this context, two case studies – that of Henri Alleg and that of Louisette Ighilahriz – are known to have included doctors administering truth drugs as part of wider efforts to extract information from them. Although some historians have commented on or acknowledged the presence of these drugs in these two accounts, little attempt has been made to systematically analyse or place them within a wider context.[83]

The fact that truth drugs were used in Algeria was well known at the time of the conflict. As Fanon stated in 1959: 'The European doctors in Algeria use the "truth serum" with staggering frequency'.[84] Alleg's account of his interrogation under its influence, which was quickly published in France as *La Question* in 1958, remains one of the best-known examples.

On the night of 12 June 1957, Henri Alleg, a French-Algerian citizen and editor of the anticolonial paper *Alger républicain*, was arrested by French police on the streets of Algiers while en route to visit the home of Maurice Audin, a fellow member of the banned Parti communiste algérien (PCA). Once in custody, Alleg was handed to a paratrooper division that had recently taken control of Algiers. Alleg was subsequently taken and held for a month at the El-Biar detention centre in a suburb of Algiers, despite having no charges brought against him.[85] During his detention, he was subjected to a variety of torture techniques at the hands of his captors: he was burnt, electrocuted, held underwater to simulate drowning and suspended from the ceiling in painful positions. Despite this treatment, Alleg refused to answer his interrogators' questions. Frustrated, one soldier told him explicitly that they had 'scientific ways [...] to make [him] talk'.[86] The following morning, Alleg was escorted to 'the infirmary', where he met a military doctor, a captain who identified himself as 'Marcel'. After explaining to Alleg that 'I shall not hurt you and I promise not to do you any harm', Marcel injected him with sodium pentothal. While Alleg was under the influence of this drug, Marcel questioned him about the location of a FLN operative. Despite the drug's influence, Alleg was able to stay silent and gave nothing away to this doctor-cum-interrogator.[87]

For decades, Alleg's account of being drugged was the best insight we had into this shadowy practice, but the example presented by Ighilahriz's 2001 memoir sheds additional light on it. Ighilahriz became the first Algerian woman to bring to the attention of the French and Algerian public the extent of France's suppression tactics in all their violence, including her testimony about being raped and tortured. Her account is valuable, not only because it provides additional insights into the French security forces' general use of torture, but also because it demonstrates their reliance on truth drugs for this purpose.

While Alleg's account offers a glimpse into how the French military used these drugs in interrogation, Ighilahriz's story elaborates on the experience of being drugged, as well as showing how FLN trained their operatives to resist their influence. In her memoir, Ighilahriz recalled talking to an 'ex-medical student' who taught her and other mujahideen 'how to act in case of arrest'. The student explained how they 'had to concentrate to try to avoid the effects of the pentothal "truth serum" that the French administered to their prisoners'.[88] Referring to the procedure as the 'injection that makes [you] talk [*la piqûre qui fait parler*]', Ighilahriz was instructed not to think about the FLN organisation or any compromising information when being interrogated with drugs. Instead, she was trained to focus on one or two people 'outside the Organisation'.[89] Ighilahriz chose to think about her father, who had already been imprisoned by the French, and Hjrissa ben Amar, another FLN *maquisard* (guerrilla), who had died a few months earlier.[90] This 'psychological training', as she called it, became invaluable when Ighilahriz was eventually captured by French security forces. While recovering in hospital from the extensive injuries she had sustained during her arrest, Ighilahriz was injected and questioned by an unknown person. Not only does she not recall who administered the injection, she also, unlike Alleg, has no memory of the questions put to her at the time. The effects of the drug were so strong that she only remembered coming to in her hospital bed, where she was assured by an unknown *maquisard* that she had not given anything away to her captors.[91] Instead, and in keeping with her training, she only talked about her father and Ben Amar.[92]

What are we to make of Alleg's and Ighilariz's respective accounts? On the one hand, they were both produced by individuals who were critical of France's conduct in the war; Ighilahriz was also an enemy combatant. As such, their testimonies require caution: their contents are difficult to prove, while the possibility cannot be ruled out that they are distorted by individual prejudice.[93] Moreover, Ighilahriz produced her story decades after the events took place and in collaboration with two others: Anne Nivat, the journalist who collected and recorded her testimony, and Ouardia, her sister who supported her as she retold her memoires and helped exorcise her trauma for the public. The product is therefore a collective endeavour, which could raise questions about the veracity of the facts being presented.[94] Nevertheless, these types of memoirs are still important tools for social historians, as they give voice to testimonies that are often missing from official accounts. In fact, this is particularly important for the subject of torture generally and the use of truth drugs specifically, as there are few solid sources to prove such techniques were used by the French.

French officials did not refer to torture by name, even when its practice became a normal part of their counterinsurgency strategy. General Massu, who used torture systematically during the Battle of Algiers in 1957, recommended 'coercive methods', while others used euphemisms such as 'professional errors' and 'certain methods peculiar to Intelligence services'.[95] Marnia Lazreg even notes that the Church developed its own 'torture vocabulary', referring to 'methods that do not respect the other' or 'intrinsically bad methods'.[96] To date, it was not possible to find any open recommendation by the French military or colonial authorities for the use of truth drugs as a technique,[97] though it should be recalled that Wuillaume suggested electrocution and water torture were the best options for police interrogators pending the introduction of lie detectors and sodium pentothal in the French legal system.[98] However, while being interviewed by Raphaëlle Branche in 2000, Dr Jean Suaud, a former military doctor, explained how his chief medical officer had permitted the use of truth drugs against Algerian detainees. According to Suaud, the chief medical officer would have some prisoners believe they were receiving a 'soothing injection' when in reality they were being injected with sodium pentothal.[99] His aim was 'to try [...] through the truth serum [...] to obtain information that others could have after physical torture'.[100] If Suaud's statement shows that some physicians did use sodium pentothal during the Algerian War, it raises questions about whether or not this was viewed as an acceptable and reliable technique at time.

Two European psychiatrists in Algeria who expressed mixed feelings about the benefits of this drug for criminal investigations were Professor Antoine Porot and Dr Charles Bardenat, who were mentioned in Chapter 2. Ever eager to promote the power of psychiatry for areas outside the clinic, these two psychiatrists published *Psychiatrie médico-légale* in 1959, which explored, among other things, the 'detection of lies [and] provocation of confession'.[101] Their assessment considered the probative value of hypnosis, mental tests, lie detectors, psychoanalysis and what they referred to as chemical narcosis techniques, that is, truth drugs. In effect, Porot and Bardenat were discussing the science of 'sincerity'.[102] While acknowledging the value of narcoanalysis for therapeutic purposes, Porot and Bardenat, like their metropolitan colleagues, were of the opinion that this technique did not necessarily produce the uncomplicated window into a suspect's soul that popular opinion believed. As they explained, individuals of a strong mindset could be troublesome: '[an] extremely resistant subject which, once having adopted a system of denial', reminiscent of Ighilahriz's training, 'will remain there for a very long time and nothing will be shaken; they will support under narcosis their false claims'.[103] Conversely, 'minds of low complexion' could easily be influenced by interrogations themselves. The psychiatrists admitted that 'the malleability of some minds indeed is considerable'.[104] Like many scientists in the late 1950s, Porot and Bardenat were of the opinion that the use of truth drugs in criminal investigations was untrustworthy. As they said, information obtained from narcoanalysis was not to be given 'too much credit'.[105]

The issue here was that some subjects could mistakenly blur facts with fantasy while under the influence of these drugs. A good example of this in the Algerian context was a case recorded by the former soldier Jean-Pierre Vittori, in *On a torturé en Algérie*. In his account, Vittori explained how he had witnessed an arrested *fellagha* (a 'bandit') being interrogated on suspicion of 'urban terrorism'. According to Vittori, a doctor was summoned to 'supervise the use of the truth serum' after other unspecified interrogation techniques had failed. Once injected, the pentothal caused the man to sink 'into a semi-comatose state', and after an initial short pause, the 'valves opened and the "patient" [started to tell] the details of an extraordinary attack perpetrated in Algiers a few weeks' before. This attack, the drugged *fellagha* claimed, had killed twenty soldiers and destroyed an entire military post. The problem, Vittori continued, was that this was complete fantasy – no such attack had ever taken place at any military post.[106] Meanwhile the prisoner continued a confused tirade against the French, explaining how he was fighting against them. 'In a way', Vittori went on, 'he takes his desires for realities and his dream is fulfilled under the influence of drugs'. The revelations of the *fellagha*'s testimony apparently left the doctor 'trembl[ing]' at the thought of what would be revealed if pentothal was 'administered to the entire [Algerian] population'.[107]

Another problem facing truth drugs at this time was the claim that their use could also be a form of abuse or torture. For example, in both the Alleg and Ighilahriz cases, as well as those mentioned by Suaud, the doctors or those administering sodium pentothal – it is not clear whether it was actually a doctor, nurse or even a soldier who injected Ighilahriz – did so without seeking the subject's consent. If Suaud is to be believed, his chief medical officer even deceived his patients. It is quite clear that the use of sodium pentothal for interrogation could not be interpreted as a therapeutic procedure, and so its use would have been a violation of the Geneva Declaration and the International Code of Medical Ethics. However, the use of truth drugs in this way was also hotly debated in French courts and European military research laboratories following the end of Second World War.

The case of significance in this context was the trial of Henri Cens, in 1948. Cens was a police officer suspected of collaborating with Nazi forces during the occupation years. However, in 1943, during a prison riot in Montpellier, Cens was accidentally shot in the head. Although he survived the incident, he was supposedly left with a form of aphasia rendering him incapable of remembering or speaking.[108] In order to establish whether he was fit to stand trial, the court appointed a board of expert psychiatrists to assess his case. During their examination, one of the psychiatrists administered sodium pentothal to Cens, telling him it was for 'therapeutic purposes'.[109] While under the drug's influence, Cens reportedly uttered one positive '*oui*' in response to the psychiatrist's questions which, they subsequently argued in court, was evidence that he was malingering and feigning his aphasia.[110] Cens was convicted. Soon after, he brought a legal case against the psychiatrists, charging them with assault and battery, illegal search and the violation of professional secrets.

Although the court decided in the favour of the psychiatrists,[111] the Cens case generated significant discussion throughout Europe. Responding to the controversy generated by the psychiatrists' conduct, the Council of the Paris Bar Association adopted a resolution opposing the use of drugs during interrogation.[112] The psychiatrists involved in the case were criticised for violations on four grounds: they had violated the article of the French Penal Code binding doctors to professional secrets; they had violated the provision on forbidding the questioning of an accused outside the presence of his advisers; they had violated the article forbidding assault and battery; and they had deprived the patient of his free will by using the truth drug.[113] Yet not all medical and legal associations were as decided on the question of this interrogation technique and the law. In March 1949, the Académie de médecine, consulted by public authorities, issued an unfavourable opinion on the legitimacy of narcoanalysis for criminal investigations as well, despite contrary opinion expressed by Professors Baudouin and Laignel-Lavastine.[114] Conversely, the Société de médecine légale de France declared narcoanalysis to be lawful for forensic evaluation, as long as it was performed by medical experts and 'strictly' in a 'medical capacity … as a means of diagnosis'.[115] With a few exceptions in both Britain and America, the feeling was largely the same: evidence obtained by way of narcoanalysis could not be trusted for criminal investigation. In Holland and Spain, the law prohibited all procedures of physical and moral coercion to provoke a confession, while in Western Germany, special precautions were put in place to protect any defendant from infringing their right to defence by techniques affecting their conscience and moral freedom.[116]

The argument that the use of these drugs was a form of torture that constituted a direct attack on human dignity was also expressed outside the courtrooms. For instance, in October 1953, Pope Pius XII grouped narcoanalysis with torture in a text he produced for the Fourth International Congress on Criminal Law.[117] In his paper, Pius denounced the whole practice of detention without trial as a mockery of the Law. He stressed, in particular, that:

> Preliminary investigation must exclude physical and mental torture and narco-analysis, firstly because they are against the natural law even if the accused is guilty. And also because very often they give the wrong results. It not infrequently happens that they produce exactly the confessions required by the court [...] not because the accused is in fact guilty but because his physical and mental energy is exhausted and he is ready to make any sort of declaration that is required. Better prison or death than such physical and mental torture![118]

In their work, Porot and Bardenat draw close attention to a whole spectrum of opinions on the moral implications of these drugs as expressed by various medical professionals, jurists and social scientists across Europe. By the late 1950s, it is clear that opinions were divided. For themselves, Porot and Bardenat concluded that 'in the judicial investigation, [the use of truth drugs] by police or magistrates is reprehensible because it constitutes a systematic and deliberate splitting of human rights by a kind of breach of conscience'.[119] However, this condemnation was limited to the use of truth drugs by non-medical individuals; Porot and Bardenat were far more ambivalent when it came to their use by medical experts. They admitted that the recourse to narcoanalysis could be useful in exceptional cases. One such case might be when narcoanalysis is called for by the defence to ascertain the mental responsibility of a defendant and their ability to stand trial. Presumably, by willingly consenting to narcoanalysis in order to strengthen the defence, the accused would not be subjected to the type of legal violations involved in the Cen's trial – their minds would not be invaded by the prosecution but willingly probed to strengthen their case. As an example, Porot and Bardenat cite the work of their colleague at the Algiers School of psychiatry, Dr J. M. Sutter, who reported on just such a case in 1951, where his use of narcoanalysis proved the inability of a suspect to stand trial due to 'obvious signs of a true psychosis'.[120] Ultimately, according to Porot and Bardenat, it seems they agreed with Sutter when he wrote that

> the truth [...] is that the doctor, and the psychiatrist more than any other, is at every moment in the presence of ethical problems of which no scale, no immutable code can bring him the solution; an uninterrupted series of cases of conscience where he must engage with all the resources of his moral dynamism.[121]

Despite providing a thorough consideration of the strengths and the various scientific, legal and ethical limitations surrounding narcoanalysis for criminal investigations, Porot and Bardenat did not address its use by doctors involved in France's counterinsurgency campaign. By the time of the publication of *Psychiatrie médico-légale* in 1959, Alleg's account had already generated significant international attention and outrage. It is curious that these two psychiatrists did not denounce such tactics, especially given that individuals like Fanon had accused the European psychiatrists, his colleagues, of being complicit in such practices.[122] The use of sodium pentothal by the French security forces in Algeria was, as with the Cens case and the views of many contemporary intellectuals, a violation of the medico-legal and ethical standards at the time. The administration of truth drugs to Alleg and Ighilahriz, in particular, was a form of assault and battery; it stripped them of their free will, contravened the privileges of the doctor–patient relationship regarding professional secrets and was administered without legal representation for the suspects. As such, these drugs represented a way in which European doctors in Algeria directly contributed their expertise to the atmosphere of violence playing out in the country. It also points to a marked difference between France's war in Algeria and the Kenya Emergency.

'Clever and unscrupulous combination of methods'

Although there is no evidence that British security forces in Kenya used truth drugs in their interrogation sessions, this does not mean this option was not considered at all. On 12 January 1955, W. F. B. Pollock-Morris, the Secretary of Defence in Kenya, sent a correspondence to the Director of Intelligence and Security in Nairobi, inquiring about a matter raised by a Dr Alfred H. Becker.[123] Becker, a controversial figure who was a Rehabilitation Officer at the detention centre on Manda Island, had written a letter on 6 January 1955 to the 'Commissioner for Community Development and Rehabilitation on the subject of applying the narco-analysis treatment in the screening of detainees'.[124] The details of Becker's original letter are currently unknown, as are the views expressed on it by Pollock-Morris and the Ministry of Defence.

If the British security forces were resistant to the idea of using truth drugs in Kenya, it was not due to any ethical or moral objections on their part. Instead, their attitudes were reflective of broader scepticism among the military and intelligence officials regarding the science of interrogation more generally. During and after the Second World War, Britain had experimented with the use of various drugs to enhance their interrogation processes. These techniques differed from the type of narcoanalysis performed in Algeria in that they were not necessarily seeking pertinent information from suspects. Instead, British experiments with these substances sought to control the minds of their subjects. Nevertheless, the arguments for their usefulness and reliability were dismissed on similar grounds to their French counterparts: the results gained from these substances were deemed unreliable and ultimately unconvincing by both British scientists and the security experts. For example, in 1940, the British military set up an interrogation centre, known as a Combined Services Detailed Interrogation Centre (CSDIC), in Cairo, where captured enemy agents were injected with amphetamines and the hormone thyroxine during interrogation sessions.[125] One interrogation office, Alexander Kennedy, a physician who would go on to become a professor of psychological medicine at the University of Edinburgh, combined these drugs with hypnosis and other stress-inducing factors, such as ambiguous sounds and visual stimuli, to produce hallucinations in his subjects. Despite attracting the curiosity of high-ranking intelligence personnel, such as Dick White, a commander of MI5's B Branch, Kennedy's techniques did not catch on. According to White, drug-assisted interrogation of this kind took too long to extract information that more direct methods could produce in hours.[126]

In the 1950s, British scientists once again explored the potential power of truth drugs as part of a joint research programme with the United States. The Cold War 'brainwashing scare' inspired a series of joint investigations between US and British scientists into possible mind-control methods being employed by the Soviets. According to the American psychiatrist Irving Janis, who was corresponding with his British counterpart, William Sargent, between 1949 and 1950, Soviet interrogators were using a mix of 'conditioning techniques' and 'drug treatments' to extort confessions.[127] Yet as Erik Linstrum has shown, scientists consulted by the War Office (and later the

Ministry of Defence) on this matter were unconvinced. This was especially the case for the Secretary of the Medical Research Council (MRC), Harold Himsworth, who argued that the communists were unlikely to deploy elaborate mind-control techniques when easier and more effective methods were already available.[128] For Himsworth, it was 'very doubtful whether we are here dealing with any strange drug such as would delight the hearts of the cheaper writers of thrillers'.[129] Far from developing a new technique that 'robs the subject of his will and allows new beliefs to be implanted in him without his being aware', it was more likely that 'the observed results can be accounted for by a clever and unscrupulous combination of methods which are well known'. These included, Himsworth suggested, 'undermining the subjects [*sic*] physical strength by under-feeding, inducing extreme fatigue by lack of sleep, the relentless maintenance of the "sword of Nemesis" atmosphere, the adroit alternation of hope and fear, and blackmail with regard to relatives and institutions to which the prisoners are devoted'.[130]

Despite Himsworth's reservations, however, further research into the novel effects of certain substances was conducted as part of a larger CIA -funded initiative. In 1951, the Harvard anaesthetist Dr Henry K. Beecher travelled to Europe in search of 'ego-depressant' drugs for enhancing interrogation as part of a top-secret US 'special interrogation programme' known as Operation Artichoke. Beecher was originally interested in the effects of what Alfred W. McCoy called 'the Gestapo's drug of choice', mescaline, but later turned his attention to hallucinatory effects of lysergic acid (LSD).[131] During his travels across Europe, Beecher tipped off the British Joint Intelligence Bureau about the powers of LSD. Although British scientists had already taken an interest in the substance's potential as an incapacitating weapon before Beecher's arrival, a more concerted research programme took place between 1953 and 1954, which saw the drug administered to unsuspecting soldiers at the British chemical and biological warfare facility at Porton Down.[132]

Despite this research, British methods of interrogation, especially in overseas territories like Kenya, did not change much over the course of the 1950s and 1960s. Notwithstanding the British government's use of psychological expertise to frame the official interpretation of and approach to the threat of Mau Mau, there is little evidence that scientists of any sort tried to develop new interrogation techniques. More often than not, the feeling was that scientific approaches, especially drug-assisted interrogation, were too slow and ineffective. In the end, it was easier to rely on the more 'traditional' types of coercive methods listed by Himsworth: controlled and restricted feeding, sleep deprivation, a persistent sense of impending judgement and an oscillating atmosphere of peril and the promise of salvation. These techniques did not require the assistance of scientific experts to implement them (though doctors like Himsworth certainly justified them); any police officer, soldier or Special Branch operative could apply them in a detention centre. However, if the Kenya Emergency was a kind of laboratory for experimenting with novel counterinsurgency techniques, then the experimenters in this case were individuals like Cowan and Gavaghan – ordinary individuals with little-to-no scientific knowledge. Yet they regarded themselves as *the* experts, often drawing on personal experience and instincts to inform their brutal methods. As Linstrum explained, 'When military and police interrogators laid claim to the language of expertise – as they habitually did – they were touting powers of intuition rather than technical knowledge'.[133] Rather than help to devise elaborate torture techniques, medical officers in Kenya merely monitored them.

Conclusion

When it came to state-sanctioned forms of torture, a range of medical expertise was utilised by the colonial authorities and security forces to help legitimise, humanise, monitor and even participate in sanctioned forms of torture. In most cases, these experts provided either scientific opinion to strengthen the official efforts to legalise torture, examined and checked the health of detainees prior to and after undergoing torture or else actively intervened in the interrogation process in order to gain operative information themselves. Despite the extraordinary circumstances and conditions these doctors were working in, they were nevertheless participating within their professional capacity as healers. Such unusual encounters between the doctor and detainee-patients raised substantial questions about the contemporary standard of international codes of medical ethics which may have influenced or at least informed their conduct.

Notes

1 Victor Hugo quoted in Edward Peters, *Torture* (Philadelphia: University of Pennsylvania Press, 1999), p. 5.
2 Kenneth Mellanby, 'Medical experiments on human beings in concentration camps in Nazi Germany', *British Medical Journal* (25 January 1947), p. 148.
3 Quote taken from 'Resolution of the Medical Chamber of Western Germany concerning the Nuremberg Trial', *World Medical Association Bulletin* 1 (April 1949), p. 12.
4 Karl-Heinz Leven, 'The invention of Hippocrates: oath, letters and Hippocratic corpus', in Trohler and Reiter-Theil (eds), *Ethics Codes in Medicine*, p. 14. See also Timmermann, 'A model for the new physician', pp. 302–324.
5 A copy of the original and updated version of the Declaration of Geneva can be found here: www.wma.net/policies-post/wma-declaration-of-geneva/
6 Here I am using the original language from the code as first published in the September 1948 Declaration of Geneva, adopted by the General Assembly of the WMA.
7 Anonymous, 'Minutes of the General Assembly in London', *World Medical Association Bulletin* 2 (1950), p. 10.
8 International Code of Medical Ethics, adopted by the Third General Assembly of the World Medical Association, London, England, October 1949.
9 The WMA was formed in 1946 to promote ties between national medical organisations and among doctors across the world. One of the primary aims of its First General Assembly was to discuss 'the principles of social security' to protect the welfare of physicians themselves. These principles were designed to support the personal and financial welfare of physicians rather than the security of patients. See George J. Annas and Michael A. Grodin, 'Medicine and human rights: reflections on the fiftieth anniversary of the Doctors' Trial', *Health and Human Right* 2 (1996), pp. 10–11.
10 Though it must be stated that the final pledge of the Declaration of Geneva is unambiguous when it binds the physician to maintaining the utmost respect for the laws of humanity.
11 Geoffrey Best, *War and Law Since 1945* (Oxford: Oxford University Press, 1994), pp. 80–81.
12 Jean S. Pictet, 'The new Geneva Conventions for the Protection of War Victims', *American Journal of International Law* 45 (1951), pp. 464–467.

13 The four conventions are: (1) Geneva Convention for the Amelioration of the Condition of the Wounded and Sick in Armed Forces in the Field; (2) Geneva Convention for the Amelioration of the Condition of Wounded, Sick and Shipwrecked Members of Armed Forces at Sea; (3) Geneva Convention relative to the Treatment of Prisoners of War; and (4) Geneva Convention relative to the Protection of Civilian Persons in Time of War.

14 Jean-Pierre Schoenholzer, 'Le médecin dans les Conventions de Genève de 1949', *Revue internationale de la Croix-Rouge et Bulletin International des Sociétés de la Croix-Rouge* 35 (1953), p. 102.

15 Schoenholzer, 'Le médecin dans les Conventions de Genève de 1949', p. 94.

16 Schoenholzer, 'Le médecin dans les Conventions de Genève de 1949', p. 103.

17 See also Fabian Klose, 'The colonial testing ground: the International Committee of the Red Cross and the violent end of empire', *Humanity: An International Journal of Human Rights, Humanitarianism, and Development* 2 (2011), p. 108.

18 Klose, 'The colonial testing ground', p. 109.

19 Article 3 of the Geneva Convention, in ICRC, ed., Geneva Convention, 24.

20 Klose, 'The Colonial Testing Ground', p. 109. See also Klose, *Human Rights in the Shadow of Colonial Violence*, pp. 38–46.

21 Klose, *Human Rights in the Shadow of Colonial Violence*, pp. 38–46.

22 Klose, 'The colonial testing ground', p. 109.

23 Klose, 'The colonial testing ground', p. 109.

24 SHD 1 H 2460/d.1. Written question produced by Monsieur Boutbien reproduced in 'Annex a la Note de Service No. 2319 en date du 3 September 1956'.

25 SHD 1 H 1492/d.2 General R. Salan, 'Camps d'Internées Militaires', 19 March 1958.

26 SHD 1 H 1492/d.2 General R. Salan, 'Camps d'Internées Militaires'.

27 To date, I have not found evidence of any real discussions or debates concerning ethical practices in relation to the colonies and colonial subjects. This absence, I would suggest, might account for why historians discussing medical conduct in these territories, such as the aforementioned Keller and Branche, have fallen into questionable assumptions about the universal meaning surrounding the Hippocratic Oath.

28 Quote taken from Anonymous, 'Declaration of Geneva', *World Medical Association Bulletin* 1 (October 1949), p. 109.

29 François Mauriac, 'La Question', reproduced in 'Algérie. Dès 1955, François Mauriac dénonçait la torture dans *L'Express*', *L'Express*, 20 December 2012.

30 According to Pierre Vidal-Naquet, the MTLD were in a state of internal chaos themselves at the time of the outbreak of war and so had nothing to do with the FLN's rebellion. See Vidal-Naquet, *Torture: Cancer of Democracy*, p. 32.
31 François Mauriac, 'La Question'.
32 Scarry, *The Body in Pain*, p. 42.
33 Vidal-Naquet, *Torture: Cancer of Democracy*, p. 32.
34 Roger Wuillaume, 'Text of the Wuillaume Report' translated and presented in the Appendix of Vidal-Naquet, *Torture: Cancer of Democracy*, p. 169.
35 Vidal-Naquet, *Torture: Cancer of Democracy*, p. 35.
36 Vidal-Naquet, *Torture: Cancer of Democracy*, pp. 170–173.
37 Vidal-Naquet, *Torture: Cancer of Democracy*, p. 175.
38 Vidal-Naquet, *Torture: Cancer of Democracy*, p. 176.
39 Vidal-Naquet, *Torture: Cancer of Democracy*, pp. 176–177.
40 Lazreg, *Torture and the Twilight of Empire*, p. 112.
41 Horne, *A Savage War of Peace*, pp. 197–207.
42 Scarry, *The Body in Pain*, p. 42.
43 Vidal-Naquet, *Torture: Cancer of Democracy*, p. 178.
44 Vidal-Naquet, *Torture: Cancer of Democracy*, p. 177.
45 Anderson, 'British abuse and torture in Kenya's counter-insurgency', p. 707.
46 Elkins, *Britain's Gulag*, pp. 319–320.
47 TNA CO 822/1251, Secret memorandum from Griffith-Jones's 'Dilution Detention Camps – Use of Force in Enforcing Discipline', June 1957, p. 3.
48 TNA CO 822/1251, Secret memorandum from Griffith-Jones's 'Dilution Detention Camps', p. 3.
49 TNA FCO 141/6303/57. Secretary of African Affairs, 'Mwea Procedure', 24 July 1957.
50 Primo Levi, *The Drowned and the Saved* (London: Abacus, 1989), p. 38.
51 TNA FCO 141/6303/7, 'Secret and Personal' letter from Baring to Lennox-Boyd, 25 June 1957, p. 1.
52 Anderson, 'British abuse and torture in Kenya's counter-insurgency', pp. 707–708.
53 TNA FCO 141/6303/7, 'Secret and Personal' letter from Baring to Lennox-Boyd, p. 2.
54 TNA FCO 141/6303/7, 'Secret and Personal' letter from Baring to Lennox-Boyd, p. 2.
55 TNA FCO 141/6303/7, 'Secret and Personal' letter from Baring to Lennox-Boyd, p. 2.

56 Elkins, *Britain's Gulag*, p. 331.
57 Josiah Mwangi Kariuki, *Mau Mau Detainee: The Account by a Kenya African of His Experience in Detention Camps 1953–60* (London: Penguin Books, 1964), p. 148.
58 Terence Gavaghan, *Of Lions and Dung Beetles* (Devon: Arthur H. Stockwell, 1999), p. 235.
59 Ekins, *Britain's Gulag*, p. 331 and Helena Coban, 'The role of mass incarceration in counterinsurgency: a reflection on Caroline Elkins's *Imperial Reckoning in Light of Recent Events*', *Radical History Review* 96 (2006), pp. 125–126.
60 Eric Morier-Genoud, 'Missions and institutions: Henri-Philippe Junod, anthropology, human rights and academia between Africa and Switzerland, 1921–1966', *Schweizerische Zeitschrift für Religions- und Kulturgeschichte* 105 (2011), p. 210.
61 Nicolas Lanza, 'Le Comité international de la Croix-Rouge et le soulèvement des Mau-Mau au Kenya, 1952–1959', *Relations internationales* 1 (2008), p. 102.
62 Klose, 'The colonial testing ground', pp. 108–111.
63 Morier-Genoud, 'Missions and institutions', p. 210.
64 TNA CO 822/1251. Griffith-Jones, '"Dilution" Detention Camps. Use of Force in Enforcing Discipline', June 1957.
65 For example, the *Parker Report* mentioned in the Introduction to this book suggested doctors be present to oversee interrogation in Northern Ireland. More recently, in Iraq and Afghanistan, the American military insisted on the presence of various clinicians when suspects underwent harsh interrogation. See Parker, *Report of the committee of Privy Counsellors Appointed to Consider Authorised Procedures for the Interrogation of Persons Suspected of Terrorism*. See also Miles, *Oath Betrayed*, p. 59–61.
66 TNA FCO 141/6568/52/2. 'The Chief Secretary's Complaints Co-Ordinating Committee. Meeting Held in the Office of the Deputy Public Prosecutor, Attorney General's Chambers at 2.15, p.m.', 8 July 1959.
67 Z detainees were those hard-core Mau Mau adherents who had previously been classified as 'black' under the original categorisation systems established at the start of the Emergency. As the Emergency wore on, the colonial authorities devised a different system for classifying Mau Mau inmates based on the level of their perceived allegiances. Z1 was reserved for senior or more determined supporters, while Z2 and Y were used to designate lesser members. Detainees would progress through these categories, ideally from higher to lower, on their way through the rehabilitation process where they would be designated as X before release.

68 The Regulation legalised definitions of 'compelling force' and 'punitive force' and allowed officers in the detention camps to use violence as a normative practice. See Anderson, 'British abuse and torture in Kenya's counter-insurgency', p. 707.

69 TNA FCO 141/6303/39/1. Commissioner of Prisons, 'Intake of Z Detainees', 25 July 1957, p. 1.

70 Implicit within these instructions is the idea that a 'stroke' is different to 'beating force'. In the former, the regulations refer to strikes as controlled and prescribed hits from a 'regulated cane', whereas the latter seems to refer to less controlled behaviour, including beating with fists or kicking a detainee. TNA FCO 141/6303/165. 'Rehabilitation Methods', 28 November 1957, pp. 1–2.

71 TNA FCO 141/6303/39/1. Commissioner of Prisons, 'Intake of Z Detainees', 25 July 1957, p. 2. See also TNA FCO 141/6303/168/2, I. P. Kelloway, Officer in Charge of Detainee Section, Special Branch to the Senior Assistant Commissioner of Police, 'Rehabilitation Methods: Mwea Camp', 28 November 1957, p. 1.

72 TNA FCO 141/6303/26, Griffith-Jones, 'Mwea Procedure', 2 July 1957, p. 1.

73 TNA FCO 141/6303/117. A. C. Small, 'Mwea Camps – Intakes', 3 October 1957.

74 TNA FCO 141/6303/117. A. C. Small, 'Mwea Camps – Intakes', 3 October 1957.

75 TNA FCO 141/6303/132. Correspondence from W. M. Campbell to the Director of Medical Services, 'Intakes – Athi River', 14 November 1957.

76 TNA FCO 141/6303/24, 'R.G. Turnball, 'Mwea Procedure', 17 July 1957, p. 1.

77 TNA FCO 141/6303/24, 'R.G. Turnball, 'Mwea Procedure', 17 July 1957, p. 2.

78 Fanon, *A Dying Colonialism*, p. 137.

79 Rejali, *Torture and Democracy*, p. 387. See also Carl N. Edwards, Samuel I. Miles, and August Piper, 'Deception: Truth serum', *Wiley Encyclopedia of Forensic Science* (2009), pp. 1–3.

80 Rejali, *Torture and Democracy*, p. 387.

81 This form of psychotherapy was used extensively during the Second World War by British and American psychiatrists seeking to help traumatised patients return to battle.

82 Alison Winter, 'The making of "truth serum"', *Bulletin of the History of Medicine* 79 (2005), p. 501.

83 For example, see footnote in Vidal-Naquet, *Torture: Cancer of Democracy*, p. 177; Franz Kaltenbeck, 'On torture and state crime',

Cardozo Law Review 24 (2002), p. 2386; Rejali, *Torture and Democracy*, p. 388; Dan Wood, 'Revisiting *La Question*: a political-phenomenological critique of Merleau-Ponty's assessment of Algerian decolonization', *Studies in Social and Political Thought* 22 (2013), p. 20.

84 Fanon, *A Dying Colonialism*, p. 137.
85 Henri Alleg, *La Question* (Paris: Les Editions de minuit, 1958), p. 7.
86 Alleg, *La Question*, p. 53.
87 Alleg, *La Question*, pp. 54–60.
88 Ighilahriz, *Algérienne*, p. 92.
89 Ighilahriz, *Algérienne*, p. 92.
90 Ighilahriz, *Algérienne*, p. 101.
91 This apparent loss of memory has been recorded in similar situations in other contexts where so-called truth serums have been used. See Schmidt, *Secret Science*, pp. 326–47.
92 Ighilahriz, *Algérienne*, pp. 105–107.
93 In an appendix to his *Torture: Cancer of Democracy*, Pierre Vidal-Naquet names Alleg's doctor-interrogator as Captain Chevrel of the Army Medical Service, who had denied Alleg's claims to having been drugged. However, Vidal-Naquet continues to state that Chevrel did not bring any evidence 'for defamation of character' against Alleg. See Vidal-Naquet, *Torture: Cancer of Democracy*, p. 177.
94 Mortimer, 'Tortured bodies, resilient souls', p. 108.
95 Lazreg, *Torture and the Twilight of Empire*, p. 114.
96 Quotes taken from Lazreg, *Torture and the Twilight of Empire*, p. 114.
97 I found one reference to drugs used for 'torture' in the appendix of a report comparing the psychological warfare approaches and methods of Western, totalitarian and communist States. Appendix II, '*Doctrine Politique Communiste*' explains how '*procédés physiques*' [physical processes] such as sleep deprivation and '*emploi de drogues Tortures*' [use of torture drugs] were thought to be used in the Soviet Union. SHD 1 H 2411/d.1/370. 'Annex 11: Doctrine politique communiste', p. 24.
98 Wuillaume, 'Text of the Wuillaume Report', p. 177.
99 Branche, *La Torture et l'armée pendant la guerre d'Algérie*, pp. 469–470.
100 SHD GR 4K 38. Interview of Jean Suaud with Raphaëlle Branche, 15 February 2000.
101 Porot and Bardenat, *Psychiatrie médico-légale*, p. 87.
102 Porot and Bardenat, *Psychiatrie médico-légale*, pp. 87–96.
103 Porot and Bardenat, *Psychiatrie médico-légale*, p. 91.

104 Porot and Bardenat, *Psychiatrie médico-légale*, p. 90.
105 Porot and Bardenat, *Psychiatrie médico-légale*, p. 90.
106 Jean-Pierre Vittori, *On a torturé en Algérie* (Paris: Editions Ramsay, 2000), p. 79.
107 Vittori, *On a torturé en Algérie,* p. 79.
108 Jean Rolin, *Police Drugs*, trans. Laurence J. Bendit (London: Hollis & Carter, 1955), p. 70.
109 Rolin, *Police Drugs*, p. 72.
110 George H. Dession, Lawrence Z. Freedman, Richard C. Donnelly and Frederick C. Redlich, 'Drug-induced revelation and criminal investigation', *The Yale Law Journal* 62 (1953), p. 316.
111 It seems the psychiatrists involved were able to persuade the court that they were only acting in accordance with routine psychiatric procedures necessary to get Cen's to answer the limited questions put to him. See Dession *et al.*, 'Drug-induced revelation and criminal investigation', p. 316.
112 This is presumably what Fanon was referring to when he wrote that 'All the Academies of Medicine of all the countries in the world have formally condemned the use of this practice for legal ends and the doctor who violates these solemn proscriptions is obviously contemptuous of the fundamental principles of medicine'. See Fanon, *A Dying Colonialism*, p. 137.
113 Dession *et al.*, 'Drug-induced revelation and criminal investigation', p. 316.
114 Porot and Bardenat, *Psychiatrie médico-légale*, p. 94.
115 Porot and Bardenat note that members of the Société de médecine légale de France later vehemently opposed the use of narcoanalysis after witnessing its abuse by Germans in the concentration camps. See Porot and Bardenat, *Psychiatrie médico-légale*, p. 94.
116 Porot and Bardenat, *Psychiatrie médico-légale*, p. 94; see also D. Colwyn William and Ilse Boon, 'The prohibition in Western Germany of the admission of evidence obtained through narco-analysis', *The British Journal of Delinquency* 2 (1951), pp. 55–57.
117 Pius is currently a controversial historical figure, as he had been well informed about the types of medical atrocities performed by German scientists during the Second World War and remained silent about them while also having close ties to the regime. See Schmidt, *Secret Science*, p. 371.
118 Quoted by Louis Allen, 'YES I SAID YES I WILL YES', *Blackfriars* 39 (1958), p. 482.
119 Porot and Bardenat, *Psychiatrie médico-légale*, p. 95.

120 Porot and Bardenat, *Psychiatrie médico-légale*, p. 95. See also J. M. Sutter, 'La subnarcose chimique', *Revue de droit canonique* (1951), pp. 679–682.
121 Porot and Bardenat, *Psychiatrie médico-légale*, p. 96.
122 Fanon, *The Wretched of the Earth*, p. 228.
123 It is not currently clear what Dr Becker's profession was before he became a Rehabilitation Officer, but he was known to be a particularly zealous character who was implicated in multiple grievances by Mau Mau detainees, including psychological and physical abusive coercion. In 1955, he was transferred from Manda Island to another unidentified camp after he stirred up controversy when he wrote letters to friends of detainees impressing on them the need to pressure the detainees into confessing.
124 TNA FCO 141/6178/66. W. F. B. Pollock Morris, 'Narco Analysis', 12 January 1955.
125 Ian Cobain, *Cruel Britannia: A Secret History of Torture* (London: Portobello Books, 2013), p. 24.
126 Cobain, *Cruel Britannia*, pp. 24–25.
127 Linstrum, *Ruling Minds*, p. 184.
128 Linstrum, *Ruling Minds*, p. 184.
129 TNA DEFE 9/37. Top Secret letter from Dr Himsworth to H. T. Tizard, 4 December 1950.
130 TNA DEFE 9/37. Top Secret letter from Dr Himsworth to H. T. Tizard, 4 December 1950.
131 Alfred W. McCoy, 'Science in Dachau's shadow: Hebb, Beecher, and the development of CIA psychological torture and modern medical ethics', *Journal of the History of Behavioural Science* 43 (2007), p. 411.
132 Ulf Schmidt has shown that further experiments took place between the late 1950s and the 1970s. See Schmidt, *Secret Science*, pp. 326–336; Dominic Streatfield, *The Secret History of Mind Control* (London: Hodder & Stoughton, 2007), pp. 71–73.
133 Linstrum, *Ruling Minds*, p. 185.

5

Bodies without evidence

In both Algeria and Kenya, the bodies of torture victims were often made to disappear in order to conceal the criminal act.[1] Alternatively, elaborate scenarios could be contrived where victims were somehow presented as being responsible for their own deaths. For instance, an individual might be shot by the security forces after they had reportedly 'tried to escape' custody.[2] The historical record is filled with such instances, most of which generated insufficient outrage to prompt formal investigations or public outcry. However, in both contexts, there were some cases that were too much to be ignored. The questions they raised drew explicit attention to the institutionalised and widespread violence in the two colonies, which had dire consequences for the colonial authorities. This chapter focuses on two important examples which not only demonstrate the ways that doctors assisted in efforts to cover up torture, but also influenced the emergencies themselves. In one case, the victim of violence was able to draw attention to herself and her plight; in the other, the sheer number of the dead was too high to be ignored.

'A most scandalous piece of professional dishonesty'

When it came to fighting subversion in the Algerian War, the military succeeded in obtaining an unprecedented transfer of power from civil justice to military justice. Article 12 of the law of 3 April 1955, which established a state of emergency in Algeria, provided for this transfer.[3] The granting of authority to hear cases which normally fell under the jurisdiction of the criminal courts was a significant step in consolidating military control over Algeria. As Sylvie Thénault put it, 'the political authorities and the army made the law into a weapon of war which they used against the Algerian freedom fighters'.[4] Rather than provide any sense of actual fairness, though, the military courts in Algeria operated as a parody of justice. In many instances, the courts already had the verdict decided before proceedings even started. This situation was described by French lawyer Jacques Vergès and the writer Georges Arnaud as 'far worse than a denial of justice, a fake justice' made up of 'sham [trials]' and 'plywood' judges where 'only the guillotine would be true'.[5] Medicine, as will be seen, played a pivotal role in supporting these performances.

On 2 June 1960, Simone de Beauvoir, the feminist intellectual and existentialist philosopher, published an article in *Le Monde* called 'Pour Djamila Boupacha'. Her article drew attention to a case which would have been disturbingly familiar to readers in Paris: a 22-year-old Muslim girl had been detained by French paratroopers in Algeria and confessed to having planted a bomb which had failed to explode in September 1959. The young woman, Djamila Boupacha, was subsequently charged with criminal conspiracy and attempted homicide, but she later filed a civil indictment against her interrogators retracting her confession, and alleged that her original statement had been extracted through torture.[6] According to de Beauvoir, Boupacha's ordeal had started on the night of 10 and 11 February 1960, when a large group of Harkis, *gardes mobiles* and police inspectors burst into the Boupacha household, where they beat up Djamila, her father and her brother-in-law, before escorting the three suspects to El-Biar detention centre.[7] Here Djamila was, as de Beauvoir said, 'given a kicking by a group of soldiers' who broke one of her ribs. Five days later, she was transferred to Hussein Dey, where her ordeal continued. Three Harkis, two soldiers and three police inspectors tortured her using electricity on her legs, face, anus and vagina and, between shocks, continued to kick her and put cigarettes out on her skin. Next, she was hanged over a bath by a pole and immersed several times.[8]

Given the content of the piece, as well as the title itself, it is clear that de Beauvoir was recalling the work of Vergès and Arnaud in the case of Djamila Bouhired, which had stirred significant outrage in France in 1957 for similar reasons.[9] There was, however, one feature of Boupacha's case that made it distinct. Several days after her abuse, her interrogators performed what they called the 'bottle treatment', in which the neck of a bottle was forced violently into the victim's vagina in order to rape her and remove her virginity.[10] This final abuse became a common form of assault during the Algerian War. Like the use of electricity, which was often targeted at the genitalia, the rape of both men and women served the purpose of not only torturing the victim, but also terrorising them and their communities. Although sometimes performed for sexual gratification by men, this was not always the aim, as Djamila Boupacha's case demonstrated. Rather, as Branche has powerfully stated, it was 'the woman herself who is the target'.[11] The assault left few physical marks, but it carried a symbolic meaning which was particularly potent within the Muslim communities in Algeria.[12] Rape was therefore used as a tool of terror and domination across the colony, since, through the victim, the soldiers could reach her family, her village and all the circles to which she belonged.[13]

While this pernicious practice was widespread, Boupacha's indictment against the French military has generated an unusual amount of material. Her case has thus been examined by historians interested in a range of questions related to gender, women's bodies and violence within the war more generally; few, however, have paid specific attention to the ways in which medicine featured in the trial.[14] This may be because the official dossier concerning her case is currently unavailable for historical research.[15] Despite this, in 1962, at the war's end, the lawyer Gisèle Halimi and de Beauvoir published *Djamila Boupacha*, which provides a detailed account of her case as it progressed through Algerian and French courts.[16] The book contains a summary of Boupacha's experiences in court provided by de Beauvoir, as well as a narrative account of the Boupacha case, official correspondences, the text for Boupacha's civil indictment, extracts of court transcripts and, most importantly, the various medical reports concerning her person. It thus remains an extensive and valuable source for assessing medical involvement in the attempted cover-up of torture and rape in the Algerian War. Her allegations show significant similarities with the case of Djamila Bouhired, mentioned above, and others who challenged the French authorities; but they go further still by showing instances where the experts themselves contradicted and invalidated one another. As such, the case of Djamila Boupacha raises questions about contested expertise in high-profile cases concerning state denial.

On 15 March 1960, thirty-five days after her arrest, Boupacha was brought before the investigating judge. It was here that she retracted her confession and indicted the soldiers who had abused her.[17] Without losing any time, the magistrate, a M. Bérard, sent her to be examined by a medical expert on the same day. Although this move might be read as a demonstration of concern for the young woman and her health, it is much more likely it was just part of a wider, well-rehearsed performance. Her examiner, Dr Jean-Claude Lévy-Leroy, appears regularly within the historical record in relation to claims of torture. It seems he was a useful candidate for this examination, as his approach to such sensitive cases was characteristically brief, descriptive and neutral in tone.[18] Lévy-Leroy was thus an ideal expert for an examination and trial which already had a foregone conclusion. Lévy-Leroy examined Boupacha's body and provided a scant report which was, as Halimi says, 'a dozen lines long, and that was all'.[19] Within this short report, Lévy-Leroy mentioned that '[Djamila Boupacha] told me she had undergone various "tortures" about a month previously. When examined completely naked, she presented no special marks or scars'.[20] This was his only acknowledgement of the girl's claims about torture, and it neither directly refutes or supports them. He went on to state that:

> All that I found was a slightly painful reaction to pressure upon the left-hand side of the rib-cage. Apart from this I found, at the upper end of the fifth (r.h.) metatarsal, a reddish patch about 1 cm in diameter, which she declares to have been caused by contact with an electrode.[21]

His examination did not suggest any alternative causes for the detainee's complaints, nor did it question their origins, though it certainly seems to play down their severity. In addition, Lévy-Leroy does not factor in the length of time that had elapsed between his patient's alleged abuse and his examination. Delaying examinations was a useful tactic for the military when it came to reports of torture, as the longer they could be delayed, the more the traces of torture would fade.[22] This was a particularly useful method for dealing with traces of electrocution, as the relatively small marks it left disappeared more quickly than lacerations or deep bruising. In fact, in an article published as early as May 1957 in the journal *Esprit*, Paul Thibaud drew attention to this feature of electric torture. In the article, Thibaud noted that 'the application of electrodes on wet skin (by sweat for example) may only cause sparks and therefore small burns, the lesions have often been noted by doctors, but they are officially attributed to "skin diseases"' such as eczema. He went on to quote a sarcastic comment by a Dr Hovnanian, according to whom this form of eczema 'would be peculiar to Algerian prisons'.[23] The military would have therefore known that, by the time Boupacha made her accusations regarding torture, most signs of this trauma would have faded from her body. But what about her rape claims? On this subject, Lévy-Leroy stated that 'It should be noted that she shows signs of acro-cyanosis of the extremities, together with certain menstrual troubles of a constitutional nature'. He went on to stress that 'On the day I examined her, there remained no trace of permanent partial disablement'.[24]

This was Lévy-Leroy's apparent clinical description of the 'bottle treatment' Boupacha claimed to have endured.[25] His descriptive account did not attempt to link the forensic evidence on her body with the narrative provided by the girl herself. Instead, he described the wounds as being of a 'constitutional nature', an unexplained expression which served no useful purpose other than to deny the possibility that Boupacha's 'troubles' had been caused by abuse. The doctor's refusal to elaborate on his findings proved useful for the French government. The day after *Le Monde* published de Beauvoir's article, the newspaper was forced to issue a communiqué 'on order of the general delegation'.[26] President Michal Debré had ordered the seizure of all copies of 'Pour Djamila Boupacha' in Algiers and issued a statement regarding the case. The statement impressed upon the public that 'even before the publication of this article information was opened to the prosecution of Algiers, on complaint of the interested [party], to determine the accuracy of the facts alleged'. To this end, the communiqué stressed, 'the results of the medical report' had not 'concluded to the reality of abuse'.[27] It is curious that the government treated Lévy-Leroy's report as a negative testimony despite it containing some references to certain anomalies in Boupacha's condition.[28] This was only possible because the doctor had failed to connect the evidence with the girl's claims, thus providing an opportunity for his findings to be used against her. It is noteworthy that Lévy-Leroy did not attempt to set the record straight. In fact, it is likely he had no interest in doing so, as there is sufficient evidence of his complicity in the government's cover-up efforts.

In his report of 15 March, Lévy-Leroy explicitly stated that he had conducted some sort of gynaecological examination on Djamila Boupacha. However, he later contradicted himself in court on 14 June 1960. While being questioned by M. Courmontagne, the *juge d'instruction* who replaced Bérard on the Boupacha case, Lévy-Leroy reportedly declared that he had not in fact examined 'the girl's genital organs, since she made no complaint of having been assaulted sexually'.[29] Moreover, while his report had indicated that Boupacha was naked during this examination, the court transcript shows that the doctor suggested she had retained her shift the whole time.[30] This statement not only denied that Boupacha had raised the rape issue at the time, it also went against the doctor's own official report. According to Halimi, Lévy-Leroy added that 'These examinations are always slightly embarrassing', in a way that trivialised the situation and demonstrated a false sense of decency regarding a sensitive matter.[31]

Lévy-Leroy's involvement in the court proceedings is a powerful example of a doctor subordinating his responsibility to the patient in order to serve a higher authority. Yet the contradiction between his report and his subsequent court statement also raises questions about his relationship to the cover-up effort. It is peculiar that the doctor should so blatantly contradict himself when the defence had access to his original report. The impression is difficult to escape that collusions between medical experts and French authorities were not necessarily straightforward but potentially messy. Nevertheless, as with the case of Djamila Bouhired before it, the military courts had no intention of offering a fair trial, and the discrepancies in Lévy-Leroy's account were not addressed by M. Courmontagne. This is not surprising. By this time, the Boupacha case had gained too much public attention and needed to be, as Halimi put it, '[wound] up as soon and as quickly as possible'.[32] For de Beauvoir, this was a serious outrage. As she stated:

> Faced with so flagrant a discrepancy in his evidence one might well be tempted to proclaim this a most scandalous piece of professional dishonesty; but for old medical hands in Algeria such a concept simply does not exist. They are there, invariably, to *deny* that maltreatment has taken place, not to confirm it: they are simply performing their allotted role.[33]

Further evidence implicating Lévy-Leroy in the cover-up emerged later in July 1960, after Boupacha officially filed her complaint against the military. In an effort to quash the claimant's allegations, Bérard, before being replaced by Courmontagne, nominated three new doctors to examine Boupacha without seeking the consent of her council. These doctors – Dr Sirot, Dr Bonafos and Dr Godard – provided another concise report. Its findings, however, corrected Lévy-Leroy on several important points.[34] According to these three doctors, 'Djamila Boupacha's body [was] marked in various places with numerous scars. These scars could have been caused either by contact with some red-hot point, or else deliberately inflicted with some sharp red-hot instrument'.[35] With regard to her claim about a broken rib, they found that 'She has a deformation at the base of the anterior extremity of the left-hand hemithorax'. Finally, on the subject of rape, they observed that 'she is no longer virgo intacta, since her hymen has been ruptured by the insertion of some hard, blunt body, e.g. an erect penis'.[36]

While this second report is just as brief as the first, the little information it does offer is in direct contrast with the findings of Lévy-Leroy's examination on 15 March. According to this later report, Boupacha's body did indeed exhibit signs of injury which clearly had a bearing on her claims. However, the gynaecological assessment was the most damning. Rather than Boupacha suffering from some vague 'menstrual troubles of a constitutional nature', the three doctors found clear evidence that she had been penetrated. Given this information and the discrepancies between his report and his statement at the hearing, the only possible conclusion is that Dr Lévy-Leroy was either an incompetent practitioner or someone determined to invalidate the plaintiff's testimony. Yet while this second report does provide some support for Boupacha's case, it remains notably shallow in its assessment. While making no recommendations for follow-up procedures to examine the nature of the scars and marks on her flesh, the report does not attempt to assess the seriousness or the possible causes of the injury to her rib.[37] In addition, the doctor's reference to an 'erect penis' would certainly suggest they were considering alternatives to the 'bottle treatment'.

Regardless of whether these experts were deliberately avoiding linking her wounds to her story, the discrepancies between their findings and Lévy-Leroy's proved useful for the defence. They allowed Halimi to arrange for a third medical examination to take place, but this time in Paris, with a set of doctors selected by the defence.[38] This was a vital development. It not only provided Boupacha with a chance to gain medical evidence to boost her claims, it also contrasted greatly with the above-mentioned case of Djamila Bouhired, where the defence lawyers were prevented from submitting counter-evidence.[39] Moreover, by transferring her to Paris for the assessment, Boupacha and her legal counsel would have been away from Algeria and the immediate point of control for the military. The final medical examination, in theory, should have been straightforward and unambiguous. However, this was not to be the case. By 1960, the Algerian War was not only a thorny political issue in Algeria; the ferocity it evoked in the more right-wing members of society had spread to the capital. Djamila Boupacha's case had essentially become a microcosm for the broader political divide surrounding the Algerian conflict. Far from being a simple and objective medical examination, then, Boupacha's body and the explanation for the marks it exhibited were now woven into this wider political fabric of unrest.

The examination took place at the infirmary in the Parisian prison of Fresnes, on 28 July 1960.[40] The doctors selected for the job included Professors Lantuejoul and Funck-Brentano, two gynaecologists from the Academy of Medicine; Professor Duperrat, a dermatologist; Professor Christiaens, an obstetrician; and Dr Hélène Michel-Wolfrom, who was commissioned for both her psychiatric and gynaecological experience at the direct request of Halimi.[41] Even at the point of examination, it is possible to detect the level of tension produced by the meeting between the doctors and their patient. According to Boupacha, all the doctors performed their tasks as quickly as they could and refused to interact with her at all. Only Dr Michel-Wolfrom engaged with the patient to any notable extent. In fact, she was the only one of the five experts to volunteer a full and unambiguous statement concerning the patient's condition and the story she professed. This was not because the other doctors were necessarily unable to confirm Boupacha's account, but because they could not agree on how best to present their findings.

Given the wider political context, it is easy to appreciate the problem. On the one hand, if the five doctors produced a report that affirmed the young woman's story, they would essentially be supporting a suspected terrorist at a time when the 'Algeria question' was becoming an increasingly heated topic in the metropole. In fact, according to Halimi, when one doctor suggested they give an unambiguous result in favour of the girl's claims, one of his/her colleagues retorted: 'Want to get yourself knocked off in the street by a bunch of hotheads?'[42] The deeply political nature of the case was clearly affecting the experts' observations and straining their professional allegiances. In this instance, rather than having their loyalty divided between the state and the patient, it was the doctors' personal safety which was the major factor. The decision to assist a suspected terrorist could make the doctors a direct target of political violence by the fanatic believers in *Algérie française*. However, to provide Boupacha with anything other than an objective medical assessment would violate the doctors' ethical responsibilities to protect their patient's best interests.

The situation provides a vital insight into the types of pressures expert witnesses can face when agreeing to take on high-profile and controversial cases. The unstable political atmosphere reveals the limits of professional objectivity. In the context of the Algerian War, the clinical encounter had become part of the theatre of conflict and was now wrapped up in the state's attempts to disavow allegations of torture. Faced with such a dilemma, the five doctors opted for a compromise. The twenty-two-page medical report submitted to M. Brossette at the Paris High Court of Justice was still neutral despite being significantly longer and more detailed than the previous two provided by the military. Dr Duperrat's dermatological findings were negative: he found no evidence that the marks on Boupacha's skin had been caused by cigarettes or electrodes, though he did not offer an alternative cause. Similarly, Dr Christiaens regarded the evidence of a 'hemithoracic deviation', her rib injury, as not significant enough to 'form the basis of any definite verdict ... since it could just as easily be rachitic in origin as due to external violence'.[43] Yet while these statements neither confirmed nor refuted Boupacha's story, a relatively conclusive diagnosis was offered regarding the gynaecological examination. Here the doctors affirmed that:

> Granted that after five months of rapid healing of vulvovaginal tissue normally makes it impossible to identify the method employed in any particular instance of defloration; and, further, bearing in mind the

> fact that we could consult no other examination of the subject's genital organs made *prior to her arrest*, our answer [is] nevertheless: *Yes, Djamila Boupacha may well have had the neck of a bottle inserted into her vaginal passage.*[44]

However, they added that, as of the date of the examination, it was 'impossible to specify either the date or the exact method of her defloration with any precision'. Despite this caveat, the doctors went on to explain that 'the tightness of the vaginal passage, the thickness of the hymen, and the narrow localization of the actual perforations [...] all might well argue *in favour of traumatic defloration*'.[45] This conclusion was significant, but it was still couched in hesitant and neutral language. The five doctors' neutrality, however, differed from previous instances. While Lévy-Leroy and even Sirot, Bonafos and Godard had issued bland descriptive statements in order to serve the interests of the military, either willingly or through pressure, neutrality in this examination was primarily a self-defence tactic, intended to protect the doctors involved from potential threats and actual violence. Yet while four of the five Parisian doctors thought it prudent to sit on the political fence and were unwilling to take a definitive stance on Boupacha's claims, Dr Michel-Wolfrom's psychiatric evaluation did answer in the affirmative.[46]

When Dr Michel-Wolfrom first examined Boupacha on 28 July 1960, she questioned the patient on her personal life, Muslim marriage customs and Algeria in general.[47] She also encouraged Boupacha to keep a diary and promised to return for a second visit in September. According to Halimi, Michel-Wolfrom became convinced that 'Djamila was quite incapable of telling a lie or pretending in any way'. This, Halimi believed, was a 'vital diagnosis' for their case.[48] Although this may be hyperbole, it was indeed Michel-Wolfrom's willingness to offer a testament to Boupacha's claims that made the difference in the end. Michel-Wolfrom's contribution to the final medical report focused on her psychological profile, presenting Boupacha as a religiously devout and obedient daughter, who was essentially sexually immature and almost naive.[49] According to this testimony, she was thus the perfect devotee for the FLN, who provided her with a cause to pursue. This was clearly an important part of the defence for Boupacha's case. Michel-Wolfrom's findings needed to provide strong evidence that Boupacha was indeed a victim of rape if she was going to add weight to the more hesitant verdicts provided by her colleagues in this third report. If this could be achieved, Boupacha's wider torture claims would also gain notable strength. Because of this, the plaintiff's character and image were just as important for her claims as the marks on her body. And as with the latter, an expert eye was needed to *prove* this. So while the army tried to portray Boupacha as a fanatical terrorist who had questionable sexual relations with her accomplices – thus invalidating her rape story – Michel-Wolfrom's psychological testimony attempted to present her as politically minded and spiritually devoted to her nationalism.[50] She was not a violent or duplicitous terrorist but a sane Muslim girl who was ultimately a virgin.

The most important point to note about Michel-Wolfrom's observations is that they invert the traditionally pejorative view of the Muslim in Algeria. As mentioned elsewhere in this book, ethnopsychiatry in Algeria played a vital role in constructing an image of the Algerian population as innately violent and religiously irrational. In fact, according to experts from the Algiers School of psychiatry, it was the Algerians' apparent religious zeal that turned the nationalists into violent terrorists in the first place. In contrast, Boupacha's religious devotion was here presented as a sign of her innocence, something that bolstered her allegations. 'Her mind', Michel-Wolfrom reported, 'seems wholly concerned with political issues, and with accomplishing such tasks as her superiors in the FLN laid down for her'.[51] This was because, Michel-Wolfrom went on, Boupacha 'had identified her personal aspirations with her sense of patriotic and religious mysticism. She is ambitious by nature; but she swears she is devoted, body and soul, to the service of her country'.[52] The girl was therefore selfless when it came to the subject of romance, apparently regarding, as Halimi added, the 'harbouring of her fighting comrades as a duty, and made a sharp distinction between the *camaraderie* engendered by war and the inclination of one's own heart'.[53]

In many ways, Michel-Wolfrom's assessment of Boupacha's devotion to political revolution matched contemporary views about the role of Algerian women in the war. Fanon dedicated a substantial portion of *A Dying Colonialism* to the subject of Algerian women and their relationship to the colonial order.[54] Rather than being passive observers of the conflict, Algerian women were active members of the FLN who, like their Mau Mau counterparts mentioned before, not only took part in combat, but also smuggled weapons and provisions to different units while helping to keep the revolutionary fires burning in the hearts of the Algerian family unit. As Fanon explained:

> It is not a war waged with an active army and reserves. Revolutionary war, as the Algerian people is waging it, is a total war in which the woman does not merely knit for or mourn the soldier. The Algerian woman is at the heart of the combat. Arrested, tortured, raped, shot down, she testifies to the violence of the occupier and to his inhumanity.[55]

This active participation in the war was routinely misunderstood by the French authorities but for individuals like Fanon, female combatants were a new form of political agent who entered the war at the same time as the FLN's 'terrorism techniques'.[56]

What both Fanon and Michel-Wolfram articulate, albeit from different perspectives, is a moment of transformation in Algerian femininity that was wrapped up with the Revolution. Within this moment, ideas about female subjugation and subjectivity were reconfigured in ways that defied contemporary expectation. As such, Boupacha's case embodied much of this social transformation; her body, and specifically the nature of her sexuality, was therefore the terrain upon which the legitimacy of this political emergence was articulated.

According to Michel-Wolfram, virginity was consequently sacred to Boupacha: 'virginity for her was a totemic symbol, with positively magical significance'.[57] Her status as a virgin was a defining psychological feature for Boupacha, according to this account. Her repeated emphasis on the Muslim nuptial ritual requirement that the bride should shed 'virgin blood during the consummation' was a strong indicator that her claims were true, at least in the eyes of her legal counsel and Michel-Wolfrom. For the latter, they were a clear psychological sign that Boupacha's 'mentality [corresponded] with that of a virgin'.[58] While it has been suggested that de Beauvoir and Halimi stressed Boupacha's femininity to gain public sympathy for the young woman's plight, this psychiatric diagnosis also utilised her religious convictions in a similar way.[59] Through this affirmative report, Boupacha gained 'scientific' support for her allegations, which, combined with the gynaecological findings, greatly enhanced her plea. Although it is unclear how the French authorities felt about this development, it appears the cumulative evidence within Boupacha's case had rattled them.

Following the submission of the report to the *juge d'instruction*, Boupacha and her legal counsel were prevented from viewing the whole dossier concerning her case. It seems M. Courmontagne in Algeria had stepped up his efforts to obfuscate the legal process. By refusing them access to this information, the magistrate directly violated their legal right to view these documents as part of the Code de procédure pénale.[60] By this stage, the dossier was replete with incriminating evidence through which the crimes committed against her could be reconstructed. Despite this, the strength of the medical report from the five Parisian doctors, along with the earlier medical discrepancies, was sufficient to get the trial adjourned and transferred to the Appeals Court in Caen, France, on 15 December 1960. Boupacha's case was thus finally removed from the jurisdiction of the Algiers Bar.[61] It was, however, not until 17 April 1961 that Boupacha finally became acquainted with the findings of the five medical examiners.[62] Although the medical report substantiated her claims and contributed to removing the case from the military's jurisdiction, the legal proceedings surrounding her case continued to drag on over the next year. The military in Algeria and their courts continued to hinder the requests for additional evidence and interviews with personnel involved in her interrogation. As the case progressed, witness testimonies from military staff and Boupacha's fellow detainees produced an increasingly damning image of the military's practices in Algeria.[63] Despite this, her torturers were never put on trial. On 29 June 1961, Boupacha was sentenced to death. In the event, however, she was amnestied on 20 March 1962, as part of the Evian Accords which brought the Algerian War to an end.

Although the scandals surrounding individuals like Djamila Bouhired, Djamila Boupacha and other high-profile Algerian nationalists contributed to the unpopularity of the conflict in France, their stories were not enough to conclude it. In fact, by the end of 1961, the French view of Algeria was less one of outrage and more one of apathy. There had been too many scandals, too many reports of torture, massacres, political intrigue and military plots.[64] As de Beauvoir had powerfully warned in her original article in *Le Monde*, 'The most scandalous part of scandal is the getting used to it'.[65] Unlike the situation in Kenya, where it is possible to identify one decisive event which signalled the end of the conflict (see below), the situation in North Africa was different. President de Gaulle had gestured for peace negotiations with the FLN as early as January 1961, but these efforts were fraught with challenges,[66] not least because violence committed by the Organisation de l'armée secrète (OAS), an extreme right-wing paramilitary group, was causing significant disruptions. The OAS took the war against the FLN into their own hands and carried out multiple bombings, torture campaigns, assassinations and disappearances against Muslims and moderate Europeans alike, in order to forestall any negotiations between de Gaulle and the rebels.[67] They even attempted a full military putsch against the President in April 1961.[68] Eventually, the violence of this civil war spilt onto the streets of Paris on 17 October 1961, when an FLN non-violent protest was met by an indiscriminately violent police crackdown under the Paris police chief, Maurice Papon.[69] On top of this, the OAS exported their terrorism to the metropole as well and brought about anarchy in the capital.

Following the Evian Accords and the continued bloody struggle between the OAS and the FLN in Algeria, the majority of the *pied-noir* population felt unsafe in the newly independent country. Independence was thus accompanied by a veritable exodus which saw both Europeans and Harki loyalists leave North Africa for the metropole. Many of the colonial doctors mentioned in this work went with them. Djamila Boupacha and her family were released from prison on 21 April 1962. The amnesty had saved her life, but it had also stripped her of the chance to prosecute her torturers or the doctors who aided them. Her case, however, remains important, for it illustrates the ways in which the state mobilised medical evidence and expert testimony to aid in its denial efforts. It speaks, moreover, to the limits of this evidence and shows how the defence could use counter-expertise to outmanoeuvre the Prosecution in an adversarial court. Finally, of course, it is worth bearing in mind the distinctiveness of Boupacha's case and the presumably much more common instances in which counter-evidence could not be deployed because the investigations into alleged violence were being conducted within a closed environment. Did Kenyan doctors play a similarly significant role in state efforts at cover-up during the Emergency? This is the question to which we now turn.

'A great administrative disaster'

In the final years of the Emergency, the Special Detainee Camp at Hola, a closed camp not far from Mombasa, near Kenya's south-eastern coast, operated as a dumping-ground for 'hard-core' Mau Mau, the more politically minded and recalcitrant rebels. According to colonial officials, these individuals were 'the worst types of detainee', beyond hope of rehabilitation.[70] As stipulated under section 22 of the Detained Persons Regulation, detainees at Hola, and other special detention camps, who were deemed to be 'fit for work' were 'employed in work which the officer-in-charge is satisfied will assist in bringing the Emergency to an end and to that end shall do such work of the nature aforesaid as [they] may be required to do by the officer-in-charge'.[71] Although this work was seen as a fundamental step in the rehabilitation process, as discussed earlier, in many instances it amounted to arduous forced labour. This was the warders' preferred punitive measure to tame the prisoners.

Since early February 1959, harsher measures had been introduced to combat the high levels of perceived malingering and resistance present at Hola.[72] In particular, John Cowan, the Senior Superintendent of Prisons and the original mastermind behind the dilution technique, recommended that the problem could 'best be solved by firmness and by intelligent cooperation between the authorities concerned'. His proposal, what became known as the Cowan Plan, was a recalibrated version of the dilution technique which recommended splitting the detainees into small, manageable groups when subjecting them to hard labour and then using 'compelling force' to coerce them to work. Although he was keen to officially state that 'This does not imply a brutal and harsh regime', the reality was very much the opposite.[73] In fact, on 17 February 1959, the Commissioner of Prisons, John Lewis, admitted in a report to the Minister of Defence that the Cowan Plan involved 'the use of a certain degree of force in which operation someone might get hurt or even killed'.[74]

On the morning of 3 March 1959, eighty-five Mau Mau detainees were taken to perform hard labour as part of the daily routine at Hola. The detainees were escorted to the surrounding fields and given tools for their job as part of an ongoing government irrigation scheme. They were ordered to begin work under the supervision of a group of African warders who greatly outnumbered them, accompanied by Michael Sullivan, the Camp Commandant, who followed in a Land Rover.[75] Despite pressure from the guards and threats from Sullivan, the detainees repeatedly refused to work. The exact details of what followed on that morning remain unclear, but it is known that the African warders, dressed in riot gear and armed with batons, beat the prisoners on Sullivan's command.[76] Despite trying to defend themselves with their labour tools, the detainees were overcome by the assault. By the end of the day, ten were dead, while many others were badly injured; another individual, Ngugi Kariti, lay dying in the hospital. He succumbed to his wounds a few days later.[77]

Prior to the incident at Hola, the British public had rarely been stirred by reports of abuse coming out of the colony. However, by the time news of the deaths reached Britain on 4 March 1959, sentiments had changed. Despite the outrage generated by what is now called the Hola Camp massacre, Governor Baring and Lennox-Boyd, back in London, were determined to protect their people in Kenya. Almost immediately after the deaths were reported to authorities in Britain, efforts to cover up the true reasons for the detainee's demise and the extent of the violence in the camp were set in motion. Baring and Lennox-Boyd, along with the then Prime Minister, Harold Macmillan, were determined to avoid a scandal during an election year.[78] Due to fervent opposition from the Labour MPs, however, the government was forced to conduct a series of inquests into the Hola incident.[79]

Public inquests investigated deaths considered to be 'unnatural', 'violent', 'sudden' or 'accidental' and involved, in normal circumstances, the findings being subjected to public inquiry by a coroner and a lay jury.[80] Within these investigations, the coroners had no formal medical training to guide their thinking but it was through them and the jury's verdict that the cause of death would be decided. This was a process that was based on a form of civic participation,[81] but at Hola, the government managed to resist the demand for an independent, and thus public, inquiry. The subsequent investigations remained internal affairs and were not as rigorous as the Opposition would have liked.[82] Moreover, the evidence gathered by colonial officers investigating the events was poorly assessed and rarely questioned by the acting government. As with the military tribunals in Algeria, what followed was a parody of justice, where the careful control of postmortem evidence and any medical-related information was crucial for sustaining the cover-up effort.

As will be shown below, although the official inquests were anaemic in their search for *truth*, their use of medical evidence reveal the same issues that occurred during most investigations into violence: the doctors involved in the investigations adopted an anodyne neutrality vis-à-vis the allegations of abuse; the experts were apparently misled by suggestions from officers involved in the incident; while a certain level of bungling further limited the impact of the findings.[83] In addition, a comparison of the inquest reports and transcripts with the debates held in the House of Commons over the Hola Camp incident reveals just how significant the medical interpretation was for both the Conservative Government and the Opposition which challenged them. This is a point of contrast with the Boupacha case, in that the findings of the inquests were discussed in Parliament, and not just in the press. Also, unlike in France, where the plaintiff's legal counsel and supporters drew explicit attention to medical complicity in the court's games, little was made in Britain of the medical professionals' involvement in the Hola inquest's cover-up efforts. This, it is argued here, was because the doctors involved were regarded as minor figures in a wider government conspiracy. The Opposition's focus on bringing down high-profile leaders in an election year afforded the same doctors a measure of protection.

As mentioned previously, medical provisions at many camps in Kenya were often limited. Hola Camp, on the other hand, housed both a sick bay and a hospital, which was about half to three-quarters of a mile from the camp. It even had a resident physician who lived on site.[84] Dr Ronald William Moyes, a young Medical Officer in his mid-twenties, had qualified as a doctor in Britain in 1956, before transferring to Kenya in July 1958. Prior to his posting at Hola, Moyes had only eleven weeks of experience with treating African patients while in Kwale, not far from Hola itself.[85] It is curious that the government would appoint someone with so little experience for monitoring the health of detainees in a camp that was regarded as the last bastion of Mau Mau resistance, though it should be admitted that, by 1959, the Colonial Officer was experiencing a serious shortage of medical staff for the colonies.[86] Moyes carried out his functions at the camp with the aid of six African dressers and one assistant.[87] In terms of medical provision, Hola was better than many camps but still extremely lacking in terms of the effective care it needed to offer detainees in a compound of that size. As such, on the morning of 3 March, Moyes was unprepared for the number of injured detainees who would flow through the hospital. Nevertheless, his account of his involvement, available in the transcripts of the subsequent inquests into the incident, is worth a detailed examination.

The first point to note in the inquests is that, when the detainee-patients started to enter the hospital on the day of the massacre, Moyes appeared unwilling to acknowledge evidence of potential abuse. According to his testimony at the first inquest on 18 March 1959, it was at 1 p.m. that Sullivan came to report that 'he had brought in some detainees some of whom were dead and he wanted me to examine them'.[88] The injured detainees, along with the six dead, were transported to the hospital in a lorry. The surviving patients were then placed in wards but soon an additional 'three batches' of injured detainees turned up at the hospital. Moyes admitted that his first concern was for the living, so he turned his attention to the injured rather than examining the bodies of the six dead detainees. At this point, another detainee died. His body was taken out to join the others.[89] The patients showed signs of 'bruising, abrasions, fractures and suspected fractures'. Some of the bruising was, as Moyes explained during the inquest, of a 'linear nature and possibly caused by sticks'. Despite this, Moyes admitted that 'I did not get the impression at that time of serious injury'.[90] Other patients were unconscious on arrival, and another died a quarter of an hour later. This detainee had black eyes and broken teeth; his death, Moyes noted, was probably due to 'internal head injury'.[91]

Soon afterwards, another two unconscious detainees were admitted to the hospital. They, Moyes thought, exhibited signs of 'aspiration of pneumonia', with water coming out of their mouths and noses. While this may have seemed a perplexing set of symptoms to be faced with in this context, Moyes suggested that he had been initially 'persuaded' by a prison officer that the detainees had been drinking heavily from a water bowser at the time when they started to collapse. Moyes appears to have been deliberately misinformed by officers involved in the event. The scenario they suggested was that the water was somehow contaminated or that the detainees' keenness to quench their thirst had caused them to drown themselves. Although the Press Office Handout which was circulated on 4 March 1959 to report on the Hola deaths did not explicitly connect the fatalities with the water, the implied causal relationship allowed it to become *the* initial explanation for the deaths at Hola.[92] It is possible that this was the preferred explanation of a government caught on the back foot by the incident. As discussed in Chapter 3, typhoid epidemics had killed detainees in camps earlier in the Emergency, notably in Manyani. By implying a connection with a 'contaminated water source', the authorities were probably trying to present the deaths as the result of negligence, rather than the more serious charge of outright abuse. It certainly seems that the colonial authorities took this explanation seriously enough to have the water, along with stomach content and liver samples from the dead detainees, examined by Mr Norman Kirby, the Government Chemist, on 6 March 1959. However, the examination found no traces of 'poisonous substances' and thus returned a negative verdict.[93]

Despite the water explanation having been rejected by the time of the first inquest in March 1959, Moyes stuck to his initial impressions with little elaboration. He, however, added more detail in a subsequent inquest held in June of that same year. This later inquest was initiated by the Macmillan government as an internal disciplinary proceeding against Sullivan and his assistant, Superintendent A. C. Coutts, who were charged with providing misleading information to the government investigators and playing down the use of force during the massacre. In particular, they were accused of trying to cover up the violence when a committee consisting of W. M. Campbell, the Acting Deputy Commissioner of Prisons, Mr A. C. Small, the Under Secretary of Defence, and Mr Garland, an Assistant Secretary in African Affairs (referred to collectively in the transcripts as 'the trio'), conducted an initial investigation into the events of 4 March 1959, the day after the massacre. In June, Moyes described the two patients as having 'bubbly chests' and that he had seen 'the water in the lorry near the mouths of the corpses'.[94] Moyes claimed he had come to this initial diagnosis through his fleeting examination of the corpses at the time, along with the oral explanations offered by prison officers. Although the drowning story had been abandoned by the government a week after it was first circulated, Moyes was still repeating it nearly four months later with little discernible effort to add clarity or to set the record straight.[95] Interestingly, in the final public report on the Hola Camp incident published in July 1959, Baring even acknowledged that Moyes had been responsible for 'exaggerating the part played by excessive consumption of water' through 'his preliminary diagnosis of the cause of death in some of the cases as aspiration pneumonia'.[96]

Yet if his account is to be believed, Moyes had been influenced and possibly misled by the prison staff who were directly involved in violence. What we are presented with is thus the image of a doctor who was either incompetent or gullible. This, however, can only be part of the explanation, since Moyes was not operating in a vacuum. His acquaintance with the other detainee-patients who were brought into the hospital on 3 March should have aroused some suspicion. In fact, this highlights a feature that is missing from his wider account: what were the testimonies and claims of the detainee-patients whom he was treating? At no point in any of the inquests does Moyes mention or show consideration for their explanations of what happened that morning or for the marks on their bodies. When the detainees' responses were discussed at all, it was generally to explain how unhelpful they were. Dr Maurice Rogoff, the government pathologist who had been called in to examine the bodies of the detainees on 4 March, described their living companions as 'bloody unhelpful' and as refusing to answer his questions about the incident.[97] It appears there was great distrust between the detainees and the doctors employed by the state to treat them, and for good reason given the common view that sick detainees were merely malingering, as discussed in Chapter 3. This is not surprising given the close relationship between the security forces and the medical officers in these camps. If the detainee-patients did not trust Moyes and his colleagues to protect them, why would they confide in them? This adds greater suspicion to Moyes's account of that day. In fact, it was only when he was directly questioned on the subject that he admitted that there had been some sort of conflict between the prison officers and the detainees. He did not volunteer the information. Apparently, he was told at some unspecified point in the afternoon of 3 March that 'non-cooperative' detainees had been 'hit', but he could not recall who had told him this. However, he said nothing more on this point and then added that, prior to that day, he had not 'seen any injuries probably the result of physical violence on any of the detainees'.[98]

Moyes's testimony, therefore, rested solely on the physical characteristics of the bodies he had examined and not the victim's own explanations. Nor did he see fit to draw attention to the reports of abuse that were circulating in the camp that day, despite clearly being aware of them. During the June Inquest, by which time the cover-up was gaining greater public scrutiny, the young doctor admitted that, when he had been questioned by 'the trio', he had failed to convey the stories about the 'fracas and melee' which he had heard on the day.[99] Instead, he stressed, 'I was not taking it on myself to mention a fracas, I was only mentioning what I saw in the hospital'.[100] This was in response to questions regarding the origins of the drowning story which was subsequently circulated by 'the trio' after their initial investigations in March. But even these medical observations were far from unambiguous. What is curious, though, is that Moyes was permitted to restrict his testimony to these purely clinical matters. Although it may not have been unusual for an ostensibly independent expert witness to be called upon to offer an interpretation of medical evidence on its own, what is suspicious is that Moyes was both offering medical evidence and an interpretation while also being involved in the events themselves.

The expert witnesses in Algeria, such as Dr Lévy-Leroy and Dr Godard, were not involved in the violent circumstances that had caused Boupacha's injuries. As such, their medical observations of her complaints were removed from the events that had caused them, even if the conclusions they drew were still shaped by the military. Yet in Kenya, a doctor who was working and living in the camp, and who had also been present on the day of the massacre, was allowed to simply state his medical observations in the inquest without being challenged. The problems presented by his dual role do not seem to have featured in any of the discussions surrounding the Hola Camp murders. The fact that Moyes's role as a witness may have interfered with his professional observations was not, it seems, even considered. Within the official inquests, Moyes is constantly above suspicion. This is to be expected, given the extent to which Macmillan's government was trying to mitigate the situation by controlling the inquest itself. The only time when suspicions were raised about Moyes's professional knowledge and role during the incident was when the findings of the June inquest were questioned in the House of Commons by the Opposition on 27 July 1959.

The subject was first broached by Sir Dingle Mackintosh Foot, the Labour MP for Ipswich, who raised the question of the Hola Camp deaths along with the 'the wider question of the detention without trial in British Dependencies of British subjects and British-protected persons'.[101] Foot was particularly unimpressed with the findings of the June inquest, which amounted to very little, save for a slight reprimand to the Commissioner of Prisons, and to Sullivan, who was 'required to retire from the service without loss of gratuity'. These were the only two individuals who were penalised in any way. As Foot noted, 'Everybody else who was concerned in this matter gets away scot-free'.[102] Of particular interest to Foot was 'the summary of the information which was given to Mr Campbell and his colleagues by Dr Moyes' . Here, Foot pointed to a 'conflict of evidence between Dr Moyes and Mr Campbell'. According to this summary, the former had reported that, on 3 March, he had admitted a number of detainees to hospital with bruises, and that there were 'two possible fractures and all had high temperatures'. The latter, on the other hand, had stated that Moyes had not told them anything 'about any other injuries' other than minor cuts and bruises. This description of the injuries was further softened in Campbell's final report, which stated that 'The Medical Officer informed us that quite a number of those in hospital were suffering from slight bruises; one man was given immediate attention on being injured in the scuffle on the way to the work site [...]'.[103] In this instance, suspicion was directed at Campbell; later in the debate, however, Barbara Castle, Labour MP for Blackburn, pointed the finger directly at Moyes:

> Let me come to the Medical Officer at Hola, Dr Moyes. Here is a man who when ten men have died gives his opinion as to the cause of death as aspiration pneumonia. I am no medical person, but I have consulted my hon. Friend the Member for Stoke-on-Trent, Central (Dr B. Stross) and, as I understand it, aspiration pneumonia is caused

> when men inhale water into the lungs as happens in drowning; and nobody at Hola had had a bath. What was really happening was that dying men were vomiting water that they had drunk, and any person fit to hold the office of medical officer in charge of detainees ought to have enough medical knowledge to be aware of that fact.

She went on to add: 'Of course, perhaps he did, but perhaps like everybody else he was "covering up"'.[104] Moyes, she suggested, was playing his part in the concealment effort. In her view, 'The most significant words of all in this business were spoken by Mr Marsden, the District Officer, at the inquest. He said: There was a general attitude amongst all Europeans not to say anything'.[105]

Yet while Moyes's testimony may have done little to illuminate the reality of violence at the camps, the government pathologist, the aforementioned Dr Rogoff, was more forthright. The postmortem evidence he presented to the first inquest in March 1959 determined that the detainees had indeed been killed by violence. Through his examination, he concluded that multiple victims died from acute pulmonary oedema.[106] He added that the symptoms of this 'may be similar' to those of 'aspirative pneumonia', as suggested by Moyes. The key point here was that the pneumonia 'resulted from material going into the lungs which should not do'.[107] Ngugi Kariti, the last victim of the Hola attack, had also died from this as well as 'acute congestive heart failure', which, Rogoff argued, was 'caused by shock and haemorrhage due to severe loss of blood caused by multiple bruising', that is, 'the result of violence'.[108] Yet while this may have appeared to be a damning indictment against those running the camp, it was itself not free from ambiguity.

Dr William Eric Laws, one of the three doctors brought in to assist Moyes following the deaths, had come up with the idea that some of the victims may have been suffering from severe scurvy. Scurvy is a vitamin C deficiency disease that, as Rogoff explained, could result in a tendency to bleed 'onto skin, bone, muscles and other parts of body'. This, he said, 'may lead to weakening of bone resulting in earlier fracture than in normal individuals'.[109] The implication was that, had the detainees been suffering from scurvy at the time of the attack on 3 March, then some of them may have had a lower 'resistance of body to shock', which would have resulted in their deaths. For Laws, the scurvy diagnosis might have helped explain the 'rather abnormal amount of bleeding particularly in the case of' Ngugi Kariti, whom Laws viewed as an exceptional case. On 9 March, Laws and his colleagues found two patients in hospital who were suffering from 'classical scurvy'. Both these individuals had been in hospital before the incident took place on 3 March. Instead of trying to carry out further investigations, however, they decided to just treat 'all the seriously ill as possible scurvies'.[110] He found that, of those in hospital after the incident, 'All the cases of haemoptysis [coughing up blood] – some 13 – which had occurred at different times had recovered from their blood spitting by the evening of 12th March 1959'.[111] However, despite this, it was still far from certain that the deceased had been suffering from the deficiency disease. In fact, Rogoff repeatedly asserted that the detainee's injuries in themselves would have been 'sufficient [...] to have caused death without involving the level of vitamin C or ascorbic acid deficiency'.[112] Even Laws had to concede that 'there is no evidence' that the eleven dead had suffered from scurvy.[113] Rogoff's conclusions were further supported by the forensic evidence supplied by Dr Geoffrey Lowe Timms, the Assistant Director of Laboratory Services in Medical Research Laboratory in Nairobi. Timms had examined the lungs of Ngugi Kariti and found evidence of severe haemorrhaging. After stating that he 'had never seen anything like it before', he admitted that such condition could be 'a result of blows on the chest wall'. Nevertheless, although he agreed with Rogoff's findings concerning the probable cause of death, he could not discount the possibility that some sort of deficiency disorder had contributed to the excessive bleeding among the various victims.[114]

The final inquest report of July 1959 accepted that 'there was almost certainly a sub-clinical state of vitamin C deficiency in Hola on 3rd March'.[115] Rogoff's reported explanation that 'the onset of scurvy is insidious and that early symptoms may be overlooked by an experienced doctor' suggested there was an error of oversight here.[116] Many of the detainees involved in the attack had an underlying deficiency disorder, which made them more likely to die from violence, but the symptoms of this disorder, at this stage, were too slight to be easily detected. Despite this, the level of violence was in itself sufficient to kill most of the victims. Moyes, therefore, was presented as not necessarily being remiss for his confusing diagnosis. The implication was that Sullivan had failed in his responsibilities and that he had tried to deliberately mislead 'the trio' when they arrived the day after the deaths to investigate the situation. However, as Barbara Castle noted in the House of Commons during the debate in June 1959, Moyes, Sullivan and the Commissioner for Prisons had all been aware of the scurvy epidemic at Hola as early as February that year. A secret report sent to the Commissioner by Sullivan on 13 February 1959, just under a month before the massacre, shows that Moyes was actively investigating the 'large numbers [of detainees who were] reporting sick, some with swollen limbs' and who were unable to work on the irrigation scheme.[117] 'Those swollen limbs', Castle explained, 'were the sign of the scurvy which was later found by the coroner to have been widespread in the camp'.[118] Rather than use this information to further condemn Sullivan or even Moyes, Castle turned her attention to 'the Commissioner of Prisons', who 'did not consider this sign of widespread sickness among co-operative detainees worthy even of comment from him, let alone investigation'.[119] In addition, Castle presented evidence that the Commissioner had ignored warnings from Sullivan that the use of the Cowan Plan in Hola was ill advised. By taking this line, Castle continued to implicate the whole colonial government and the Colonial Office in negligence and efforts to cover up the extent of violence in the camp and the colony more generally.[120]

By concentrating on the colonial powers that be, Castle took the focus away from the doctor in this instance. Moyes thus escaped any further scrutiny into his role in the cover-up efforts. He continued to serve as the resident doctor at the camp and, after the Emergency came to an end and Kenya received its independence, he was a registered medical practitioner in Kenya up to as late as 1964.[121] In the end, it seems, the Opposition were not willing to expend energies to pursue one doctor who may have colluded with the security forces to disguise the violence at Hola. What they were really after were the officials who had conspired to bury the evidence more generally. Why would they be worried about individual cogs when they were trying to bring down the vast engine of indiscriminate violence in the detention camps?

The Hola Camp massacre was to be the decisive event in Kenya's road to independence.[122] It expedited the emptying and closing of the detention camps and finally brought the Emergency to an end in 1960.[123] After this, as Anderson says, 'there was no way back'. Even members of the Tory party presented the events at Hola and the subsequent whitewashing efforts as a disgrace. Famously, the young Enoch Powell stated in the July debate at the House of Commons that the whole thing was 'a great administrative disaster'.[124] Regarding the standard of treatment in Kenya, he added: 'We cannot say, "We will have African standards in Africa, Asian standards in Asia and perhaps British standards here at home." We have not that choice to make. We must be consistent with ourselves everywhere'.[125] If this was not possible, he argued, then Britain should divest itself of its empire. On 12 January 1960, the Kenya Emergency was officially lifted. Ian Macleod, Lennox-Boyd's replacement as Secretary of State for the Colonies, then started the transition process to give Kenya a constitution and a majority black rule.[126] Independence was eventually granted on 12 December 1963. The end of the Mau Mau rebellion was thus largely brought about by the excessive use of violence that had characterised the British counterinsurgency campaign throughout the 1950s. Unlike in Algeria, and despite their involvement in the Emergency, many colonial doctors continued to live and serve in the newly independent nation along with other wealthy settlers. Medical collusion or complicity with violence and torture were tacitly forgotten as part of President Jomo Kenyatta's more general 'forgive and forget' policy.[127] There would be no investigations or prosecutions into any act of violence during the rebellion, nor would any European doctor attempt to break the deep culture of silence that continued to surround these events.

Conclusion

This chapter has examined the various ways that physicians reacted to torture and the damaged or deceased bodies it produced. It did so by focusing on two extreme case studies where medical expertise and opinion were sought by the colonial governments or the security forces to help conceal evidence of abuse. In both cases, it is not easy to identify whether doctors willingly colluded with torture or whether they were caught up in what were otherwise extremely complicated and politically charged situations with few obvious answers. However, collectively, the actions taken by the doctors in these two case studies do shine important light on the ways that medical expertise could help cover up abuse by, for want of a better word, 'fudging' their duties during investigations into abuse in order to obfuscate the truth.

The court trial of Djamila Boupacha in Algeria and the Hola Camp massacre in Kenya not only provide details on the atmosphere of collusion and confusion present in both contexts, but they also help to bring the narratives concerning these two emergencies to an end. While it is well known that the military manipulated the law in Algeria in order to hold show trials that legitimised the execution of captured FLN rebels, the case of Djamila Boupacha represents a rare instance where a range of medical expertise was used to undermine the plaintiff's accusations. In this case, Dr Lévy-Leroy appears as an unambiguous offender who purposefully underplayed Boupacha's injuries, especially those related to her rape claims, as well as openly lying during court. As has been suggested here, this is either a sign of an incompetent doctor or one who was deliberately trying to dismiss her case. Yet the extent to which his report conflicts with that of Drs Sirot, Bonafos and Godard highlights an almost careless effort to participate in this cover-up effort, which may itself tell us something about the messy nature of such collaborations between the medical community and the military. Nevertheless, these contradictions allowed Boupacha's counsel to secure a transfer to the metropole, where she could be examined by five practitioners who were beyond the military's reach. But even in Paris, the examination of Boupacha's body was not free from political pressures. In fact, this chapter has argued that, by this stage in the War, Boupacha's case had become a microcosm of the wider political instabilities surrounding this conflict and so an affirmative or negative report was itself a contentious and politically charged act which could put the safety of the examining physicians into question. Ultimately, it was Dr Michel-Wolfrom's affirmative psychological and carefully worded gynaecological report which made the difference. Using language that presented the young woman as a naive virgin and a religiously devout nationalist, Michel-Wolfrom was able to vindicate Boupacha's claims. Despite this, Boupacha did not receive justice for her case, nor was she ever put on trial, as the amnesty introduced at the end of the Algerian War removed her chance of pursuing her torturers.

Finally, the death of eleven detainees during the Hola Camp massacre represents the last significant scandal in the Kenya Emergency, which led directly to the end of the detention process and Kenya's subsequent independence. This case, it has been shown, brings together many elements of the types of ineffective medical reporting that characterised other investigations into abuses in Kenya. Despite the Opposition's efforts back in Parliament to have the incident subject to an independent investigation, the actual inquests were organised by a government determined to protect the staff involved in the violence. During these inquests, the resident Medical Officer for Hola Camp, Dr Moyes, functioned simultaneously as a material witness and expert, which raised few objections from either examining magistrates or the Opposition in the House of Commons. The testament Moyes offered was confused and unclear, especially as he seemed initially to suggest the detainees had died from drowning or contaminated water. He was also reticent for the most part when it came to the rumours about the violence that had taken place on the morning of 3 March, pointing out that he had relied on information gathered from other staff to shape his verdict. Moyes had direct access to the detainees who witnessed the attacks, but he paid them little attention. As such, the detainee-patients were not permitted to provide their own account of what happened to their bodies. As with the case of Djamila Boupacha in Algeria, the medical findings were crucial for dictating the trajectory of the investigation, but in the end the pathologist's findings were not definitive enough for any serious criminal charges to be brought against those involved. The Opposition scrutinised the details of inquest reports but, so this chapter has argued, any potential evidence of collusion between the medical staff at Hola and the wider cover-up effort were of secondary importance when the overall aim was to topple the Government itself.

Notes

1 For Kenya, see David M. Anderson and Paul J. Lane, 'The unburied victims of Kenya's Mau Mau Rebellion: where and when does the violence end?', in Jean-Marc Dreyfus and Elisabeth Anstett (eds), *Human Remains in Society: Curation and Exhibition in the Aftermath of Genocide and Mass-Violence* (Manchester: Manchester University

Press, 2016), pp. 14–37; for Algeria, see Klose, *Human Rights in the Shadow of Colonial Violence*, pp. 185–186.

2 Richard Evans, *Law and Disorder: or Scenes of Life in Kenya* (Bath: The Pitman Press, 1956), pp. 188–189.

3 It stated that 'When the state of emergency is established in part or the entirety of a department, a decree issued at the behest of the Minister of Justice and the Minister of Defence may authorise military courts to hear crimes and related felony cases that [normally] fall under the department's appellate court'. These powers were later extended by the law of 23 April 1955, which provided an extensive list of crimes that could now be prosecuted by military courts. These included a variety of petty crimes, as well as those more directly related to terrorism. See Sylvie Thénault, 'Armée et justice en guerre d'Algérie', *Vingtième siècle. Revue d'histoire* 57 (1998), p. 106.

4 Thénault, *Une drôle de justice*, p. 9.

5 George Arnaud and Jacques Vergès, *Pour Djamila Bouhired* (Paris: Les Editions de minuit, 1957), p. 8.

6 Simone de Beauvoir, 'Pour Djamila Boupacha', *Le Monde*, 2 June 1960. www.lemonde.fr/archives/article/1960/06/02/pour-djamila-boupacha_2092987_1819218.html [Accessed 12 January 2018].

7 De Beauvoir, 'Pour Djamila Boupacha'.

8 De Beauvoir, 'Pour Djamila Boupacha'.

9 On 11 July 1957, Djamila Bouhired and Djamila Bouazza were the first two women to appear before the Permanent Armed Forces Tribunal [*le tribunal permanent des forces armées*] in Algeria. Both young women were accused of helping to organise or executing bomb attacks against Europeans earlier that year. Bouazza was accused of planting a bomb on a coffee table in Coq Hardi in Algiers, which killed multiple people and injured dozens more. Bouhired was a twenty-six-year-old Algerian militant supporter of the FLN. She was arrested on 26 April 1957, after being found carrying important correspondences intended for two leaders of the rebellion, Yacef Saadi and Ali Ammar (otherwise known as Ali la Pointe). Bouazza had also told the court that Bouhired had actively planted bombs. While the case seemed damning, it was not straightforward. Firstly, Bouazza was thought to be mentally unstable and so her allegations were suspect, while Bouhired had also alleged that she had been tortured while in custody. Despite many complaints from their legal representatives, the military court would not allow the defence to provide any counter-evidence to support their case and ultimately sentenced the two women to death on 15 July 1957, four days after the trial started. In response, Vergès and Arnaud published *Pour Djamila Bouhired*,

which contained the first public denunciation of military's use of torture in North Africa and the irregularities in court procedure taking place in its defence.

10 De Beauvoir, 'Pour Djamila Boupacha'.

11 Raphaëlle Branche, 'Des viols pendant la guerre d'Algérie', *Revue d'histoire* 75 (2003), p. 128.

12 Lazreg, *Torture and the Twilight of Empire*, pp. 154–160.

13 Branche, 'Des viols pendant la guerre d'Algérie', p. 128.

14 One exception to this is a short analysis of the two doctors involved in the Boupacha case by Branche. See Branche, *La Torture et l'armée pendant la guerre d'Algérie*, pp. 474–476. Others who have discussed her case more generally include Marnia Lazreg, 'Chapter 6. Women: between torture and military feminism', in *Torture and the Twilight of Empire*, pp. 145–169; Ryan Kunkle, ' "We must shout the truth to the rooftops": Gisèle Halimi, Djamila Boupacha, and sexual politics in the Algerian War of Independence', *Iowa Historical Review* 4 (2013), pp. 5–24; and Judith Surkis, 'Ethics and violence: Simone de Beauvoir, Djamila Boupacha, and the Algerian War', *French Politics, Culture & Society* 28 (2010), pp. 38–55.

15 It was not possible to consult the documents related to this case as part of this study. This is because they are currently covered by the seventy-five-year restriction period without special derogation.

16 Simone de Beauvoir and Gisèle Halimi, *Djamila Boupacha: The Story of the Torture of a Young Algerian Girl Which Shocked Liberal French Opinion*, trans. Peter Green (Paris: Gallimard, 1962).

17 Anonymous, 'Le Cas de Djamila Boupacha signalé à la Commission de sauvegarde', *Le Monde*, 27 May 1960. www.lemonde.fr/archives/article/1960/05/27/le-cas-de-djamila-boupacha-signale-a-la-commission-de-sauvegarde_2089098_1819218.html [Accessed 15 July 2019].

18 Branche, *La Torture et l'armée pendant la guerre d'Algérie*, pp. 474–475.

19 De Beauvoir and Halimi, *Djamila Boupacha*, p. 52.

20 Dr Lévy-Leroy's medical examination of Djamila Boupacha, 15 March 1960, reproduced in de Beauvoir and Halimi, *Djamila Boupacha*, pp. 105–106.

21 De Beauvoir and Halimi, *Djamila Boupacha*, pp. 105–106.

22 A similar tactic was used in the case of Djamila Bouhired, who was not examined by the military doctor until a month had passed following her complaints. In this time, her wounds had more or less healed, presenting the doctor with an opportunity to produce a negative report. See Arnaud and Vergès, *Pour Djamila Bouhired*, pp. 77–78.

23 Paul Thibaud, 'Comment fonctionne la justice en Algérie', *Esprit* 250 (1957), p. 863.
24 Dr Lévy-Leroy's medical examination of Djamilia Boupacha, 15 March 1960, reproduced in de Beauvoir and Halimi, *Djamila Boupacha*, pp. 105–106.
25 De Beauvoir and Halimi, *Djamila Boupacha*, pp. 105–106.
26 Anonymous, 'Un article sur le cas de Djamila Boupacha provoque la saisie du "Monde" à Alger et un communiqué du gouvernement', *Le Monde*, 3 June 1960. www.lemonde.fr/archives/article/1960/06/03/un-article-sur-le-cas-de-djamila-boupacha-provoque-la-saisie-du-monde-a-alger-et-un-communique-du-gouvernement_2093607_1819218.html [Accessed 15 July 2019].
27 Anonymous, 'Un article sur le cas de Djamila Boupacha'.
28 De Beauvoir and Halimi, *Djamila Boupacha*, p. 67.
29 Dr Lévy-Leroy's statement in court, quoted in de Beauvoir and Halimi, *Djamila Boupacha*, p. 52.
30 De Beauvoir and Halimi, *Djamila Boupacha*, p. 52.
31 De Beauvoir and Halimi, *Djamila Boupacha*, p. 106.
32 Gisèle Halimi's narrative of the Boupacha case, in de Beauvoir and Halimi, *Djamila Boupacha*, p. 106.
33 Simone de Beauvoir, 'Introduction', in de Beauvoir and Halimi, *Djamila Boupacha*, p. 12 (emphasis in original).
34 It should be noted that there is a high chance Dr Godad is the same medical expert who examined Djamila Bouhired in 1957 when she made her allegations of torture. According to Vergès, Bouhired was examined by a Dr Goddard, who provided a similarly scant and inconclusive account of her wounds. In fact, he recorded a festering bullet wound which had been kept open by subsequent beatings as being 'fistula of tuberculous origin', while another wound that had already closed was described as an 'old tuberculous fistula'. See Arnaud and Vergès, *Pour Djamila Bouhired*, pp. 77–78.
35 The medical report produced by Drs Sirot, Godard and Bonafos as reproduced in de Beauvoir and Halimi, *Djamila Boupacha*, p. 104 (emphasis in original text).
36 De Beauvoir and Halimi, *Djamila Boupacha*, p. 104.
37 De Beauvoir and Halimi, *Djamila Boupacha*, p. 116.
38 Anonymous, 'CINQ MEDECINS SONT DESIGNES POUR EXAMINER EN METROPOLE DJAMILA BOUPACHA', *Le Monde*, 19 July 1960. www.lemonde.fr/archives/article/1960/07/19/cinq-medecins-sont-designes-pour-examiner-en-metropole-djamila-boupacha_2102119_1819218.html [Accessed 15 July 2019].

39 Arnaud and Vergès, *Pour Djamila Bouhired*, pp. 40–41, 90–91.
40 De Beauvoir and Halimi, *Djamila Boupacha*.
41 Confusingly, *Le Monde* referred to Professor Christiaens as 'expert in forensic medicine' and not an obstetrician. See Anonymous, 'CINQ MEDECINS SONT DESIGNES POUR EXAMINER EN METROPOLE DJAMILA BOUPACHA'.
42 One of the five doctors quoted in de Beauvoir and Halimi, *Djamila Boupacha*, p. 124.
43 Extract of the medical report of the five doctors examining Djamila Boupacha, quoted in de Beauvoir and Halimi, *Djamila Boupacha*, p. 125.
44 De Beauvoir and Halimi, *Djamila Boupacha*, p. 125 (emphasis in the original text).
45 De Beauvoir and Halimi, *Djamila Boupacha*, pp. 125–126 (emphasis in the original text).
46 Although it cannot be ruled out that the doctors involved in her previous examinations were not subjected to threats from the military either.
47 De Beauvoir and Halimi, *Djamila Boupacha*, p. 120.
48 De Beauvoir and Halimi, *Djamila Boupacha*, p. 123.
49 See the extract of Dr Michel-Wolfrom's contribution to the five doctor's medical report, reproduced de Beauvoir and Halimi, *Djamila Boupacha*, p. 123.
50 In July 1960, the military circulated a photo of Boupacha in the company of several FLN soldiers in an attempt to discredit her image. The images were given to multiple right-wing magazines, which used them to portray the girl as having questionable sexual relationships with the soldiers. See de Beauvoir and Halimi, *Djamila Boupacha*, p. 87.
51 De Beauvoir and Halimi, *Djamila Boupacha*, p. 126.
52 De Beauvoir and Halimi, *Djamila Boupacha*, 126.
53 De Beauvoir and Halimi, *Djamila Boupacha*, p. 126.
54 Fanon, *A Dying Colonialism*, pp. 35–67.
55 Fanon, *A Dying Colonialism*, p. 66.
56 Jeffrey Louis Decker, 'Terrorism (un)veiled: Frantz Fanon and the women of Algiers', *Cultural Critique* (1990), p. 180.
57 De Beauvoir and Halimi, *Djamila Boupacha*, p. 126.
58 De Beauvoir and Halimi, *Djamila Boupacha*, p. 126.
59 Surkis, 'Ethics and violence', p. 44.
60 De Beauvoir and Halimi, *Djamila Boupacha*, p. 128.
61 Anonymous, 'A LA COUR DE CASSATION: LA PLAINTE POUR SERVICES DE MLLE BOUPACHA SERA INSTUITE

A CAEN ET NON PLUS A ALGER', *Le Monde*, 17 December 1960. www.lemonde.fr/archives/article/1960/12/17/la-plainte-pour-sevices-de-mlle-boupacha-sera-instruite-a-caen-et-non-plus-a-alger_2105512_1819218.html [Accessed 15 July 2019].

62 De Beauvoir and Halimi, *Djamila Boupacha*, p. 135.

63 In a letter addressed to 'Monsieur le Général Cdt. La R.T. et le C.A. d'Oran', the Général de Corps d'Armée and Commandant Supérieur des Forces en Algérie, Ailleret, showed considerable concern for the revelations made regarding named soldiers involved in Boupacha's case. Although I have not been able locate a response to this letter, his concerns reveal the extent to which the military were becoming increasingly rattled by her case. See SHD 1 H 1246/d.2. See also Anonymous, 'L'INSTRUCTION DE L'AFFAIRE BOUPACHA', *Le Monde*, 1 July 1961. www.lemonde.fr/archives/article/1961/07/01/l-instruction-de-l-affaire-boupacha_2265228_1819218.html [Accessed 15 July 2019].

64 The scandals of the Algerian War were greeted with the same type of detachment by the French as more modern versions have in recent years, such as Guantanamo Bay, Abu Ghraib and Baghram. See Surkis, 'Ethics and violence', p. 38.

65 De Beauvoir, 'Pour Djamila Boupacha'.

66 On 8 January 1961, de Gaulle organised a referendum where voters were asked to respond to questions about self-determination for the Algerian people. See Droz and Lever, *Histoire de la guerre d'Algérie, 1954–1962*, p. 297.

67 Evans, *Algeria*, pp. 291–292.

68 Benjamin Stora, *La Gangrène et l'oubli* (Paris: La Découverte, 1998), pp. 204–205.

69 Josh Cole, 'Remembering the Battle of Paris: 17 October 1961 in French and Algerian Memory', *French Politics, Culture & Society* 21 (2003), p. 24.

70 TNA FCO 141/5651, p. 2. J. Hayden Lewis, Commissioner of Prisons, 'Directive for use of force in detention camps', 10 September 1957.

71 TNA CO 542/52. Section 22 of the Emergency (detained persons) Regulation, 1954.

72 TNA FCO 141/5651. J. B. T. Cowan, Senior Superintendent of Prisons, 'Discipline – Hola Camp', 11 February 1959.

73 As discussed in the previous chapter, from July 1957, torture in the form of the dilution technique was officially sanctioned within the Kenya detention camps. This provided prison staff with the legal justification for extreme acts of violence, especially if it led to a prisoner's confession. In addition to this, the prison staff were issued a series of

directives which permitted the use of force in certain conditions, such as in self-defence, during prison riots, attempted escapes or to overcome 'violence or resistance'. The loose language surrounding the 'use of force' meant Hola Camp could operate with the type of impunity that characterised the detention process. See TNA FCO 141/5651. J. Hayden Lewis, Commissioner of Prisons, 'Directive for use of force in detention camps', 10 September 1957.

74 TNA CO 822/1267. Records of the Proceedings of an Enquiry Under Colonial Regulation 60 into charges against Superintendent M. G. Sullivan, M.B.E., and Assistant Superintendent A. C. Coutts, both of the Kenya Prisons Service', p. 23.

75 David M. Anderson, 'Mau Mau in the High Court and the "lost" British Empire archives: colonial conspiracy or bureaucratic bungle?', *The Journal of Imperial and Commonwealth History* 39 (2011), p. 705.

76 Elkins, *Britain's Gulag*, pp. 346–347; Anderson, 'Mau Mau in the High Court and the "lost" British Empire archives', p. 705.

77 Anonymous, 'Inquest on 11 Mau Mau: HAD BEEN "PREVAILED ON" TO WORK', *Manchester Guardian*, 19 March 1959.

78 Elkins, *Britain's Gulag*, p. 349.

79 Elkins, *Britain's Gulag*, p. 349.

80 Ian Adnan Burney, 'Viewing bodies: medicine, public order, and English inquest practice', *Configurations* 2 (1994), p. 33.

81 Burney, 'Viewing bodies', p. 33.

82 Elkins, *Britain's Gulag*, p. 349.

83 In early 1959, a security guard called Samual Githu was sentenced by the Attorney General with mere assault after he beat a prisoner to death. During the inquest, a Dr Hadman investigating allegedly bungled the process by not only leaving the body for several days but also recording the wrong cause of death. The frequency of such 'inept' or unwilling medical examinations of the victims of torture became so frustrating that, on 24 February 1959, Reginald Paget, the MP for Northampton stated in Parliament that 'this is the sixth case of which I am aware where no murder charge has been brought each time one is told that it is very unfortunate and that a man did fire a revolver but, unfortunately, the damage done to the heart of the deceased was such that it was impossible for the doctor to say that the heart might not previously have had some natural defect from which the chap might have died, and that therefore a charge of murder cannot be brought and the Government are very reluctantly obliged to accept the plea of common assault'. For Githu's case, see TNA FCO 141/5668/50. 'Meeting Held in the Office of the Deputy Public Prosecutor', 1 January 1959. For the discussion in Parliament, see Hansard. Parliamentary

Debate, 'Prisons and Detention Camps, Kenya', Reginald Paget MP, 24 February 1959, paragraphs 1025–1026.

84 TNA CO 822/1267. 'Records of the Proceedings of an Enquiry Under Colonial Regulation 60 into charges against Superintendent M. G. Sullivan, M.B.E., and Assistant Superintendent A. C. Coutts, both of the Kenya Prisons Service', p. 43. See also the oral evidence given by Dr Ronald William Moyes in the same source on 8 June 1959. Elkins, *Britain's Gulag*, p. 71.

85 Anonymous, 'The "unco-operative" beaten: Inquest on Mau Mau detainees', *Manchester Guardian*, 25 March 1959.

86 Hansard. House of Commons Debate, 'Doctors', Mr Blenkinsop MP, 17 June 1958, paragraphs 887–888.

87 TNA CO 822/1267. 'Records of the Proceedings of an Enquiry Under Colonial Regulation 60 into charges against Superintendent M. G. Sullivan, M.B.E., and Assistant Superintendent A. C. Coutts, both of the Kenya Prisons Service', p. 55. See also Anonymous, 'The "unco-operative" beaten: Inquest on Mau Mau detainees'.

88 TNA FCO 141/5651. Dr Ronald William Moyes's witness statement in 'Inquest on Eleven Persons who Died in the Hola District, Coast Province, on or about 3rd March, 1959. Vol. 1', p. 39.

89 TNA FCO 141/5651. Dr Ronald William Moyes's witness statement, p. 40.

90 TNA FCO 141/5651. Dr Ronald William Moyes's witness statement, p. 40.

91 TNA FCO 141/5651. Dr Ronald William Moyes's witness statement, p. 40.

92 The Press Office Handout, 'Death of Ten Detainees at Hola', states that 'The deaths occurred after they had drunk water from a water cart which was used by all members of the working party and by their guards'. TNA FCO 141/5651. 'Hola Inquest Case No. 1 of 1959. Exhibit No. X: Kenya News: Press Office Handout No. 142: Deaths of Ten Detainees at Hola', 4 March 1959.

93 TNA FCO 141/5651. Norman Kirby's witness statement in 'Inquest on Eleven Persons who Died in the Hola District, Coast Province, on or about 3rd March, 1959. Vol. 1', p. 10.

94 TNA CO 822/1267. Oral evidence from Dr Ronald William Moyes, 8 June 1959 as part of 'Records of the Proceedings of an Enquiry Under Colonial Regulation 60 into charges against Superintendent M. G. Sullivan, M.B.E., and Assistant Superintendent A. C. Coutts, both of the Kenya Prisons Service', p. 71.

95 Although Kirby's report contributed to the water story being dropped, there were other reasons. Barbra Castle had also received evidence from

D. N. Prit, the left-wing QC who was representing the detainees in Kenya. According to an interview Castle later gave, Prit had managed to obtain the autopsy reports of the eleven dead detainees which showed the extent of violence used to kill them. Elkins, *Britain's Gulag*, p. 345.

96 Evelyn Baring, 'Despatches from Governor, Kenya to Secretary of State for the Colonies', in *Further Documents Relating to the Deaths of Eleven Mau Mau Detainees at Hola Camp in Kenya* (London: Her Majesty's Stationery Office, 1959), p. 7.

97 CO 822/1267. Dr Rogoff had also worked on the case of Kamau Gichina, a Kikuyu detainee who died in police custody, as the government pathologist, p. 50.

98 TNA CO 822/1267. Oral evidence from Dr Ronald William Moyes, pp. 43, 53.

99 CO 822/1267. Dr Moyes's testimony when re-examined on the subject of violence in the camp, p. 73.

100 CO 822/1267. Dr Moyes's testimony when re-examined, p. 73.

101 Hansard. House of Commons Debate, 'Hola Camp, Kenya (Report)', Mr Dingle Foot MP, 27 July 1959, paragraphs 181–182.

102 Hansard. House of Commons Debate, 'Hola Camp, Kenya (Report)', paragraphs 181–182.

103 Hansard. House of Commons Debate, 'Hola Camp, Kenya (Report)', paragraphs 183–185.

104 Hansard. House of Commons Debate, 'Hola Camp, Kenya (Report)', Barbara Castle MP, 27 July 1959, paragraphs 231–232.

105 Hansard. House of Commons Debate, 'Hola Camp, Kenya (Report)', paragraphs 231–232.

106 FCO 141/5651. Statement by Dr Rogoff, pp. 25–39.

107 FCO 141/5651. Statement by Dr Rogoff, p. 38.

108 FCO 141/5651. Statement by Dr Rogoff, p. 34.

109 FCO 141/5651. Statement by Dr Rogoff, pp. 36–37.

110 FCO 141/5651. Statement by Dr Rogoff, p. 45.

111 FCO 141/5651. Statement by Dr Rogoff, p. 45.

112 FCO 141/5651. Statement by Dr Rogoff.

113 FCO 141/5651. Statement by Dr Rogoff, p. 46.

114 FCO 141/5651. Testimony of Dr Geoffrey Lowe Timms, p. 47.

115 *Further Documents Relating to the Deaths of Eleven Mau Mau Detainees at Hola Camp in Kenya*, p. 46.

116 *Further Documents Relating to the Deaths of Eleven Mau Mau Detainees at Hola Camp in Kenya*, p. 46.

117 FCO 141/5656. Copy of M. G. Sullivan's telegram to The Commissioner of Prisons, 13 February 1959 in 'Decypher telegram to Secretary of State', 12 June 1953.

118 Hansard. House of Commons Debate, 'Hola Detention Camp', Barbara Castle MP, paragraphs 301–302.
119 Hansard. House of Commons Debate, 'Hola Detention Camp', paragraphs 301–302.
120 Hansard. House of Commons Debate, 'Hola Detention Camp', paragraphs 300–306.
121 Though it must be stated that the 'List of Registered Medical Practitioners and Dentists' described him as being 'out of the Country' in Sept. 1964. *The Kenya Gazette*, 16 September 1964, p. 1015.
122 Anderson, *Histories of the Hanged*, p. 326.
123 Following the final inquest, a small Committee, headed by R. D. Fairn, one of Her Majesty's Prison Commissioners, carried out an investigation into the remaining camps. The advice of the Fairn Committee was responsible for putting an end to the use of 'lawless violence' in the camps, especially that related to the dilution technique. See Rosberg and Nottingham, *The Myth of Mau Mau*, p. 346.
124 Hansard. House of Commons Debate, 'Hola Camp, Kenya (Report)', Enoch Powell MP, paragraphs 237–238.
125 Hansard. House of Commons Debate, 'Hola Camp, Kenya (Report), paragraphs 237–238.
126 Elkins, *Britain's Gulag*, p. 353.
127 A year after coming into office, on 20 October 1964, Kenyatta broadcast the following message: 'Let this be the day on which all of us commit ourselves to erase from our minds all the hatreds and the difficulties of those years which now belong to the history. Let us agree that we shall never refer to the past. Let us instead unite, in all our utterances and activities, in concern for the reconstruction of our country and the vitality of Kenya's future'. Quoted in Elkins, *Britain's Gulag*, p. 360.

Concluding thoughts

This study's comparative discussion has highlighted several important themes common to both the Algerian and the Kenyan colonial contexts. These include the role medical professionals played in the French and British conquest and occupation of the two territories during the nineteenth and early twentieth centuries. Medical professionals, moreover, were deeply rooted into the colonies' economic, political and social order, which, unwittingly or otherwise, contributed to the rise of violent nationalism. European psychiatrists, as well as other scientists of the mind, offered expertise to both 'diagnose' and 'treat' the collective psychological causes that produced the FLN, Mau Mau and their violent ways. These experts represented the 'terrorist' organisations as consisting of 'brainwashed' religious fanatics. Some prominent medical practitioners among the European settler communities became personally involved in violence when the state's management of the perceived anticolonial threat seemed ineffective; doctors helped to justify or add a humane appearance to certain torture techniques. They also aided with their administration by treating and dealing with the consequences of these methods. Sometimes this led them wilfully to conceal or manipulate records and reports in order to deny or play down evidence of torture.

Although these shared themes and features have been useful for framing this analysis, local and national peculiarities were no less important. They played a fundamental role in shaping and influencing, not only the reasons for how and why torture was practised, but also the specific ways that doctors participated in it. Ultimately, the histories of medical participation in violence in Algeria and Kenya, the ways that it evolved and the types of individuals who participated in it varied, due to a range of important temporal and contextual factors peculiar to the wider histories of the two colonies. For instance, during the early stages of both conflicts, colonial doctors featured prominently among the settlers who were attacked and often killed by the insurgents. Yet while this was common to both Algeria and Kenya, a closer examination of these murdered or targeted doctors revealed a wealth of information about not only the place of medicine within the colonial order, but the factors that contributed to the rise of violent anticolonial movements in both colonies. Chapter 1 of this book explored this point. It showed that, in colonial Algeria, the administration of medicine meant that civilian and military medical practices were perceived to be more intimately entangled than in Kenya, where a distinction existed between the CMS and medical missionaries. Despite being a central symbol of the European civilising mission in both colonies, medicine and its benefits were rarely extended to local people in the same way as settlers. In fact, France's failure to provide adequate healthcare for the Algerians allowed the FLN to create their own competing health system in the form of the Croissant-Rouge algérien, once the Algerian War started. This was in contrast to the situation in Kenya, where Mau Mau were not able to present themselves as a proto-authority in the same way as their North African counterparts.

The behaviour and activities of some doctors in Kenya had more directly fostered anticolonial sentiments among the Kikuyu. The controversy surrounding the clitoridectomy scandal served as a distinct rallying point for Kenyan nationalists, but it also highlighted an important instance where medical ideals merged with or became confused with religious ones. Doctors were also among some of the wealthier landowners in both colonies, but in Kenya, there is currently more evidence that shows the extent to which these settlers benefitted from this situation, something which helps account for why doctors were among the first to be attacked by Mau Mau. Once hostilities erupted in both countries, the psychiatric and psychological expertise mobilised by colonial authorities drew on established perceptions of the indigenous populations that represented them as mentally unstable, inferior and ultimately prone to hysterical violence. In North Africa, the Algiers School of psychiatry, which had historical connections with the French military, used its expertise to present the FLN as Islamic extremists whose innate criminality led them to commit heinous mutilations and acts of terrorism.

For their part, their Mau Mau counterparts were understood by ethnopsychiatrists and anthropologists as expressing a form of collective madness provoked by acculturation.[1] Ultimately, ideas about 'collective insanity' provided local explanations that fed off a wider international faith in the powers of the science of the mind in the postwar period, as well as contemporary fears about the Cold War and the threat of communist subversion and brainwashing techniques.[2]

These scientists' expertise helped inform and structure the colonial authorities' programmes to 're-educate' (Algeria) or 'rehabilitate' (Kenya) the indigenous populations and treat their perceived 'sickness'. In practice, these policies relied on detention centres, concentration camps and resettlement villages to divide the population and cut the insurgents off from their supply chains. These camps, as has been known for some time, were not only the sites of extraordinary violence but were also inhospitable locations that were often cramped, primitive and rife with disease. Behind their barbed wire perimeters, the detainees' lives were organised and overseen by prison wardens or military officers, as well as doctors who were supposed to treat their wounds and monitor their health. However, despite being formally required to be present within the camp system and to carry out a duty of care for the detainees, these professionals were often ineffective. The reasons for this vary between Kenya and Algeria, but in general there appears to have been a mixture of negligence and potential prejudice, but also more mundane issues related to understaffing and an inability to keep doctors employed on site. This meant that detainees could go weeks without seeing a doctor. In Algeria, the situation was made more confusing as the camp administration system was split between civilian facilities and military camps, the latter of which were often more hostile and unhealthier than their civilian counterparts. Due to the poor conditions within the Kenya pipeline and the network of camps in Algeria, infectious diseases like tuberculosis and dysentery were a persistent concern. Yet Kenya appears to be the only context where an epidemic became a significant crisis for the colonial authorities. In Algeria, the climate, especially within the deserts, was a persistent source of suffering and ill health for the detainees.

Besides demonstrating the important role doctors and medicine played within the everyday administration of life and suffering within the camps, this book has also shone light on the functions physicians performed when torture became an established practice in these punitive environments. In particular, it has shown how both the French and British colonial authorities sought medical participation in (or validation of) specific techniques, such as water torture in Algeria or the dilution technique in Kenya, to add a humane and scientific sheen to their justifications. While British medical officers were officially required to monitor the health of detainees before and after a dilution intake, it does not seem that the French made such a stipulation in Algeria. Regardless, French military doctors were just as likely to be in close proximity to abuse. In fact, while there is at present no evidence suggesting that British medical officers took any active role in torture, the use of truth drugs by French military physicians represented just that. This is one of the most significant distinctions in this study. Although scholars have been aware that these drugs were used by the French in Algeria for some time, this study has expanded our understanding of this underexplored feature of the Algerian War. Not only did French military physicians use these tools to actively participate in coercive interrogation, they also used them to compete with their soldier colleagues. This highlights an interesting social dynamic between military medical staff and the regiments they served. Moreover, knowledge of their use was so widespread that the FLN combatants undertook special training in order to resist their influence. This contrasted greatly with the situation in Kenya. As this book has shown, the reasons the British security forces did not use truth drugs against Mau Mau had to do with the demands of the rehabilitation process and with perceptions of narcoanalysis more generally. Whereas the French military sought to extract operative information from FLN suspects through narcoanalysis, the British resorted mainly to coercive techniques to extract confessions. Moreover, there appears to have been a general distrust among British military and defence scientists of the drugs' effectiveness. In the end, the British preferred more tried and tested techniques, such as sleep deprivation, starvation and extreme isolation in conjunction with the dilution technique.

At the same time that torture was becoming a staple of life within the detention camps of North and Eastern Africa, Britain and France were playing prominent roles in shaping a new era of international ethics. Along with the rise of the human rights regime, these international guides to medical ethical conduct were produced in the hope they would prevent a repeat of the Nazi regime's murderous excesses, especially in relation to medical atrocities and human experimentation.[3] However, the WMA's Declaration of Geneva and the International Code of Medical Ethics, created for this purpose, lacked relevant language for doctors faced with the realities of torture. Moreover, they were not enforceable. In the end, it seems that British and French doctors operating in and around the detention centres in Kenya and Algeria had to rely on their own judgement. Demands posed by the need for information and the counterinsurgency strategy of mass detention, coupled with understaffed and ill-equipped facilities, often meant that military and medical officers alike were faced with dilemmas that could not easily be resolved through recourse to such codes of practice. In fact, there is currently little evidence informing us as to what types of ethical or moral ideas these doctors evoked in their work or whether they regarded their practices as unethical in any way. Nor is there any indication that had there been a more concrete set of principles, such as those that would eventually form the WMA's Declaration of Tokyo on torture, that this would have made any material difference to these conflicts. After all, the existence of this code from 1975 has not stopped doctors from participating in torture.[4]

The final chapter of this book addressed the ways that doctors helped, intentionally or otherwise, with wider efforts to conceal evidence of mistreatment. Be it by providing misleading pathology or medical reports, or intentionally playing down the severity of direct evidence of torture, doctors in both Algeria and Kenya aided wider efforts to deny or conceal abuse. This was shown through a comparison of two important cases in France and Britain, which focused public attention on the use of torture in these conflicts. While these two cases highlight how medical evidence and testimony could be used to deny allegations of abuse in the detention camps, the types of allegations and the general situations surrounding them vary greatly. The case of Djamila Boupacha illustrated the ways in which medicine and the law could be instrumentalised by the French authorities in order to deny justice to the rebels as well as legitimising their execution. What made this case significant was that the claimant was alive and able to draw public attention to her situation. This was in direct contrast to the situation in Kenya, where the Hola Camp incident drew public attention because of the sheer number of detainees killed by the dilution technique. While Boupacha's trial highlights the strategic value medical evidence could play for either the defence or the prosecution in an adversarial military court, the Hola Camp incident exemplified deep issues surrounding criminal investigations into allegations of abuse during the Emergency, as well as the government's tactics for covering them up.

Boupacha's trial brought into focus a range of medical activities that helped deny the torture and rape allegations she made against the military. Doctors working for the army appear to have deliberately provided ineffective and incomplete medical assessments of the complainant's body to undermine her case. Yet these slim medical reports raised more questions than they answered, allowing the defence to have her case adjourned and moved to France, away from the military's immediate spheres of influence. This chapter, however, tried to caution against overstating the power of medical evidence in this case. Although a significant amount of the narrative presented by de Beauvoir and Halimi revolved around the findings of the various medical examinations Boupacha was subjected to, it is arguable they would not have amounted to much had her counsel not succeeded in drawing public attention to her plight. It was their ability to keep the case in the public domain which ultimately prevented her allegations from being quashed by the military courts as others had been many times before. Nevertheless, the role of the doctors hired by Boupacha's counsel reveals the extent to which the application of medicine to a terrorist suspect could be seen as a controversial and politically dangerous move. Rather than carrying out a purely objective practice, the five medical experts who examined her wounds in Paris appear to have couched their report in neutral terms to avoid committing themselves to a politically contentious verdict.

The story of concealment in Kenya, on the other hand, did not take place within the courts but through inquests and parliamentary debates to impede efforts to investigate allegations of abuse or to quell questions from the Opposition. The disappearance or invalidation of medical evidence appeared to be part of a wider effort within the Kenya Home Guard, the screening teams and the government more generally to conceal signs of torture. While there were some efforts to prosecute individuals for clear cases of excessive force, it seems the pathology reports were often too inconclusive to convict the accused of murder. It was argued that the Hola Camp massacre represents a clear instance in which the inquests commissioned by the government were designed to avoid exposing the pervasive atmosphere of violence that took place behind the barbed wire in many detention camps in Kenya. Rather than admit that the eleven detainees had been killed through violent means, the initial explanation suggested that they had either drowned themselves or else been poisoned by a contaminated water source. Once this was dismissed, the doctor in residence at the camp was actually consulted as both an expert witness and a material witness for the case, despite having been involved in the incident on the day. Yet while the inquest was unprepared to question the doctor's participation in this investigation, the Opposition raised questions about it in the House of Commons. Eventually, the evidence provided by Dr Rogoff was sufficient to prove that the eleven detainees at Hola Camp had been killed through the use of force. This, however, proved insufficient to pin charges on any individuals, while the Opposition failed to pursue Dr Moyes for his role in the whole affair. In the end, the Opposition's real aim, it was argued, was not the subordinates but the whole government.

The conclusion that doctors' participation in abuse was contingent upon a complicated interaction between local and historically specific factors may not appear especially groundbreaking at first. However, the findings of this research challenge the standard psychological explanations employed by the medical experts and organisations who have studied other contexts where doctors participated in torture.[5] It is not possible to simply regard the doctors within this study as immoral or cruel in all instances, nor can we regard them as passive agents of corrupt or shoddy colonial regimes. Although Chapters 3 to 5 have certainly revealed cases where physicians showed little regard for the victims of torture or actively participated in violence, there are plenty of other situations where doctors behaved more ambiguously or even attempted to help victims of torture. This should not be surprising given that, as demonstrated throughout this book, medicine in the colonial context was not a homogenous practice constituted by a unified set of professionals serving the same ends or indeed the same clients.

Instead, the doctors discussed here were themselves complicated agents with varied professional backgrounds, loyalties and social roles within the colonial setting. The subject of professional loyalty has thus formed a theme that weaves together multiple strands of this book. In particular, it has been used to examine the types of social, cultural, political and economic factors that may have influenced a given doctor's activities or behaviours. It has also helped to elicit tensions between the role of the medical profession within its clinical and therapeutic capacities, as well as helping to identify the beliefs and ideals of the same professionals as individuals situated in the colonial order. By conceiving of these professionals as dynamic and complicated historical agents in their own right, with varying levels of commitment to the survival of the colonies and competing personal interests, it is possible to question the effectiveness of some modern perspectives on doctors and their professional loyalties. For instance, the BMA recently argued that an answer to the modern dual-loyalty dilemma rests in affording the medical profession greater freedom from government agencies.[6] Yet the results of this study have shown that both government-employed and private doctors were capable of actively participating and perpetrating abuse if they deemed it necessary to defend their personal interests or fulfil their political aims. We should therefore be careful about relying on overly generalised or simplistic explanations for doctors' participation in human rights violations.

What can be concluded, however, is that scholars have much to gain by looking beyond the simple interface where doctors became entangled with military or security-run interrogation operations. By comparing and understanding the contexts within which the doctors discussed here lived and worked, as well as the types of personal commitments they had to the colonies, historians can access greater information about the beliefs, ideas and attitudes that they espoused. Moreover, as this study has paid consideration to wider international forces generated in the immediate postwar period, it has broadened the historical study of decolonisation in the Cold War. In particular, it has shone greater light on the role of medical and human sciences in relation to counterinsurgency and torture. The application of this approach to other wars of decolonisation or counterinsurgency operations could yield greater information about the ways in which medical practitioners and scientists participated in violence. As mentioned in the Introduction, scholars such as Erik Linstrum and Darius Rejali have developed thoughtful accounts of the ways that human scientists and other experts were employed in counterinsurgency and torture activities, respectively. These studies have debunked the idea that scientists provided sophisticated and scientifically calibrated techniques to produce the 'truth' in interrogations. However, there is still a lot more to be learnt from examining groups of experts involved in such practices to understand what they thought they were doing and why. As Marnia Lazreg has argued when discussing the French approach to torture, while it is important to examine what people *did* in terms of supporting torture, it is also necessary to understand what they thought about what they were doing.[7] There are still questions to be answered about the ways the medical community more generally thought about their responsibilities, ethical obligations and abilities when working within highly violent contexts. Such studies could contribute to a greater understanding of the ways that different expertise became entangled with counterinsurgency activities, how local and international ideas about medical conduct impacted on their motivations or resistance, and how they reconciled any dilemmas.

Notes

1 Anderson, *Histories of the Hanged*, pp. 279–284.

2 As mentioned in Chapter 2, the subject of 'brainwashing' has recently received focused attention from scholars working on the Wellcome Trust-funded project, Hidden Persuaders.

3 Annas and Michael, 'Medicine and human rights'.

4 For the full text of the Declaration of Tokyo, see www.wma.net/policies-post/wma-declaration-of-tokyo-guidelines-for-physicians-concerning-torture-and-other-cruel-inhuman-or-degrading-treatment-or-punishment-in-relation-to-detention-and-imprisonment/ [Accessed 13 December 2019].

5 British Medical Association, *Medicine Betrayed*; Lifton, *The Nazi Doctors*; Lifton, 'Doctors and torture'; Miles, *Oath Betrayed.*

6 Julian Sheather, Rhian Beynon, Tom Davis and Kamran Abbasi, 'Torture and doctors' dual obligation', *British Medical Journal* 350 (2015), p. 1.

7 Lazreg, *Torture and the Twilight of Empire*, p. 3.

Bibliography

Primary sources

British newspapers

Anonymous, 'Clarke wants terrorists treated like victims of cult brainwashing', *Daily Telegraph*, 2 October 2005.
Anonymous, 'Inquest on 11 Mau Mau: HAD BEEN "PREVAILED ON" TO WORK', *Manchester Guardian*, 19 March 1959.
Anonymous, 'Knife attack repulsed: Man's Escape from Mau Mau', *Manchester Guardian*, 21 September 1954.
Anonymous, 'Mau Mau Shoot Africa's Churchill', *Daily Mail*, 8 October 1952.
Anonymous, 'Search for Murderers of British Family', *Manchester Guardian*, 26 January 1953.
Anonymous, 'SURVIVOR'S STORY OF MAU MAU RAID: Seven Kikuyu Charged with Murder', *Manchester Guardian*, 23 January 1953.
Anonymous, 'The "Unco-operative" beaten: Inquest on Mau Mau detainees', *Manchester Guardian*, 25 March 1959.

French newspapers

Anonymous, 'A LA COUR DE CASSATION: LA PLAINTE POUR SERVICES DE MLLE BOUPACHA SERA INSTUITE A CAEN ET NON PLUS A ALGER', *Le Monde*, 17 December 1960. www.lemonde.fr/archives/article/1960/12/17/la-plainte-pour-sevices-de-mlle-boupacha-sera-instruite-a-caen-et-non-plus-a-alger_2105512_1819218.html [Accessed 15 July 2019].
Anonymous, 'Un article sur le cas de Djamila Boupacha provoque la saisie du "Monde" à Alger et un communiqué du gouvernement', *Le Monde*,

3 June 1960. www.lemonde.fr/archives/article/1960/06/03/un-article-sur-le-cas-de-djamila-boupacha-provoque-la-saisie-du-monde-a-alger-et-un-communique-du-gouvernement_2093607_1819218.html [Accessed 15 July 2019].

Anonymous, 'CINQ MEDECINS SONT DESIGNES POUR EXAMINER EN METROPOLE DJAMILA BOUPACHA', *Le Monde*, 19 July 1960. www.lemonde.fr/archives/article/1960/07/19/cinq-medecins-sont-designes-pour-examiner-en-metropole-djamila-boupacha_2102119_1819218.html [Accessed 15 July 2019].

Anonymous, 'DES REBELLES HARCELENT SOUK-AHRAS', *Le Monde*, 9 January 1957. www.lemonde.fr/archives/article/1957/01/09/des-rebelles-harcelent-souk-ahras_2329536_1819218.html [Accessed 17 November 2017].

Anonymous, 'Le Cas de Djamila Boupacha signalé à la Commission de sauvegarde', *Le Monde*, 27 May 1960. www.lemonde.fr/archives/article/1960/05/27/le-cas-de-djamila-boupacha-signale-a-la-commission-de-sauvegarde_2089098_1819218.html [Accessed 15 July 2019].

Anonymous, 'LE SUICIDE DANS SA CELLULE DE LARBI BEN M'HIDI EST ATTRIBUE A L'ETAT DE DEPRESSION OU LE CHEF F.L.N, SE SERAIT TROUVE', *Le Monde*, 7 March 1957. www.lemonde.fr/archives/article/1957/03/07/le-suicide-dans-sa-cellule-de-larbi-ben-m-hidi-est-attribue-a-l-etat-de-depression-ou-le-chef-f-l-n-se-serait-trouve_2332479_1819218.html [Accessed 26 June 2019].

Anonymous, 'LES MEDECINS MILITAIRES et l'assistance médicale gratuite en Algérie', *Le Monde*, 28 August 1957. www.lemonde.fr/archives/article/1957/08/28/les-medecins-militaires-et-l-assistance-medicale-gratuite-en-algerie_2326178_1819218.html [Accessed 17 November 2017].

Anonymous, 'L'INSTRUCTION DE L'AFFAIRE BOUPACHA', *Le Monde*, 1 July 1961. www.lemonde.fr/archives/article/1961/07/01/l-instruction-de-l-affaire-boupacha_2265228_1819218.html [Accessed 15 July 2019].

Anonymous, 'Une patrouille ouvre le feu dans la Casbah d'Alger CINQ MORTS, TRENTE-SEPT BLESSES, *Le Monde*, 28 February 1958. www.lemonde.fr/archives/article/1957/02/28/une-patrouille-ouvre-le-feu-dans-la-casbah-d-alger-cinq-morts-trente-sept-blesses_3134093_1819218.html [Accessed 19 March 2018].

Anonymous, 'QUARANTE BANDITS EN ARMES ont attaqué le petit village de Pasteur', *Le Monde*, 17 November 1954. www.lemonde.fr/archives/article/1954/11/17/quarante-bandits-en-armes-ont-attaque-le-petit-village-de-pasteur_2026138_1819218.html [Accessed 17 November 2017].

De Beauvoir, Simone, 'Pour Djamila Boupacha', *Le Monde*, 2 June 1960. www.lemonde.fr/archives/article/1960/06/02/pour-djamila-boupacha_2092987_1819218.html [Accessed 12 January 2018].

Mauriac, François, 'La Question', reproduced in 'Algérie. Dès 1955, François Mauriac dénonçait la torture dans *L'Express*', *L'Express*, 20 December 2012. www.lexpress.fr/actualite/monde/afrique/algerie-des-1955-francois-mauriac-denoncait-la-torture-dans-l-express_1201581.html [Accessed 16 July 2018].

Hansard

House of Lords Debate, vol. 84 cols 305–320, 'Kenya Land Commission', 4 May 1932.
House of Commons Debate, vol. 233 cols 581–616, 'Colonial Policy in Relation to coloured races', 11 December 1929.
House of Commons Debate, vol. 527 cols 1234–1235, 'Kenya (anti-Mau Mau operations)', 28 April 1954.
House of Commons Debate, vol. 531 cols 1192–1193, 'Manyani Camp', 20 October 1954.
House of Commons Debate, vol. 545 cols 176–184, 'Kamau Case (Police Organisation)', 26 October 1955.
House of Commons Debate, vol. 589 cols 887–888, 'Doctors', 17 June 1958.
House of Commons Debate, vol. 589 cols 853–864, 'Kenya (Prisoners, Lokitaung)', 16 June 1958.
House of Commons Debate, vol. 600 cols 1019–1078, 'Prisons and Detention Camps, Kenya', 24 February 1959.
House of Commons Debate, vol. 607 cols 248–384, 'Hola Detention Camp', 16 June 1959.
House of Commons Debate, vol. 610 cols 181–262, 'Hola Camp, Kenya (Report)', 27 July 1959.

International Committee of the Red Cross Archives, Geneva

ACICR, B AG 225 008-002; ACICR B AG 251 108-007; ACICR B AG 255 008-004; ACICR, B AG 255-008-032.

Kenya National Archives (KNA), Nairobi

MSS/3/479/91

London School of Tropical Medicine Archives, London

GB 0809 Nutrition/17/01/04/02

Service historique de la Défense (SHD), Paris

Series H: Outre-mer de 1830 à 1973

1 H 1240/8; 1 H 1246/d.2; 1 H 1492/d.2; 1 H 2409/d.1; 1 H 2411/d.1; 1 H 2460/d.1; 1 H 2524/d.1; 1 H 2573/d.1; 1 H 2584/d2; 1 H 2584/d.5.

GR 4K 38. Interview of Jean Suaud with Raphaëlle Branche, 15 February 2000.

SOAS Special Collections, London

Conference of British Missionary Society Archives CBMS A 14/5

The National Archives (TNA), London

CO 542/52; CO 822/489; CO 822/794; CO 822/801; CO 822/1251; CO 822/1267; CO 822/1267.

FCO 141/5651; FCO 141/5656; FCO 141/5666; FCO 141/5667; FCO 141/5668; FCO 141/5877; FCO 141/6166; FCO 141/6178; FCO 141/6303; FCO 141/6324; FCO 141/6510; FCO 141/6519; FCO 141/6540; FCO 141/6568; FCO 141/6750; FCO 141/6777.

WO 291/1670.

World Medical Association Archives

Refshauge, William, 'Statement from the Secretary General to the 29th World Medical Assembly', 1975.

Memoirs

Askwith, Thomas, *From Mau Mau to Harambee: Memoirs and Memoranda of Colonial Kenya* (Cambridge: University of Cambridge, African Studies Centre, 1995).

Aussaresses, Paul, *The Battle of the Casbah: Terrorism and Counter-Terrorism in Algeria, 1955–1957*, trans. Robert L. Miller (New York: Enigma Books, 2004).

Blundell, Michael, *So Rough a Wind* (London: Weidenfeld and Nicolson, 1964).

Carman, John, *A Medical History of the Colony and Protectorate of Kenya: A Personal Memoir* (London: Rex Collings, 1976).

Gavaghan, Terence, *Of Lions and Dung Beetles* (Devon: Arthur H. Stockwell, 1999).

Henderson, Ian, *The Hunt for Kimathi* (London: Hamish Hamilton, 1958).

Hewitt, Peter, *Kenya Cowboy: A Police Officer's Account of the Mau Mau Emergency in Kenya* (London: Avon Books, 1999).

Ighilahriz, Louisette, *Algérienne. Récit recueilli par Anne Nivat* (Paris: Fayard/Calmann-Lévy, 2001).

Kariuki, Josiah Mwangi, *Mau Mau Detainee: The Account by a Kenya African of His Experience in Detention Camps 1953–60* (London: Penguin Books, 1964).
Massu, Jacques, *La Vraie Bataille d'Alger* (Paris: Plon, 1971).
Massu, Jacques, *Le Torrent et la digue* (Paris: Plon, 1972).
Rawcliffe, D. H., *The Struggle for Kenya* (London: Victor Gollancz, 1954).

Other published books and articles

Ainsworth, Mary D., and Leonard H. Ainsworth, 'Acculturation in East Africa. IV. Summary and discussion', *The Journal of Social Psychology* 57 (1962), pp. 417–432.
Ainsworth, Leonard H., and Mary D. Ainsworth, 'Acculturation in East Africa. I. Political awareness and attitudes toward authority', *The Journal of Social Psychology* 57 (1962), pp. 391–399.
Alleg, Henri, *La Question* (Paris: Les Editions de minuit, 1958).
Allen, Louis, 'YES I SAID YES I WILL YES', *Blackfriars* 39 (1958), pp. 474–487.
Anonymous, 'Cruel treatment', *British Medical Journal*, 9 August 1975.
Anonymous, 'Declaration of Geneva', *World Medical Association Bulletin* 1 (October 1949), pp. 108–109.
Anonymous, *The Gangrene*, trans. Robert Silvers (New York: Lyle Stuart, 1960).
Anonymous, 'Obituary', *British Medical Journal*, 28 February 1953, p. 513.
Anonymous, 'Obituary', *British Medical Journal*, 29 May 1954, pp. 1270–1271.
Anonymous, 'Statement by the International Preparatory Commission of the International Congress on Mental Health' (1948), pp. 65–99.
Arnaud, George, and Jacques Vergès, *Pour Djamila Bouhired* (Paris: Les Editions de minuit, 1957).
Arthur, John W., '"Female Circumcision" among the Kikuyu', *British Medical Journal*, 24 October 1942, p. 498.
Baldwin, William, *Mau Mau Man-Hunt: The Adventures of the Only American Who Has Fought the Terrorist in Kenya* (New York: Dutton, 1957).
Barnett, Homer G., 'Acculturation: an exploratory formulation. The Social Science Research Council Summer Seminar on Acculturation, 1953: Comment', *American Anthropologist* 56 (1954), pp. 1000–1002.
Barrat, Robert, and Denise Barrat, *Algérie, 1956. Livre blanc sur la répression* (La Tour-d'Aigues: Editions de l'aube, 2001).
Carothers, John Colin, *The African Mind in Health and Disease: A Study in Ethnopsychiatry* (Geneva: World Health Organization, 1953).
Carothers, John Colin, 'Frontal lobe function and the African', *Journal of Mental Science* 97 (1951), pp. 12–48.

Camus, Albert, 'Misère de la Kabylie', in Albert Camus, *Actuelles III. Chronique algérienne, 1939–1958* (Paris: Gallimard, 1958).

Camus, Albert, *The Outsider* (London: Penguin Books, 2013).

De Beauvoir, Simone, and Gisèle Halimi, *Djamila Boupacha: The Story of the Torture of a Young Algerian Girl Which Shocked Liberal French Opinion*, trans. Peter Green (Paris: Gallimard, 1962).

Dession, George H., Lawrence Z. Freedman, Richard C. Donnelly and Frederick C. Redlich, 'Drug-induced revelation and criminal investigation', *The Yale Law Journal* 62 (1953), pp. 315–347.

Evans, Richard, *Law and Disorder: or Scenes of Life in Kenya* (Bath: The Pitman Press, 1956).

Fanon, Frantz, *A Dying Colonialism*, trans. Haakon Chevalier (New York: Grave Press, 1965).

Fanon, Frantz, *The Wretched of the Earth*, trans. Constance Farrington (London: Penguin Books, 2001).

Faure, J., 'Problèmes d'éthique posés au médecin par la torture. A propos d'une expérience personnelle', *Droits de l'homme et contrainte de la personne, XI congrès de l'Académie internationale de médecine légale et de médecine sociale, Acta medicinae legalis et socialis* 30 (1980), pp. 71–74.

Fletcher, Eileen, *The Truth About Kenya: An Eye Witness Account* (London: Movement for Colonial Freedom, 1956).

Gallais, P., and L. Planques, 'Etude sur les déficiences mentales dans les territoires d'Outre-Mer. Perspectives ethnopsychiatriques dans l'Union Française', *Médecine tropicale* 11 (1951), pp. 5–30.

Hafid, Keramane, *La Pacification. Livre noir de six années de guerre en Algérie* (Paris: Les Petits Matins, 2013).

Hunter, Edward, *Brain-Washing in Red China: The Calculated Destruction of Men's Minds* (New York: The Vanguard Press, 1953).

Kenyatta, Jomo, *Facing Mount Kenya* (London: Secker & Warburg, 1974).

Le Bon, Gustave, *The Psychology of Revolution*, Project Gutenberg www.gutenberg.org/cache/epub/448/pg448-images.html [24.05.2018].

Leakey, Lewis S. B., *Defeating Mau Mau* (London: Methuen, 1954).

Leakey, Lewis S. B., *Mau Mau and the Kikuyu* (London: Methuen, 1952).

Lagrot, F., and J. Greco, 'Les Mutilations facials au cours du terrorisme en Algérie et leur réparation', *La Presse médicale* 51 (1956), pp. 1193–1198.

Lartéguy, Jean, *The Centurions* (London: Penguin Books, 2015).

Levi, Primo, *The Drowned and the Saved* (London: Abacus, 1989).

Lewis, W. Arthur, Michael Scott, Martin Wight and Colin Legum, *Attitude to Africa: A Survey of the Main Problems of British Africa, Suggesting the Lines of Policy That Any British Government Should Follow in the Years Ahead* (Middlesex: Penguin Books, 1951).

Pictet, Jean S., 'The New Geneva Conventions for the Protection of War Victims', *American Journal of International Law* 45 (1951), pp. 462–475.

Pierson, C. A., 'Paléophrénie réactionnelle. Physiopathologie de l'impulsion morbide en milieu nord-africain', *Maroc médical* 360 (1955), pp. 642–647.

Porot, Antoine, 'Notes de psychiatrie musulmane', *Annales médico-psychologiques* 74 (1918), pp. 377–384.

Porot, Antoine, and Don Côme Arrii, 'L'Impulsivité criminelle chez l'indigène algérien. Ses facteurs', *Annales médico-psychologiques* 14 (1932), pp. 588–611.

Porot, Antoine, and Charles Bardenat, *Anormaux et malades mentaux devant la justice pénale* (Paris: Maloine, 1960).

Porot, Antoine, and Charles Bardenat, *Psychiatrie médico-légale* (Paris: Maloine, 1959).

Porot, Antoine and Jean Stutter, *Le "Primitivisme" des indigènes nord-africains, ses incidences en pathologie mentale, par le professeur* (Marseille: Impr. marseillaise, 1939).

Rees, J. R., 'The International Congress on Mental Health', *British Medical Bulletin*, 6 (1949).

Robe, Eugène, *La Propriété immobilière en Algérie, commentaire de la loi du 26 juillet 1873* (Algiers: Juillet St Lager, 1875).

Rolin, Jean, *Police Drugs*, trans. Laurence J. Bendit (London: Hollis & Carter, 1955).

Sartre, Jean-Paul, *Colonialism and Neocolonialism*, trans. Azzedine Haddour, Steve Brewer and Terry McWilliams (London and New York: Routledge, 2001).

Schoenholzer, Jean-Pierre, 'Le médecin dans les Conventions de Genève de 1949', *Revue internationale de la Croix-Rouge et Bulletin International des Sociétés de la Croix-Rouge* 35 (1953), pp. 94–126.

Solzhenitsyn, Aleksandr, *The Gulag Archipelago, 1918–1956: An Experiment in Literary Investigation*, trans. Thomas P. Whitney (New York: Harper & Row, 1974).

Stora, Benjamin, *La Gangrène et l'oubli* (Paris: La Découverte, 1998).

Sutter, J. M., 'La subnarcose chimique', *Revue de droit canonique* (1951), pp. 679–682.

Thibaud, Paul, 'Comment fonctionne la justice en Algérie', *Esprit* 250 (1957), pp. 859–873.

Trinquier, Roger, *Modern Warfare: A French View of Counterinsurgency*, trans. Daniel Lee (Westport and London: Praeger Security International, 2006).

Tse-Tung, Mao, *On Guerrilla Warfare* (Chicago: University of Illinois Press, 1961).

Vergès, Jacques, Michel Zavrian and Maurice Courrégé, *Les Disparus. Le Cahier vert* (Lausanne: La Cité, 1959).

Vidal-Naquet, Pierre, *Torture: Cancer of Democracy*, trans. Barry Richard (Middlesex: Penguin Books, 1963).

Vint, F. W., 'The brain of the Kenya native', *Journal of Anatomy* 68 (1934), pp. 216–223.

Watkins, O. F., 'The Report of the Kenya Land Commission', *Journal of the Royal African Society* 33 (1933), pp. 207–216.

Wilkinson, John, 'The Mau Mau movement: some general and medical aspects', *The East African Medical Journal* 31 (1954), pp. 295–314.

William, D. Colwyn and Ilse Boon, 'The prohibition in Western Germany of the admission of evidence obtained through narco-analysis', *The British Journal of Delinquency* 2 (1951), pp. 55–57.

Wiseman, Robert Howitt, 'Mau Mau', *British Medical Journal*, 7 March 1953, p. 65.

Worsley, Peter, 'The anatomy of Mau Mau', *The New Reasoner* 1 (1957), pp. 13–25.

Wuillaume, Roger, 'Text of the Wuillaume Report', translated and presented in the Appendix of Pierre Vidal-Naquet, *Torture: Cancer of Democracy*, trans. Barry Richard (Middlesex: Penguin Books, 1963), pp. 169–179.

Publications of the British government

Carothers, John Colin, *The Psychology of the Mau Mau* (London: Government Printer, 1954).

Compton, Edmond, *Report of the Enquiry into Allegations Against the Security Forces of Physical Brutality in Northern Ireland Arising out of Events on the 9th August, 1971* (London: Her Majesty's Stationery Office, 1971).

Corfield, F. D., *Historical Survey of the Origins and Growth of Mau Mau* (London: Her Majesty's Stationery Office, 1960).

Further Documents Relating to the Deaths of Eleven Mau Mau Detainees at Hola Camp in Kenya (London: Her Majesty's Stationery Office, 1959).

Parker, Hubert Lister, *Report of the Committee of Privy Counsellors Appointed to Consider Authorised Procedures for the Interrogation of Persons Suspected of Terrorism* (London: Her Majesty's Stationery Office, 1972).

United Kingdom Parliament. *Report of the Kenya Land Commission* (London: Her Majesty's Stationery Office, 1933).

The Kenya Gazette

'List of Registered Medical Practitioners and Dentists', *The Kenya Gazette*, 16 September 1964, pp. 1010–1020.

'The Prisons Ordinance (Cap. 78)', *The Kenya Gazette*, 23 September 1958, p. 1091.

Secondary sources

Agamben, Giorgio, *Homo Sacer: Sovereign Power and Bare Life*, trans. Daniel Heller-Roazen (Stanford: Stanford University Press, 1998).

Ahmed, Shahab, *What Is Islam? The Importance of Being Islamic* (Princeton and Oxford: Princeton University Press, 2016).
Aldrich, Robert, *Greater France: A History of French Overseas Expansion* (Basingstoke: Macmillan Press, 1996).
Alexander, Martin S., Martin Evans and J. F. V. Keiger, 'The "war without a name", the French Army and the Algerians: recovering experiences, images and testimonies', in Martin S. Alexander, Martin Evans and J. F. V. Keiger (eds), *The Algerian War and the French Army, 1954–62: Experiences, Images and Testimonies* (Basingstoke: Palgrave Macmillan, 2002), pp. 1–39.
Allhoff, Fritz, 'Physician involvement in hostile interrogations', *Cambridge Quarterly of Healthcare Ethics* 15 (2006), pp. 392–402.
Allhoff, Fritz, 'Introduction', in Fritz Allhoff (ed.), *Physicians at War: The Dual-Loyalties Challenge* (Dordrecht: Springer, 2008).
Amnesty International, *Report on Torture* (London: Duckworth in association with Amnesty International Publications, 1973).
Amnesty International Medical Commission and Valérie Marange, *Doctors and Torture: Collaboration or Resistance?* (London: Bellew Publishing, 1991).
Amrith, Sunil S., *Decolonizing International Health: India and Southeast Asia, 1930–65* (Basingstoke: Palgrave Macmillan, 2006).
Anderson, David, *Eroding the Commons: Politics of Ecology in Baringo, Kenya, 1895–1963* (Oxford: James Currey, 2002).
Anderson, David, *Histories of the Hanged: The Dirty War in Kenya and the End of Empire* (New York and London: W. W. Norton & Company, 2005).
Anderson, David M., 'British abuse and torture in Kenya's counter-insurgency, 1952–1960', *Small Wars & Insurgencies* 23 (2012), pp. 700–719.
Anderson, David M., 'Mau Mau in the High Court and the 'lost' British Empire archives: colonial conspiracy or bureaucratic bungle?', *The Journal of Imperial and Commonwealth History* 39 (2011), pp. 699–716.
Anderson, David M., and Paul J. Lane, 'The unburied victims of Kenya's Mau Mau Rebellion: where and when does the violence end?', in Jean-Marc Dreyfus and Elisabeth Anstett (eds), *Human Remains in Society: Curation and Exhibition in the Aftermath of Genocide and Mass-Violence* (Manchester: Manchester University Press, 2016), pp. 14–37.
Anderson, Warwick, *The Cultivation of Whiteness: Science, Health & Racial Destiny in Australia* (Melbourne: Melbourne University Press, 2005).
Annas, George J., and Michael A. Grodin, 'Medicine and human rights: reflections on the fiftieth anniversary of the Doctors' Trial', *Health and Human Rights* 2 (1996), pp. 6–21.
Annas, George J., and Michael A. Grodin (eds), *The Nazi Doctors and the Nuremberg Code: Human Rights in Human Experimentation* (New York and Oxford: Oxford University Press, 1992).

Amster, Ellen J., *Medicine and the Saints: Science, Islam, and the Colonial Encounter in Morocco, 1877–1956* (Austin: University of Texas Press).
Applebaum, Anne, *Gulag: A History of Soviet Camps* (London and New York: Penguin Books, 2003).
Arnold, David, *Colonizing the Body: State Medicine and Epidemic Disease in Nineteenth-Century India* (Berkeley: University of California Press, 1993).
Badger, Anthony, 'Historians, a legacy of suspicion and the "Migrated Archives"', *Small Wars & Insurgencies* 23 (2012), pp. 799–807.
Baggallay, A. R., 'Myths of Mau Mau expanded: rehabilitation in Kenya's detention camps, 1954–60', *Journal of Eastern African Studies* 5 (2011), pp. 553–578.
Baldwin-Ragaven, Laurel, Jeanelle de Gruchy and Leslie London (eds), *An Ambulance of the Wrong Colour: Health Professionals, Human Rights and Ethics in South Africa* (Cape Town: University of Cape Town Press, 1999), pp. 91–112.
Beck, Ann, *A History of the British Medical Administration of East Africa* (Cambridge, MA: Harvard University Press, 1970).
Beck, Ann, 'Medical administration and medical research in developing countries: remarks on their history in colonial East Africa', *Bulletin of the History of Medicine* 46 (1972), pp. 349–358.
Beckett, Ian F. W., *Modern Insurgencies and Counterinsurgencies: Guerrillas and Their Opponents Since 1750* (London and New York: Routledge, 2001).
Bégué, Jean-Michel, 'French psychiatry in Algeria (1830–1962): from colonial to transcultural', *History of Psychiatry* 7 (1996), pp. 533–548.
Bennett, Huw, 'The other side of the COIN: Minimum and exemplary force in British Army counterinsurgency in Kenya', *Small Wars and Insurgencies* 18 (2007), pp. 638–664.
Bennoune, Mahfoud, *The Making of Contemporary Algeria, 1830–1987* (Cambridge: Cambridge University Press, 2002).
Berman, Bruce J., and John M. Lonsdale, 'Lewis Leakey's Mau Mau: a study in the politics of knowledge', *History and Anthropology* 5 (1991), pp. 143–204.
Bernault, Florence, 'The shadow of rule: Colonial power and modern punishment in Africa', in Frank Dikötter and Ian Brown (eds), *Cultures of Confinement: A History of the Prison in Africa, Asia, and Latin America* (Ithaca: Cornell University Press, 2007), pp. 71–72.
Best, Geoffrey, *War and Law Since 1945* (Oxford: Oxford University Press, 1994).
Bloch, Sidney, and Peter Reddaway, *Soviet Psychiatric Abuse: The Shadow over World Psychiatry* (London: Gollancz, 1984).
Bloche, M. G., 'Uruguay's military physicians: cogs in a system of state terror', *JAMA* 255 (1986), pp. 2788–2793.

Bonnichon, Philippe, Pierre Geny and Jean Nemo (eds), *Présences françaises outre-mer (XVIe–XXIe siècles). Science, religion et culture* (Paris: Editions Karthala, 2012).

Bourke, Joanna, *The Story of Pain: From Prayer to Painkillers* (Oxford: Oxford University Press, 2014).

Branch, Daniel, *Defeating Mau Mau, Creating Kenya: Counterinsurgency, Civil War, and Decolonisation* (Cambridge: Cambridge University Press, 2009).

Branch, Daniel, 'Imprisonment and colonialism in Kenya, *c.* 1930–1952: escaping the carceral archipelago', *The International Journal of African Historical Studies* 38 (2005), pp. 239–265.

Branche, Raphaëlle, 'Des viols pendant la guerre d'Algérie', *Revue d'histoire* 75 (2003), pp. 123–132.

Branche, Raphaëlle, 'The French in Algeria: can there be a prisoner of war in a "domestic" operation?', in Sibylle Scheipers (ed.), *Prisoners in War* (Oxford: Oxford University Press, 2010), pp. 178–179.

Branche, Raphaëlle, *La Torture et l'armée pendant la guerre d'Algérie: 1954–1962* (Paris: Gallimard, 2001).

Branche, Raphaëlle, 'Torture of terrorists? Use of torture in a "war against terrorism": justifications, methods and effects: the case of France in Algeria, 1954–1962', *International Review of the Red Cross* 89 (2007), pp. 543–560.

Branche, Raphaëlle and Jim House, 'Silences on state violence during the Algerian War of Independence: France and Algeria, 1962–2007', in Efrat ben-Zeer, Ruth Ginio and Jay Winter (eds), *Shadow of War: A Social History of Silence in the Twentieth Century* (Cambridge: Cambridge University Press, 2010), pp. 115–137.

Brennan, T. A., and R. Kirscher, 'Medical ethics and human rights violations: the Iraqi occupation of Kuwait and its aftermath', *Annals of Internal Medicine*, 117 (1992), pp. 78–82.

British Medical Association, *Medicine Betrayed: The Participation of Doctors in Human Rights Abuses* (London: Zed Books, 1992).

Browning, Christopher R., *Ordinary Men: Reserve Police Battalion 101 and the Final Solution in Poland* (New York: HarperCollins, 1998).

Bruce-Lockhart, Katherine, '"Unsound" minds and broken bodies: the detention of "hardcore" Mau Mau women at Kamiti and Gitamayu detention camps in Kenya, 1954–1960', *Journal of Eastern African Studies* 8 (2014), pp. 590–608.

Bullard, Alice, 'The critical impact of Frantz Fanon and Henri Collomb: race, gender, and personality testing of North and West Africans', *Journal of the History of the Behavioural Sciences* 41 (2005), pp. 225–248.

Burney, Ian Adnan, *Bodies of Evidence: Medicine and the Politics of the English Inquest, 1830–1926* (Baltimore and London: The Johns Hopkins University Press, 2000).

Burney, Ian Adnan, 'Viewing bodies: medicine, public order, and English inquest practice', *Configurations* 2 (1994), pp. 33–46.

Burrows, Mathew, '"Mission civilisatrice": French cultural policy in the Middle East, 1860–1914', *The Historical Journal* 29 (1986), pp. 109–135.

Campbell, Chloe, *Race and Empire: Eugenics in Colonial Kenya* (Manchester: Manchester University Press, 2007).

Chakrabarti, Pratik, *Medicine & Empire, 1600–1960* (Basingstoke: Palgrave Macmillan, 2014).

Chopin, Charlotte Ann, 'Embodying "the new white race": colonial doctors and settler society in Algeria, 1878–1911', *Journal for the Social History of Medicine* 29 (2015), pp. 1–20.

Clark, Hannah-Louise, 'Doctoring the *Bled*: Medical Auxiliaries and the Administration of Rural Life in Colonial Algeria, 1904–1954' (Unpublished dissertation, Princeton University, 2014).

Clark, Hannah-Louise, 'Expressing entitlement in colonial Algeria: villages, medical doctors, and the state in the early 20th century', *International Journal of Middle East Studies* 48 (2016), pp. 445–472.

Clayton, Anthony, *The Wars of French Decolonization* (London and New York: Longman, 1994).

Coban, Helena, 'The role of mass incarceration in counterinsurgency: a reflection on Caroline Elkins's *Imperial Reckoning in Light of Recent Events*', *Radical History Review* 96 (2006), pp. 112–136.

Cobain, Ian, *Cruel Britannia: A Secret History of Torture* (London: Portobello Books, 2013).

Cobain, Ian, *The History Thieves: Secrets, Lies and the Shaping of a Modern Nation* (London: Portobello Books, 2016).

Cohen, Deborah, 'Comparative history: buyer beware', *Bulletin of the GHI Washington* 29 (2001), pp. 23–33.

Cohen, Stanley, *States of Denial: Knowing About Atrocities and Suffering* (Cambridge and Malden, MA: Polity Press, 2001).

Cohen, W. B., 'The legacy of empire: the Algerian connection', *Journal of Contemporary History* 15 (1980), pp. 97–123.

Cole, Joshua, 'Massacres and their historians: recent histories of state violence in France and Algeria in the twentieth century', *French Politics, Culture & Society* 28 (2010), pp. 106–126.

Cole, Joshua, 'Remembering the Battle of Paris: 17 October 1961 in French and Algerian memory', *French Politics, Culture & Society* 21 (2003), pp. 21–50.

Connelly, Matthew, *A Diplomatic Revolution: Algeria's Fight for Independence and the Origins of the Post-Cold War Era* (Oxford: Oxford University Press, 2002).

Crosby, Alfred W., *Ecological Imperialism: The Biological Expansion of Europe 900–1900* (Cambridge: Cambridge University Press, 1993).

Crowder, Michael, 'The Second World War: prelude to decolonisation in Africa', in Michael Crowder (ed.), *The Cambridge History of Africa Volume 8: From c. 1940 to c. 1975* (Cambridge: Cambridge University Press, 1984), pp. 8–51.

Crozier, Ann, 'The Colonial Medical Officer and Colonial Identity: Kenya, Uganda and Tanzania Before World War Two' (Doctoral thesis, University College London, 2005).

Crozier, Anna, *Practising Colonial Medicine: The Colonial Medical Services in British East Africa* (London: I. B. Tauris, 2005).

Darwin, John, *The End of the British Empire: The Historical Debate* (Oxford: Basil Blackwell, 1991).

Dawson, Marc H., 'Socioeconomic change and disease: smallpox in colonial Kenya, 1880–1920', in Steven Feierman (ed.), *The Social Basis of Health and Healing in Africa* (Berkeley and Oxford: University of California Press, 1992), pp. 90–103.

Decker, Jeffrey Louis, 'Terrorism (un)veiled: Frantz Fanon and the women of Algiers', *Cultural Critique* (1990), pp. 177–195.

Dixon, Paul, '"Hearts and minds"? British counter-insurgency from Malaya to Iraq', *Journal of Strategic Studies* 32 (2009), pp. 353–381.

Donzelot, Jacques, *The Policing of Families*, trans. Robert Hurley (New York: Pantheon, 1979).

Doyle, Shane, 'Social disease and social science: the intellectual influence of non-medical research on policy and practice in the Colonial Medical Services in Tanganyika and Uganda', in Anna Greenwood (ed.), *Beyond the State: The Colonial Medical Services in British Africa* (Manchester: Manchester University Press, 2016), pp. 126–152.

Dubin, Martin David, 'The League of Nations Health Organization', in Charles Webster and Charles Rosenberg (eds), *International Health Organisations and Movements, 1918–1939* (Cambridge: Cambridge University Press, 1995), pp. 56–80.

Duder, C. J. D., '"Men of the officer class": the participants in the 1919 Soldier Settlement Scheme in Kenya', *African Affairs* 92 (1993), pp. 69–87.

Duder, C. J. D., 'The Soldier Settlement Scheme of 1919 in Kenya' (Doctoral thesis, University of Victoria, 1978).

Droz, Bernard, and Evelyne Lever, *Histoire de la guerre d'Algérie 1954–1962* (Paris: Editions du Seuil, 1991).

Eckart, Wolfgang U. (ed.), *Man, Medicine, and the State: The Human Body as an Object of Government Sponsored Medical Research in the 20th Century* (Stuttgart: Franz Steiner Verlag, 2006).

Edgerton, Robert B., *Mau Mau: An African Crucible* (New York: Free Press, 1989).

Edwards, Carl N., Samuel I. Miles and August Piper, 'Deception: Truth serum', *Wiley Encyclopedia of Forensic Science* (2009), pp. 1–13.

Elkins, Caroline, 'Alchemy of evidence: Mau Mau, the British Empire, and the High Court of Justice', *Journal of Imperial and Commonwealth History* 39 (2011), pp. 731–748.

Elkins, Caroline, *Britain's Gulag: The Brutal End of Empire in Kenya* (London: Jonathan Cape, 2005).

Elkins, Caroline, *Legacy of Violence: A History of the British Empire* (London: Bodley Head, 2022).

Elkins, Caroline, 'Looking beyond Mau Mau: archiving violence in the era of decolonization', *The American Historical Review* 120 (2015), pp. 852–868.

Elkins, Caroline, 'The struggle for Mau Mau rehabilitation in late colonial Kenya', *The International Journal of African Historical Studies* 33 (2000), pp. 25–57.

Evans, Martin, *Algeria: France's Undeclared War* (Oxford: Oxford University Press, 2012).

Evans, Richard J., *Telling Lies About Hitler: The Holocaust, History and the David Irving Trial* (London and New York: Verso, 2002).

Fitzsimmons, Michael, 'Hard hearts and open minds? Governance, identity and the intellectual foundations of counterinsurgency strategy', *Journal of Strategic Studies* 31 (2008), pp. 337–365.

Fortier, Bénédicte, 'L'Indigène algérien. Du sujet au citoyen (1944–1947)', *Le Genre humain* 32 (1997), pp. 53–61.

Foucault, Michel, *Birth of the Clinical Gaze: An Archaeology of Medical Perception*, trans. A. M. Sheridan-Smith (New York: Vintage, 1973).

Foucault, Michel, *Discipline and Punish: The Birth of the Prison*, trans. A. M. Sheridan (London: Penguin Books, 1977).

Foucault, Michel, *Madness and Civilization: A History of Insanity in the Age of Reason*, trans. Richard Howard (London and New York: Routledge, 1989).

Frémeaux, Jacques, 'Les SAS (sections administratives spécialisées)', *Guerres mondiales et conflits contemporains* 208 (2002), pp. 55–68.

French, David, *The British Way in Counter-Insurgency, 1945–67* (Oxford: Oxford University Press, 2011), pp. 59–60.

French, David, 'Nasty not nice: British counter-insurgency doctrine and practice, 1945–1967', *Small Wars & Insurgencies* 23 (2012), pp. 744–761.

Frewer, Andreas, and Markus Rothhaar, 'Medicine, human rights and ethics: paths to universal rights', *Medical Health Care Philosophy* 13 (2010), pp. 247–249.

Gallois, William, *The Administration of Sickness: Medicine and Ethics in Nineteenth-Century Algeria* (Basingstoke: Palgrave Macmillan, 2008).

Gallois, William, 'Local responses to French medical imperialism in late nineteenth-century Algeria', *Social History of Medicine* 20 (2007), pp. 315–331.

Good, Charles M., 'Pioneer medical missions in colonial Africa', *Social Science and Medicine* 32 (1991), pp. 1–10.

Greenwood, Anna (ed.), *Beyond the State: The Colonial Medical Services in British Africa* (Manchester: Manchester University Press, 2016).

Greenwood, Anna, and Harshad Topiwala, 'The maintenance of hegemony: the short history of Indian doctors in the Colonial Medical Services,

British East Africa', in Anna Greenwood (ed.), *Beyond the State: The Colonial Medical Services in British Africa* (Manchester: Manchester University Press, 2016), pp. 64–84.

Grimal, Henri, *Decolonisation: The British, French, Dutch and Belgian Empires* (London and Henley: Routledge & Kegan Paul, 1978).

Hansen, Jonathan M., 'Development at the Margins: Missionaries, the State, and the Transformation of Marsabit, Kenya in the Twentieth Century' (Unpublished thesis, Vanderbilt University, 2015).

Hardiman, David, 'Introduction', in David Hardiman (ed.), *Healing Bodies, Saving Souls: Medical Missions in Asia and Africa* (Amsterdam and New York: Clio, 2006), pp. 5–58.

Harrison, Mark, 'Medicine and the management of modern warfare', *History of Science* 34 (1996), pp. 379–410.

Harrison, Mark, 'Medicine and the management of modern warfare: an introduction', in Roger Cooter, Mark Harrison and Steve Sturdy (eds), *Medicine and Modern Warfare* (Amsterdam: Editions Rodopi, 1999), pp. 1–28.

Harrison, Mark, *Medicine in an Age of Commerce and Empire* (Oxford: Oxford University Press, 2010).

Hartwig, Gerald W., and Karl D. Paterson, *Disease in African History: An Introductory Survey and Case Studies* (Durham: Duke University Press, 1978).

Hasian Jr, Marouf, 'The development of ethnographic science and psychological warfare during the suppression of the Mau Mau Rebellion', *Journal of Medical Humanities* 34 (2013), pp. 329–345.

Headrick, Daniel R., *The Tools of Empire: Technology and European Expansion in the Nineteenth Century* (Oxford: Oxford University Press, 1981).

Hokkanen, Markku, 'The government medical service and British missions in colonial Malawi, *c.* 1911–1940: crucial collaboration, hidden conflicts', in Anna Greenwood (ed.), *Beyond the State: The Colonial Medical Services in British East Africa* (Manchester: Manchester University Press, 2016), pp. 39–63.

Holmes, Marcia, 'Edward Hunter and the origins of 'brainwashing', www.bbk.ac.uk/hiddenpersuaders/blog/hunter-origins-of-brainwashing/ [Accessed 28 August 2019].

Horne, Alistair, *A Savage War of Peace: Algeria 1954–1962* (New York: New York Review Books, 2006).

Howard-Jones, Norman, *The Scientific Background of the International Sanitary Conferences 1851–1938* (Geneva: World Health Organization, 1975).

Huggins, Matha K., Mika Haritos-Fatouros and Philip G. Zimbardo, *Violence Workers: Police Torturers and Murderers Reconstruct Brazilian Atrocities* (Berkeley: University of California Press, 2002).

Hughes, Geraint, 'Militias in internal warfare: from the colonial era to the contemporary Middle East', *Small Wars and Insurgencies* 24 (2016), pp. 196–225.

Hurst, Mark, *British Human Rights Organizations and Soviet Dissent 1965–1985* (London and New York: Bloomsbury, 2016).

Jennings, Michael, 'Healing bodies, salvation of souls': missionary medicine in colonial Tanganyika, 1870s–1939', *Journal of Religion in Africa* 38 (2008), pp. 27–56.

Johnson, Jennifer, *The Battle for Algeria: Sovereignty, Health Care, and Humanitarianism* (Philadelphia: University of Pennsylvania Press, 2016).

Jones, Heather, *Violence Against Prisoners of War in the First World War: Britain, France and Germany, 1914–1920* (Cambridge: Cambridge University Press, 2011).

Kahn, Paul W., *Sacred Violence: Torture, Terror, and Sovereignty* (Ann Arbor: University of Michigan Press, 2008).

Kaltenbeck, Franz, 'On torture and state crime', *Cardozo Law Review* 24 (2002), pp. 2381–2391.

Katz, Jay, 'The consent principle of the Nuremberg Code: its significance then and now', in George J. Annas and Michael A. Grodin (eds), *The Nazi Doctors and the Nuremberg Code: Human Rights in Human Experimentation* (New York and Oxford: Oxford University Press, 1992), pp. 227–239.

Katz, Jay, 'Human sacrifice and human experimentation: reflections at Nuremberg', *Yale Journal of International Law* 22 (1997), pp. 401–418.

Katz, Jay, 'The Nuremburg Code and the Nuremberg Trial: a reappraisal', *JAMA* 276 (1996), pp. 1662–1666.

Katz, Jonathan G., *Murder in Marrakesh: Emile Mauchamp and the French Colonial Adventure* (Bloomington and Indianapolis: Indiana University Press, 2006).

Keller, Richard C., 'Clinician and revolutionary: Frantz Fanon, biography, and the history of colonial medicine', *Bulletin of the History of Medicine* 81 (2007), pp. 823–841.

Keller, Richard C., *Colonial Madness* (Chicago and London: Chicago University Press, 2008).

Keller, Richard C., 'Madness and colonization: psychiatry in the British and French empires, 1800–1962', *Journal for Social History* 35 (2001), pp. 295–326.

Keller, Richard C., 'Taking science to the colonies: psychiatric innovation in France and North Africa', in Sloan Mahone and Megan Vaughan (eds), *Psychiatry and Empire* (Basingstoke: Palgrave Macmillan, 2007), pp. 17–40.

Khalili, Laleh, 'Thinking about violence', *International Journal of Middle East Studies* 45 (2013), pp. 791–794.

King, Nicholas B., 'Security, disease, commerce: ideologies of postcolonial global health', *Social Studies of Science* 32 (2002), pp. 763–789.

Klose, Fabian, 'The colonial testing ground: the International Committee of the Red Cross and the violent end of empire', *Humanity: An International Journal of Human Rights, Humanitarianism, and Development* 2 (2011), pp. 107–26.

Klose, Fabian, *Human Rights in the Shadow of Colonial Violence: The Wars of Independence in Kenya and Algeria*, trans. Dona Geyer (Philadelphia: University of Pennsylvania Press, 2013).

Koerner, Francis, 'Le Mouvement nationaliste algérien (Nov. 1942–mai 1945)', *Revue d'histoire de la Deuxième Guerre mondiale* 93 (1974), pp. 45–64.

Kunkle, Ryan, '"We must shout the truth to the rooftops": Gisèle Halimi, Djamila Boupacha, and sexual politics in the Algerian War of Independence', *Iowa Historical Review* 4 (2013), pp. 5–24.

Laberge, Marie-France, 'Les Instituts Pasteur du Maghreb. La recherche médicale dans le cadre de la politique coloniale', *Revue française d'histoire d'outre-mer* 74 (1987), pp. 27–42.

Lanza, Nicolas, 'Le Comité international de la Croix-Rouge et le soulèvement des Mau-Mau au Kenya, 1952–1959', *Relations internationales* 1 (2008), pp. 91–110.

Lazrag, Marnia, *Torture and the Twilight of Empire: From Algiers to Baghdad* (Princeton and Oxford: Princeton University of Press, 2009).

Le Cour Grandmaison, Olivier, *Coloniser. Exterminer. Sur la guerre et l'Etat colonial* (Paris: Fayard, 2005).

Le Cour Grandmaison, Olivier, *L'Empire des hygiénistes. Faire vivre aux colonies* (Paris: Fayard, 2014).

Le Cour Grandmaison, Olivier, 'The exception and the rule: on French colonial law', *Diogenes* 212 (2006), pp. 34–53.

Leven, Karl-Heinz, 'The invention of Hippocrates: oath, letters and Hippocratic corpus', in U. Trohler and S. Reiter-Theil (eds), *Ethics Codes in Medicine: Foundations and Achievements of Codification Since 1947* (Farnham: Ashgate Publishing, 1998), pp. 3–23.

Lifton, Robert Jay, 'Doctors and torture', *The New England Journal of Medicine* 351 (2004), pp. 415–416.

Lifton, Robert Jay, *Home From the War: Vietnam Veterans: Neither Victims nor Executioners* (London: Wildwood House, 1974).

Lifton, Robert Jay, *The Nazi Doctors: Medical Killing and the Psychology of Genocide* (New York: Basic Books, 2000).

Linstrum, Erik, 'Facts about atrocity: reporting colonial violence in postwar Britain', *History Workshop Journal* 84 (2017), pp. 108–127.

Linstrum, Erik, *Ruling Minds: Psychology in the British Empire* (Cambridge, MA and London: Harvard University Press, 2016).

London, Leslie, Leonard S. Rubenstein, Laurel Baldwin-Ragaven and Adriaan Van Es, 'Dual loyalty among military health professionals:

human rights and ethics in times of armed conflict', *Cambridge Quarterly of Healthcare Ethics* 15 (2006), pp. 381–391.

Lonsdale, John, 'Mau Maus of the mind: making Mau Mau and remaking Kenya', *The Journal of African History* 31 (1990), pp. 392–421.

Macey, David, 'The Algerian with a knife', *Parallex* 4 (1998), pp. 159–167.

Macias, Teresa, '"Tortured bodies": the biopolitics of torture and truth in Chile', *The International Journal of Human Rights* 17 (2013), pp. 113–132.

McCoy, Alfred W., 'Science in Dachau's shadow: Hebb, Beecher, and the development of CIA psychological torture and modern medical ethics', *Journal of the History of Behavioural Science* 43 (2007), pp. 401–417.

McCollock, Jock, *Colonial Psychiatry and 'the African Mind'* (Cambridge: Cambridge University Press, 1995).

Macleod, R., and M. Lewis (eds), *Disease, Medicine and Empire: Perspectives on Western Medicine and the Experience of European Expansion* (London: Routledge, 1988).

McMahon, Robert J., 'Introduction' in Robert J. McMahon (ed.), *The Cold War in the Third World* (Oxford: Oxford University Press, 2002), pp. 1–10.

Macmaster, Neil, 'The torture controversy (1998–2002): towards a "new history" of the Algerian war?', *Modern & Contemporary France* 10 (2002), pp. 449–459.

Mahone, Sloan, 'East African psychiatry and the practical problems of empire', in Slone Mahone and Megan Vaughan (eds), *Psychiatry and Empire* (Basingstoke: Palgrave Macmillan, 2007), pp. 41–66.

Mahone, Sloan, 'The psychology of rebellion: colonial medical responses to dissent in British East Africa', *The Journal of African History* 47 (2006), pp. 241–258.

Marcovich, Anne, 'French colonial medicine and colonial rule: Algeria and Indochina', in R. Macleod and M. Lewis (eds), *Disease, Medicine and Empire: Perspectives on Western Medicine and the Experience of European Expansion* (London: Routledge, 1988), pp. 103–115.

Marks, Shula, 'What is colonial about colonial medicine? And what has happened to imperialism and health?', *Social History of Medicine* 10 (1997), pp. 205–219.

Mathu, Mohamed, recorded by Don Barnett, *Urban Guerrilla: The Story of Mohamed Mathu* (Richmond, BC: LSM Press, 1974).

Mellanby, Kenneth, 'Medical experiments on human beings in concentration camps in Nazi Germany', *British Medical Journal* (25 January 1947), pp. 148–150.

Melley, Timothy, 'Brain warfare: the covert sphere, terrorism, and the legacy of the Cold War', *Grey Room* 45 (2011), pp. 18–40.

Meloni, Giulia and Johan Swinnen, 'The rise and fall of the world's largest wine exporter – and its institutional legacy', *Journal of Wine Economists* 9 (2014), pp. 3–33.

Menozzi, Filippo, 'Fanon's letter: between psychiatry and anticolonial commitment', *Interventions* 17 (2015), pp. 360–377.

Miles, Steven H., *Oath Betrayed: Torture, Medical Complicity and the War on Terror* (New York: Random House, 2006).

Mockaitis, Thomas R., 'The origins of British counter-insurgency', *Small Wars & Insurgencies* 1 (1990), pp. 209–225.

Monnais, Laurence, 'Which medications did they trust? The role of French colonialism in Vietnamese attitudes towards pharmaceuticals, 1858–1939', Paper presented at Princeton Workshop in the history of science, 'Science across Cultures – Historical and Philosophical Perspectives', Princeton University, 24 October 2003.

Moore, Karl, and David Charles Lewis, 'Globalization and the Cold War: the Communist dimension', *Management & Organizational History* 5 (2013), pp. 5–17.

Morier-Genoud, Eric, 'Missions and institutions: Henri-Philippe Junod, anthropology, human rights and academia between Africa and Switzerland, 1921–1966', *Schweizerische Zeitschrift für Religions- und Kulturgeschichte* 105 (2011), pp. 193–219.

Mortimer, Mildred, 'Tortured bodies, resilient souls: Algeria's women combatants depicted by Danièle Djamila Amrane-Minne, Louisette Ighilahriz, and Assia Djebar', *Research in African Literatures* 43 (2012), pp. 101–117.

Morton, Stephen, *States of Emergency: Colonialism, Literature and Law* (Liverpool: Liverpool University Press, 2013).

Nowak, Manfred, 'What practices constitute torture? US and UN standards', *Human Rights Quarterly* 28 (2006), pp. 809–841.

Nutton, Vivian, 'Beyond the Hippocratic Oath', in Andrew Wear, Johanna Geyer-Kordesh and Roger French (eds), *Doctors and Ethics: The Earlier Historical Setting of Professional Ethics* (Amsterdam and Atlanta: Rodopi, 1993), pp. 10–37.

Ocobock, Paul, 'Spare the rod, spoil the colony: corporal punishment, colonial violence, and generational authority in Kenya, 1897–1952', *The International Journal of African Historical Studies* 45 (2012), pp. 29–56.

Onyedum, Jennifer Johnson, '"Humanize the conflict": Algerian health care organizations and propaganda campaigns, 1954–62', *Journal of Middle East Studies* 44 (2012), pp. 713–731.

Osborne, Michael A., 'Acclimatizing the world: a history of the paradigmatic colonial science', *Osiris* 15 (2000), pp. 135–151.

Osgood, Kenneth, *Total Cold War: Eisenhower's Secret Propaganda Battle at Home and Abroad* (Lawrence: University of Kansas Press, 2006).

Packard, Randall, 'Visions of postwar health and development and their impact on public health interventions in the developing world', in Frederick Cooper and Randall Packard (eds), *International Development and the Social Sciences: Essays on the History and Politics of Knowledge* (Berkeley: University of California Press, 1997), pp. 93–115.

Peters, Edward, *Torture* (Philadelphia: University of Pennsylvania Press, 1985).

Pick, Daniel, *The Pursuit of the Nazi Mind: Hitler, Hess and the Analysts* (Oxford: Oxford University Press, 2012).

Pringle, Yolana, 'Crossing the divide: medical missionaries and government service in Uganda, 1897–1940', in Anna Greenwood (ed.), *Beyond the State: The Colonial Medical Services in British Africa* (Manchester: Manchester University Press, 2016), pp. 19–38.

Rabinow, Paul, *French Modern: Norms and Forms of the Social Environment* (Cambridge, MA: MIT Press, 1998).

Rayner, Mary, *Turning a Blind Eye: Medical Accountability for Torture in South Africa* (Washington, DC: American Association for the Advancement of Science, 1987).

Rejali, Darius, *Torture and Democracy* (Princeton and Oxford: Princeton University Press, 2009).

Roelcke, Volker, and Giovanni Maio (eds), *Twentieth Century Ethics of Human Subjects Research: Historical Perspectives on Values, Practices, and Regulations* (Stuttgart: Franz Steiner Verlag, 2004).

Rosberg, Carl, and John Nottingham, *The Myth of Mau Mau: Nationalism in Kenya* (London: Pall Mall Press, 1966).

Ruedy, John, *Modern Algeria: The Origins and Development of a Nation* (Bloomington and Indianapolis: Indiana University Press, 2005).

Sato, Shohei, '"Operation Legacy": Britain's destruction and concealment of colonial records worldwide', *The Journal of Imperial and Commonwealth History* 45 (2017), pp. 697–719.

Scarry, Elaine, *The Body in Pain: The Making and Unmaking of the World* (Oxford: Oxford University Press, 1985).

Scheipers, Sibylle, 'The use of camps in colonial warfare', *The Journal of Imperial and Commonwealth History* 43 (2015), pp. 678–698.

Schmidt, Ulf, *Justice at Nuremburg: Leo Alexander and the Nazi Doctors' Trial* (Basingstoke: Palgrave Macmillan, 2004).

Schilling, Donald G., 'Local Native Councils and the politics of education in Kenya, 1925–1939', *The International Journal of African Historical Studies* 9 (1976), pp. 218–247.

Schmidt, Ulf, 'Medical ethics and human experimentation at Porton Down: informed consent in Britain's biological and chemical warfare experiments', in Ulf Schmidt and Andreas Frewer (eds), *History and Theory of Human Experimentation: The Declaration of Helsinki and Modern Medical Ethics* (Stuttgart: Steiner, 2007), pp. 283–313.

Schmidt, Ulf, *Secret Science: A Century of Poison Warfare and Human Experiments* (Oxford: Oxford University Press, 2015).

Seed, David, 'Brainwashing and Cold War demonology', *Prospects* 22 (1997), pp. 535–573.

Sheather, Julian, Rhian Beynon, Tom Davis and Kamran Abbasi, 'Torture and doctors' dual obligation', *British Medical Journal* 350 (2015), pp. 1–2.

Shephard, Ben, *A War of Nerves* (London: Jonathan Cape, 2000).
Shipway, Martin, 'Algeria and the "official mind": the impact of North Africa on French colonial policy south of the Sahara, 1944–58', in Martin S. Alexander, Martin Evans and J. F. V. Keiger (eds), *The Algerian War and the French Army, 1954–62: Experiences, Images, Testimonies, 2002* (New York: Palgrave Macmillan, 2002), pp. 61–75.
Smith, Simon, 'General Templer and counter-insurgency in Malaya: hearts and minds, intelligence, and propaganda', *Intelligence and National Security* 16 (2001), pp. 60–78.
Streatfield, Dominic, *The Secret History of Mind Control* (London: Hodder & Stoughton, 2007).
Stoler, Ann Laura, 'Imperial debris: reflections on ruins and ruination', *Cultural Anthropology* 23 (2008), pp. 191–219.
Stoler, Ann Laura, *Race and the Education of Desire: Foucault's History of Sexuality and the Colonial Order of Things* (Durham and London: Duke University Press, 1995).
Stover, E., *The Open Secret: Torture and the Medical Profession in Chile* (Washington, DC: American Association for the Advancement of Science, 1987).
Stover, E., and E. O. Nightingale (eds), *The Breaking of Bodies and Minds: Torture, Psychiatric Abuse and the Health Professions* (New York: W. H. Freeman, 1985).
Surkis, Judith, 'Ethics and violence: Simone de Beauvoir, Djamila Boupacha, and the Algerian War', *French Politics, Culture & Society* 28 (2010), pp. 38–55.
Sutphen, Mary P. and Bridie Andrews (eds), *Medicine and Colonial Identity* (London and New York: Routledge, 2003).
Thénault, Sylvie, 'Armée et justice en guerre d'Algérie', *Vingtième siècle. Revue d'histoire* 57 (1998), pp. 104–114.
Thénault, Sylvie, *Une drôle de justice. Les Magistrats dans la guerre* (Paris: Découverte, 2001).
Thénault, Sylvie, 'L'Internement en France pendant la guerre d'indépendance algérienne', *Recueil Alexandries*, 15 (2008). reseau-terra.eu/article917.html [Accessed 21 August 2018].
Thénault, Sylvie, 'Personnel et internés dans les camps français de la guerre d'Algérie. Entre stéréotypes coloniaux et combat pour l'indépendance', *Politix* 1 (2005), pp. 63–81.
Thénault, Sylvie, *Violence ordinaire dans l'Algérie colonial. Camps, internements, assignations à résidence* (Paris: Odile Jacob, 2012).
Thénault, Sylvie and Raphaëlle Branche, 'Le Secret sur la torture pendant la guerre d'Algérie', *Matériaux pour l'histoire de notre temps* 58 (2000), pp. 57–63.
Thompson, Robert, *Defeating Communist Insurgency* (London: Chatto & Windus, 1966).

Timmermann, Carsten, 'A model for the new physician: Hippocrates in interwar Germany', in David Cantor (ed.), *Reinventing Hippocrates* (Aldershot: Ashgate, 2002), pp. 302–324.

Tröler, U., and S. Reiter-Theil (eds), *Ethics Codes in Medicine* (Farnham: Ashgate, 1998).

Vaughan, Megan, *Curing Their Ills: Colonial Power and African Illness* (Stanford and Cambridge: Stanford University Press, 1991).

Vaughan, Megan, 'Introduction', in Sloan Mahone and Megan Vaughan (eds), *Psychiatry and Empire* (Basingstoke: Palgrave Macmillan, 2007), pp. 1–16.

Villatoux, Maria-Catherine, 'Traitement psychologique, endoctrinement, contre-endoctrinement en guerre d'Algérie. Le cas des camps de détention, *Guerres mondiales et conflits contemporains* 208 (2002), pp. 45–54.

Villatoux, Paul, 'L'Institutionnalisation de l'arme psychologique pendant la guerre d'Algérie au miroir de la guerre froide', *Guerres mondiales et conflits contemporains* 208 (2002), pp. 35–44.

Vittori, Jean-Pierre, *On a torturé en Algérie* (Paris: Editions Ramsay, 2000).

Vogel, H., 'Torture', *Encyclopaedia of Forensic Science* (2013), pp. 123–132.

Waddington, Keir, *An Introduction to the Social History of Medicine* (Basingstoke: Palgrave Macmillan, 2011).

Walter, Diek, *Colonial Violence: European Empires and the Use of Force* (London: Hurst, 2017).

Weil, Patrick, 'Le Statut des musulmans en Algérie colonial', *Histoire de la justice* 16 (2005), pp. 93–109.

Weissbrodt, David, and Cheryl Heilman, 'Defining torture and cruel, inhuman, and degrading treatment', *Law and Inequality* 29 (2011), pp. 343–394.

Winter, Alison, 'The making of "truth serum"', *Bulletin of the History of Medicine* 79 (2005), pp. 500–533.

Wood, Dan, 'Revisiting *La Question*: a political-phenomenological critique of Merleau-Ponty's assessment of Algerian decolonization', *Studies in Social and Political Thought* 22 (2013), pp. 11–29.

Worboys, Michael, 'Colonial medicine', in Roger Cooter and John V. Pickstone (eds), *Companion to Medicine in the Twentieth Century* (London: Routledge, 2003), pp. 67–80.

Worboys, Michael, 'The emergence of tropical medicine: a study in the establishment of a scientific speciality', in Gerard Lemaine, Roy Macleod, Michael Mulkay and Peter Weingart (eds), *Perspectives on the Emergence of Scientific Disciplines* (Berlin and Boston: De Gruyter Mouton, 1976), pp. 76–98.

Worboys, Michael, 'Science and British Colonial Imperialism: 1895–1940' (DPhil thesis, University of Sussex, 1979).

Yarwood, Lisa, 'Defining torture: the potential for abuse', *Journal of the Institute of Justice and International Studies* 8 (2008), pp. 324–339.

Young, Charles S., *Name, Rank, and Serial Number: Exploiting Korean War PoWs at Home and Abroad* (Oxford: Oxford University Press, 2012).

Zack, Lizabeth, 'Early origins of Islamic activism in Algeria: the case of Khaled in post-World War I Algiers', *Journal of North African Studies* 11 (2006), pp. 205–217.

Index

EU authorised representative for GPSR:
Easy Access System Europe, Mustamäe tee 50,
10621 Tallinn, Estonia
gpsr.requests@easproject.com

www.ingramcontent.com/pod-product-compliance
Ingram Content Group UK Ltd.
Pitfield, Milton Keynes, MK11 3LW, UK
UKHW021834100926
8556IPUK00004B/332
* 9 7 8 1 5 2 6 1 6 7 5 1 4 *